KATHARINE F. WELLS, Ph.D.

Visiting Associate Professor Retired,
Department of Health, Physical Education and Recreation,
Mary Washington College of the University of Virginia

Formerly Associate Professor
Department of Hygiene and Physical Education
Wellesley College

FIFTH EDITION

KINESIOLOGY

THE SCIENTIFIC BASIS OF HUMAN MOTION

W. B. SAUNDERS COMPANY — Philadelphia · London · Toronto

W. B. Saunders Company: West Washington Square
Philadelphia, Pa. 19105

12 Dyott Street
London, WC1A 1DB

833 Oxford Street
Toronto 18, Ontario

Listed here is the latest translated edition of this book together with the language of the translation and the publisher.

Japanese (3rd Edition) — Baseball magazine Sha, Tokyo, Japan.

Kinesiology   ISBN   0-7216-9217-6

Print No.:   9   8   7   6   5   4

PREFACE TO THE FIFTH EDITION

The two chief objectives in the preparation of this fifth edition of *Kinesiology* were (1) to bring the contents up to date, and (2) to try to make this book a more useful tool for student and instructor alike. The preliminary work for bringing a textbook of this type up to date consists of reading the pertinent literature that has appeared since the preparation of the preceding edition and, in doing this, to note the new findings or views concerning the anatomic and mechanical aspects of human motion in general and of specific activities or motor skills. The research investigations and articles which appear to be of particular interest and significance are then briefly summarized for incorporation into the text.

The tasks involved in achieving the goal of increasing the usefulness of the book are less clearly defined. Extensive reading of professional literature, attending professional conferences, and engaging in discussions with one's colleagues and students all help, but for real inspiration one depends to a large extent upon a "sixth sense."

The major changes made in this 1971 edition consist of the following:

Summaries of recent research investigations have been added and some of the old summaries have been deleted, especially those that had to do with variations in bone structure and those which have been superseded by newer ones using more modern techniques.

Based on new findings in recent electromyographic investigations, a few revisions have been made in regard to muscular actions.

The principles of stability and the principles of motion have been combined in one chapter.

Detailed anatomic analyses of sport skills have been dropped or only briefly summarized.

A discussion of trampolining has been added.

A new chapter on basic anatomic concepts has been included. This is presented in the form of a glossary and is for the convenience of students who may want to brush up on such concepts without having to refer to an anatomy text.

The chapter on the Applications of Kinesiology to Motor Learning and Performance has been replaced by a new chapter on Implications for Teaching. This is placed at the end of the book and is intended to aid the individual in making the transition from student to teacher, especially with reference to kinesiology. It is hoped that he will not look upon this course merely as one which is now over and done with, but rather as a helpful storehouse of information upon which he can constantly draw to aid him in the teaching of sports, dance and other physical education activities.

As in the earlier editions, the author has sought in this one also to arouse in the student a true appreciation of the potentialities of the body for performing almost unbelievable feats of skill. One does not need to go to the circus to see such feats; he may see them in the school gymnasium or wherever high school gymnasts are performing on the high balance beam, the trampoline, or the uneven parallel bars.

I would like to express my appreciation to Dr. Janet A. Wessel, Professor of Physical Education at Michigan State University, for her many helpful suggestions in the preparation of this revision, such as placing greater emphasis on the various principles of activity, reorganizing portions of the material in Parts One and Three, planning Appendices C, E and G, and providing the first drafts from which the drawings were made for Appendix G.

My special thanks go to Miss Judi Ford, Miss America, 1969, and to her mother, Mrs. Virgil Ford, for giving so generously of their time and energy in order to provide pictures of trampolining that would show particular aspects of twist movements that I wanted illustrated.

I am also grateful to the authors and publishers who graciously gave permission to quote passages and reproduce illustrations from their publications. Finally, I would like particularly to express my gratitude to the editorial and production staffs of the W. B. Saunders Company for their continued helpfulness throughout the preparation of this edition and for the excellent drawings they prepared for Appendix G.

Katharine F. Wells

Needham, Massachusetts

PREFACE TO
THE FIRST EDITION

This book is intended as a kinesiology text both for the teacher and for the student. The book is divided into four parts. The first part deals with the basic mechanics of human motion, the second with the action of the joints and muscles, the third with major types of motor skills, and the fourth with the applications of kinesiology to physical education activities, to the techniques of physical and occupational therapy, and to daily life skills. For those who like to teach the anatomic aspects of movements before the mechanical, Parts I and II may easily be used in the reverse order. Also, the topics in the anatomic section itself may be taken up in any order the instructor desires. Some may prefer to start with the upper extremity, some with the lower. The arrangement of this text need not deter the instructor from following the order of his preference.

It is believed that there is enough material in this book to use it as a text for a full year's course, yet, at the same time, by judicious selection of the subject matter, by omission of the supplementary material and by the substitution of classroom demonstrations for some of the laboratory exercises, the book should serve equally well as a text for a one semester course in kinesiology. It is left to the discretion of the instructor to select the material that meets his particular needs.

In its original form this textbook was an unpublished handbook-laboratory manual. It was used by the author in her kinesiology classes for three years before it was expanded to its present form. The original manual did not serve as an independent textbook. It was intended to be used as a companion book to a kinesiology or anatomy text. Since this limited its usefulness, however, it was decided to expand it to what is intended as a complete and independent textbook. For those who like to use a single textbook for a course it should suffice. To help the student (and the instructor) in his collateral reading, most chapters in this text contain a comprehensive bibliography. In many cases there is also a list of readings which are particularly recommended. These bibliographies and reading lists provide a rich source of information for the inquiring student.

In regard to the value of laboratory exercises and projects as a means of learning, James B. Stroud, in his book *Psychology in Education*, points out that "Effectiveness of instruction is not determined so much by what the teacher does, as by what he leads the pupils to do. . . ." Again, "Perhaps one of the most successful procedures for infusing learning with significance has been the [educational method known as] constructive activities. . . . The activity is thus a means of making learning meaningful and of giving it a purpose." In accord with this point of view numerous laboratory exercises are suggested. In conformity to the same principle, only a few complete analyses of skills are presented, for it is the writer's contention that the student will gain far more from making one complete analysis himself than from reading a dozen or more ready-made analyses.

As a further means of enriching the kinesiology course a number of the chapters include supplementary material in the form of brief descriptions of research projects in the field of anatomy and kinesiology. A few of these were carried out by the author, but the majority were conducted by other investigators and reported in the professional journals. The purpose of including this material is to broaden the instructor's background and to provide supplementary reading assignments for advanced students.

It has been the intention of the author to write simply and to use non-technical terminology whenever this conveyed the meaning as clearly and specifically as technical terms. The latter have been used, however, whenever they served to avoid ambiguity. For instance, terms like "proximal" (meaning nearest to the body) and "distal" (meaning farthest from the body) have been used in preference to the terms "upper" and "lower," which might easily be misinterpreted. While it is desirable for the kinesiology student to enlarge his scientific vocabulary, a text which confronts him with a staggering list of new and strange words defeats its purpose. Textbooks should stimulate the curiosity of their readers, not frighten them with a forbidding vocabulary. For the same reason the use of mathematical formulae has been studiously avoided. True, these might clarify certain explanations for the mathematically trained reader, but they tend to confuse and discourage the uninitiated.

The author acknowledges her indebtedness to many individuals without whose help it is doubtful if this book could have been written. She wishes to express her grateful appreciation particularly to Professor C. H. McCloy of the State University of Iowa for his continued guidance, encouragement and criticism, also for his generous permission to use material from his course in The Mechanical Analysis of Motor Skills; to Marjorie D. Sanger and Evelyn K. Dillon for their critical reading of the manuscript and for their constant help and encouragement throughout its preparation; to Constance K. Greene, Ada R. Hall and Mary E. Nesbitt for their helpful advice concerning the sections on neuromuscular action and physical therapy; and finally to the students in her kinesiology classes of the last three years who served patiently as "guinea pigs" and who made many constructive suggestions concerning the laboratory exercises.

For the illustrations, which add immeasurably to the usefulness of the text, grateful acknowledgment is made to Miss Mildred Codding, who made the anatomic drawings; to Mrs. George Homans, who printed the labels for these; to Mrs. Margareta F. Lyons, who made most of the non-anatomic sketches; to Dale Ballantyne, whose illustrations for the author's doctoral dissertation served as the basis for several of the sketches in this book; and to Miss Irene MacLaurin, who took a number of photographs specifically for this text. Many of the anatomic sketches are adapted from illustrations in standard texts by Braus, Bresnahan and Tuttle, Brubaker, Gray, Molliere, Ranson, Sobotta and Spalteholtz.

The author is under obligation to a number of individuals for the use of photographs and to several publishers for permission to reproduce copyrighted materials. To all writers and teachers from whom the author, either wittingly or unwittingly, has derived ideas which have provided the necessary background for the writing of this book she humbly acknowledges her indebtedness.

KATHARINE F. WELLS

CONTENTS

Introduction to
the Study of Kinesiology

Kinesiology, as it is known in physical education, orthopedics and physical medicine, is the study of human movement from the point of view of the physical sciences. The study of the human body as a machine for the performance of work has its foundations in three major areas of study, namely, mechanics, anatomy and physiology; more specifically, biomechanics, musculoskeletal anatomy and neuromuscular physiology. The majority of courses in kinesiology are based primarily on the first two of these and a separate course, physiology of muscular activity, covers much of the third. There is some overlapping, however, as there are certain physiologic concepts which even the most elementary course in kinesiology cannot afford to ignore.

In the early days of physical education, when few activities were taught other than gymnastics and the dance, the content of a course in kinesiology was confined chiefly to functional anatomy. Gradually, as sports assumed a more important place in the curriculum, the concept of kinesiology was broadened to include the study of the mechanical principles which apply to sport techniques. The principles were applied not only to the movements of the body itself, but also to the movements of the implements, balls and other equipment used for the sport in question. In like manner, the development of the kinesiology course in schools of physical therapy and occupational therapy has kept pace with the development of their expanded curricula. Having started as "muscle reeducation," it has come to include the application of mechanical principles to postural adjustments, to the gait, to the use of tools and household implements, and to the modifications of vocational and homemaking activities necessitated by limitations in neuromuscular capacity and skeletal structure.

Some authorities refer to kinesiology as a science in its own right; others claim that it should be called a study rather than a true science because the principles on which it is based are derived from basic sciences such as anatomy, physiology and physics. In any event, its

1

unique contribution is that it selects from many sciences those principles which are pertinent to human motion and systematizes their application. However it may be categorized, to the inquiring student it is a door opening into a whole new world of discovery and appreciation. Human motion, which most of us have taken for granted all our lives, is seen through new eyes. One who gives it any thought whatever cannot help being impressed not only by the beauty of human motion, but also by its apparently infinite possibilities, its meaningfulness, its orderliness, its adaptability to the surrounding environment. Nothing is haphazard; nothing is left to chance. Every structure that participates in the movements of the body does so in obedience to physical and physiologic principles. The student of kinesiology, like the student of anatomy, physiology, psychology, genetics and other biological sciences, can only look with reverent wonder at the intricate mechanism of the body and in the words of the psalmist exclaim to his creator, "I will praise thee, for I am fearfully and wonderfully made."

But kinesiology is not studied merely for the purpose of inciting our interest in a fascinating and mysterious subject. It has a useful purpose. We study kinesiology in order to learn how to analyze the movements of the human body and to discover their underlying principles. The study of kinesiology is an essential part of the educational experience of students of physical education and physical medicine. For the physical educator it has a dual purpose: on the one hand, the purpose of perfecting performance in motor skills, and on the other, the purpose of perfecting the performer, himself. Kinesiology helps to prepare the physical educator to teach effective performance in both fundamental and specialized motor skills. Furthermore, it enables him to evaluate exercises and activities from the point of view of their effect on the human structure. As Dr. William Skarstrom used to say to his kinesiology students, the human machine has this advantage over the manufactured machine: Whereas the latter wears out with use, the former improves with use (within limits), *provided it is used in accordance with the principles of efficient human motion.* The function of kinesiology, therefore, is to contribute not only to *successful participation* in various physical activities, but also to the *improvement* of the human structure through the intelligent selection of activities and the efficient use of the body.

For the physical therapist and the occupational therapist the purpose of studying kinesiology (whether called by that name or by some other) is not unlike that of the physical education teacher. The difference is in emphasis, rather than in purpose. The therapist is primarily concerned with the effect that exercises and other techniques of physical medicine have upon the body. He—or she—is concerned particularly with the restoration of impaired function and with methods of compensating for lost function. Effective performance is a goal for the therapist as it is for the physical educator, but to the therapist "effective performance" refers not so much to *skillful* performance in athletic activities, as to *adequate* performance in the activities associated with daily living. Whereas the educator applies his knowledge of kinesiology chiefly to the movements of the normal body, the therapist is concerned with the movements of a body which has suffered an impairment in function.

The educator and the therapist have at least one purpose in common in studying kinesiology. Both are concerned with posture and body mechanics, hence both are interested in discovering the anatomic and mechanical bases for training in this area. Both apply their knowledge of kinesiology to analyzing the postural needs of others, to the intelligent selection of posture exercises based on individual need and to the mechanically efficient methods of using the body in daily life skills.

The most satisfactory way of studying kinesiology is by supplementing book study with laboratory experimentation. It is a truism that we learn best by doing. When time must be conserved; demonstration may be substituted for some of the experimental work, but it should never replace it entirely.

The use of motion picture films is another good device for supplementing book study. It is particularly helpful if a hand projector is used, or a projector which can be stopped at will, thus making it possible to analyze positions and body relationships.

Whatever method of teaching or of study is employed it is well for the student to keep in mind the aims of a kinesiology course and the applications he intends to make of what he learns. He must remember that the analysis of motion is not an end in itself, but rather a means to the learning of new movement patterns and the improvement of old ones. This is as true for the physical therapist teaching amputees and paraplegics to walk again as it is for the physical educator teaching a sport technique. Finally, he must remember that the skill itself is of less importance than the one who practices it. Kinesiology serves only half its purpose when it provides the background for learning or teaching motor skills. It must also serve to lay the foundation for perfecting, repairing and keeping in good condition that incomparable mechanism—the human body.

DEMONSTRATIONS AND LABORATORY EXERCISES

Purpose. To familiarize the student with the method of observing and palpating muscles.

1. Have the subject bend his arm at the elbow while you resist the action by holding his wrist. With your other hand, feel the subject's forearm flexors (biceps and brachialis). While his arm is bent, release and reapply the resistance several times so that he will alternately relax and contract his muscles.

2. Have the subject bend his head to the right and turn his chin to the left, while you resist both motions with your hands. Observe the long muscle going from behind the ear diagonally downward

and forward to the sternum. This is the sternocleidomastoid muscle. It bends the head to the same side and rotates it to the opposite side.

3. Have the subject raise his arm sideward against resistance. Observe and feel the bulky muscle (the deltoid) on the upper part of the arm, just below the shoulder.

4. Have the subject lower his arm sideward against resistance. Observe and feel the tendons forming the anterior and posterior borders of the axilla. The former is part of the pectoralis major, and the latter of the latissimus dorsi.

5. Have the subject rise on his toes. Observe and feel the muscle in the calf of the leg. This is the gastrocnemius.

PART ONE

The Mechanics of Human Motion

INTRODUCTION TO PART ONE

The human body as seen by the kinesiologist is a highly complex machine constructed of living tissue. As such, it is subject to both mechanical and biological principles.

Part I, which is devoted to the mechanical aspects of human movement, opens with a chapter on mechanical concepts that are basic to the study of kinesiology. Following this is a discussion of the mechanics of both joint and muscular action, a brief presentation of the three simple machines found in the musculoskeletal structure, and a simplified discussion of the manner in which the principles of stability, laws of motion, and effects of forces upon bodies apply to this human machine.

The last three chapters are devoted to a discussion of the chief types of activities which can be performed by the musculoskeletal machine. These are: (1) the movements of the body in different media, without particular reference to external objects; (2) the variety of ways of giving impetus to external objects; and (3) the receiving of impetus, both that of one's own body and that of external objects. Although it might seem that activities such as landing from a jump or a fall should be discussed separately from activities such as catching or stopping balls and other moving objects, nevertheless, as both types of activity involve the reception of impetus, they are governed by the same principles. To discuss them separately would be unnecessarily repetitious.

CHAPTER 1

Basic Mechanical Concepts

If the study of kinesiology is to be meaningful to the student, it is essential that he grasp certain concepts, for without an understanding of these he is likely to get lost in ambiguities. If we are to understand one another we must talk the same language, use the same vocabulary. We must agree on basic definitions and points of reference.

Starting Positions. Except when analyzing upper extremity movements, the *fundamental standing position* is the one usually accepted as the point of reference. In this position the individual stands erect with the feet slightly separated and parallel, the arms hanging easily at the sides, palms facing the body (Fig. 1–1, A). This is the position usually assumed for gymnastic exercises. The military and the old-fashioned formal gymnastic positions are more vigorous and tense variations of this.

The *anatomic standing position* is the one usually depicted in anatomy textbooks. The individual is erect with the elbows fully extended and the palms facing forward. The legs and feet are the same as in the fundamental standing position (Fig. 1–1, B). When making a kinesiologic analysis of the fundamental movements of the forearm, hand, and fingers, the anatomic position is the one accepted as the point of reference.

The Center of Gravity. The center of gravity is defined as "an imaginary point representing the weight center of an object"; also as "that point in a body about which all the parts exactly balance each other"; and as "the point at which the entire weight of the body may be considered as concentrated." In a perfect sphere or cube the weight center coincides with the geometric center. Its precise location in the human body depends upon the individual's anatomic structure, posture, position and whether he is supporting external weights. In a person of average build, standing erect with the arms hanging at the sides, the center of gravity is located in the pelvis in front of the upper part of the sacrum. It is usually lower in women than in men because of their heavier pelves and thighs and shorter legs.

The Line of Gravity. The line of gravity is an imaginary vertical line which, by definition, passes through the center of gravity. Hence

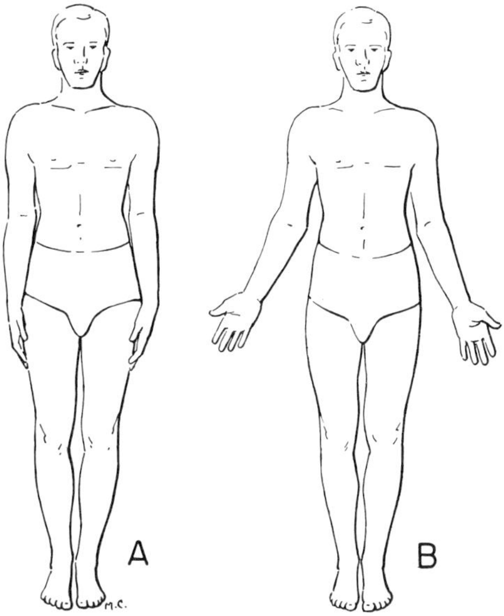

Figure 1–1. Standing positions.
A, Fundamental standing position.
B, Anatomic standing position.

its location is dependent upon the position of the center of gravity. It
is a simple matter to determine experimentally the location of an
individual's line of gravity with reference to his base of support.
Directions for a common method of doing this are given in the Supplementary Material section in this chapter.

Orientation Planes of the Body and Axes of Motion. There are
three planes, corresponding to the three dimensions of space. Each
plane is perpendicular to each of the other two. There are likewise
three axes of motion, each perpendicular to the plane in which the
motion occurs. The planes and axes of the body are defined as follows:

PLANES (Fig. 1–2, A, B, C.)

1. The sagittal, anteroposterior, or median plane is a vertical
plane passing through the body from front to back, dividing it into
right and left halves.

2. The frontal, lateral, or coronal plane is a vertical plane passing
through the body from side to side, dividing it into anterior and
posterior halves.

3. The horizontal or transverse plane is a horizontal plane which
passes through the body, dividing it into upper and lower halves.

Since each plane bisects the body, it follows that each plane must
pass through the center of gravity. Hence the center of gravity may
be defined as the point at which the three planes of the body intersect one another, and the line of gravity as the vertical line at which
the two vertical planes intersect each other. When describing a movement in terms of a plane, such as "a movement of the forearm in the
sagittal plane," we mean that the movement occurs in a plane parallel
with the sagittal plane. It does not necessarily imply that the move-

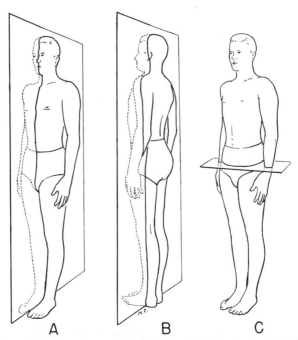

Figure 1–2. The planes of the body. *A*, Sagittal or anteroposterior plane; *B*, frontal or lateral plane; *C*, horizontal or transverse plane.

ment occurs in a plane passing through the center of gravity. If the latter is intended, the term "cardinal plane" is used. Thus nodding the head is a movement occurring in the cardinal sagittal plane.

AXES

1) The vertical axis is perpendicular to the ground.

2) The frontal or lateral horizontal axis passes horizontally from side to side.

3) The sagittal or anteroposterior horizontal axis passes horizontally from front to back.

A rotatory (axial, angular) movement of a segment of the body occurs *in* a plane, and *around* an axis. The axis around which the movement takes place is always at right angles to the plane in which it occurs.

Basic Movements of the Major Body Segments. The human body, being a multijointed structure, consists of many movable segments. When we watch a skillful acrobat, dancer or basketball player it might seem like a hopeless task to try to organize these movements into a meaningful classification. The task is greatly simplified, however, when we consider one segment at a time and visualize each movement as though it were performed from the anatomic standing position. This may take a bit of imagination, but knowing ahead of time the movements of which each joint in the body is capable is nine tenths of the battle. These are described in Part II in the systematic discussions of the regions of the body. The information given below is basic to understanding the movements of specific joints and segments. *Note:* The anatomic standing position is the point of reference for these movements.

MOVEMENTS IN THE SAGITTAL PLANE ABOUT A FRONTAL-HORIZONTAL AXIS. (Fig. 1–3, A.) Viewed from the side.

Flexion. The angle at the joint diminishes.

Examples:

a. The forward and backward tipping of the head.

b. Lifting the foot and leg backward from the knee.

c. Raising the entire lower extremity forward-upward as though kicking.

d. With the upper arm remaining at the side, raising the forearm straight forward (Fig. 1–3, A).

e. With the elbow straight, raising the entire upper extremity forward-upward. The "diminishing angle" is hard to see in this movement until one views the raising of the arm from the shoulder in the same way that he views the raising of the thigh from the hip joint. In the latter, one automatically notices the angle that appears between the top of the thigh (i.e., the anterior surface) and the trunk, or *the part of the body that lies above the hip joint.* Similarly, when raising the arm, the angle to look for is the angle between the top of the arm and the neck-head segment, *not* the angle between the underside of the raised arm and the trunk. It is necessary to train oneself to view the sagittal plane movements of the arm at the shoulder as being similar to those of the thigh at the hip joint.

Extension. The return movement from flexion.

Hyperflexion. This term refers only to the movement of the upper arm. When the arm is flexed beyond the vertical, it is considered to be hyperflexed. In other joints of the body flexion is terminated by contact of the moving segment with another part of the body, e.g., the forearm against the upper arm, the lower leg against the thigh, or by structural limitations of the joints themselves, e.g., flexion of the thoracic and lumbar spine.

Hyperextension. The continuation of extension beyond the starting position, or beyond the straight line.

Examples:

a. Hyperextension of the upper arm is said to occur when the arm is extended backward beyond the body.

b. The forearm is considered to be hyperextended when the angle at the elbow joint has exceeded 180 degrees.

Reduction of hyperextension. Return movement from hyperextension. This could also be called flexion to the starting position, i.e., the fundamental or the anatomic starting position, as the case may be.

Movements of the extremities in the sagittal plane. In viewing these movements, instead of using the body itself as the stationary point of reference, especially for the movements of the upper arm and thigh, it may help to use an imaginary vertical midline which is extended well above the level of the head. The similarity between upper and lower extremity flexion should then be easier to perceive. For general purposes the upper arm may be considered fully flexed when it has reached the overhead vertical position. Later, when the role of the shoulder girdle in arm movements has been studied, it will be seen that the elevation of the arm does not take place solely at the shoulder joint. The movements of the scapula and clavicle are an important part of the total arm movement. Strictly speaking, the shoulder joint is in a fully flexed position when the humerus is raised until it is parallel with the long axis of the scapula (i.e., when it is in the same plane as the scapula). For the present, however, the upper arm will be considered fully flexed when it has been raised forward-upward until it has reached the vertical position, and hyperflexed when it passes beyond this.

MOVEMENTS IN THE FRONTAL PLANE ABOUT A SAGITTAL-HORIZONTAL AXIS. (Fig. 1–3, *B*.) Viewed from the front or back.

Abduction. Sideward movement away from the midline or sagittal plane, or, in the case of the fingers, away from the midline of the hand. This term is used most commonly for sideward movements of the upper arm away from the trunk—in other words, sideward

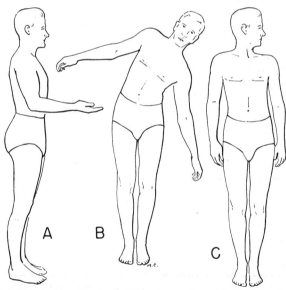

Figure 1–3. Movements of the body in the three planes. *A*, Movement of the forearm in the sagittal plane around a frontal-horizontal axis. *B*, Movement of the trunk in the frontal plane around a sagittal-horizontal axis. *C*, Movement of the head in the horizontal plane around a vertical axis.

elevation of the arm—and for sideward elevation of the lower extremity. The jumping jack exercise involves both of these.

Adduction. The return movement from abduction.

Lateral flexion. This refers to the lateral bending of the head or trunk. It may also be used for sideward movements of the middle finger, but the more specific terms, radial or ulnar flexion, are usually used for these.

Hyperabduction. Like hyperflexion, this term usually refers to the upper arm when the latter is abducted beyond the vertical, as seen from the front or back.

Hyperadduction. The trunk blocks hyperadduction of the upper extremity and the presence of the supporting lower extremity blocks hyperadduction of the other lower extremity. By combining slight flexion with hyperadduction, the upper extremities can move across the front of the body and one lower extremity can move across in front of the supporting one.

Reduction of hyperadduction. The return movement from hyperadduction.

Reduction of lateral flexion. The return movement from lateral flexion.

MOVEMENTS IN THE HORIZONTAL PLANE ABOUT A VERTICAL AXIS. (Fig. 1–3, C.) Viewed or visualized from overhead or from directly beneath, e.g., through a glass platform. The point of reference for all rotations of the upper extremities is the midposition as in the fundamental (not anatomic) standing position.

Rotation left and right. Applies to rotation of the head or neck in such a way that the anterior aspect turns respectively to the left or to the right.

Outward (lateral) and inward (medial) rotation. Applies to rotation of the thigh, the upper arm, or to the upper or lower extremity as a whole in such a way that the anterior aspect of the segment turns laterally or medially.

Supination and pronation. Apply respectively to outward (lateral) and inward (medial) rotation of the forearm.

Reduction of outward rotation, inward rotation, supination or pronation. Rotation of the segment back to the midposition.

MOVEMENTS IN AN OBLIQUE PLANE ABOUT AN OBLIQUE AXIS. Many movements take place in planes between the sagittal and frontal planes, the sagittal and horizontal planes, and the frontal and horizontal planes. These are oblique planes and the axes about which the movements occur are oblique axes. Whatever the degree of obliquity of the plane, the axis for a movement in that plane is always perpendicular to it. Although it is possible to define the obliquity precisely in terms of the number of degrees that it deviates from the fundamental planes, for general purposes descriptive terms are adequate.

A familiar example of an oblique plane movement is raising the arm between the straight forward and straight sideward directions. A golf swing and a tennis serve are also examples of arm movements that take place in oblique planes. Lower extremity examples include the frog kick in swimming and a deep knee bend performed with the heels together and the knees separated.

Circumduction. An orderly sequence of the movements which occur in the sagittal, frontal and intermediate oblique planes so that the segment as a whole describes a cone.

CLASSIFICATION OF FUNDAMENTAL MOTOR SKILLS

The types of joint movements defined previously constitute the basis of all the motor skills experienced by man. By combining flexion, extension, abduction, adduction and rotation of various segments of the body in different patterns and sequences, skills such as walking, throwing, kicking, catching a ball and turning a somersault are performed. Just as in the written language there is first the alphabet, then the vocabulary, then the thought expressed in one or more sentences, and finally the complete essay or story, so in physical activities there is first the category of movements available to the various body segments, then the motor skills consisting of selected segmental movements coordinated in such a way that a purposeful act is executed, then a series of such acts or skills, one following the other in logical sequence, leading to the attainment of a meaningful objective (such as, in baseball, the skills of hitting, running, sliding, and eventually crossing home plate to attain the objective of a run), and then finally, the complete game.

There are many bases for classifying motor skills. The important thing is to select, or to devise, a classification that is meaningful to the person who is going to use it. The one that follows is organized on the basis of the primary objectives of the skills and on the immediate environment and the unique circumstances under which they are performed.

FUNDAMENTAL MOTOR SKILLS

I. Skills of handling one's own body
  A. On land or other solid surface
    1. Maintaining and regaining equilibrium
    2. Locomotion
    3. Movements of the trunk and extremities within a limited area (e.g., in calisthenics or fitness exercises)
    4. Rotatory movements of the body as a whole (e.g., forward rolls or cartwheels)
    5. Receiving the impetus of one's own body (e.g., landing from jumps or falls)
  B. In water
    1. Swimming
    2. Aquatic stunts

      3. Boating

  C. In suspension

      1. Swinging activities on trapeze, flying rings, or similar equipment

      2. Hand traveling on traveling rings or horizontal ladder

  D. In the air

      1. Diving

      2. Trampoline activities, acrobatics

II. Skills of handling external objects

  A. Giving impetus

      1. Pushing, pulling, thrusting, lifting

      2. Throwing with hand or implement

      3. Striking, hitting, kicking

  B. Receiving impetus

      1. Catching and trapping

      2. Receiving performer (e.g., spotting in stunts and apparatus events)

One advantage to a grouping of fundamental motor skills, such as the above, is that it makes it easier to recognize the elements common to several activities. For instance, chopping a tree, batting a baseball and throwing a discus may seem like completely unrelated skills, yet each is a form of giving impetus to an external object. As such, they are based on the same underlying principles. Familiarity with one particular skill in a group, therefore, gives an advantage in learning another skill in the same group. Understanding the major principles that apply make it much easier to learn the new skill, even though the precise methods of applying the principles differ.

It is undoubtedly apparent to the reader that many familiar activities involve more than one skill. For example, a running high jump includes skills of horizontal locomotion, jumping, balancing and receiving the impetus of one's own body in landing. Similarly, the activities involved in carpentry may include skills of locomotion, balance and the giving of impetus to an object by means of striking. Any physical activity, whether from the area of sport, industry, gardening or homemaking, may be analyzed into its constituent elements or skills and the appropriate principles identified.

This chapter on basic concepts has presented, as it were, the alphabet and the vocabulary of human movement together with what might be called some ground rules. To carry this analogy a step further, we might say that before we can proceed to the construction of sentences it is essential to learn basic grammar. Otherwise the words that we put together may be meaningless. In the field of movement this means exploring certain anatomic and mechanical factors. We consider the nature of the segments to be moved and the leverage that is involved and whether it favors force or range; we consider the joint at which each movement occurs and the kinds of motions it permits; we consider the force needed to perform the movements and whether the muscular strength available is adequate; we consider the external forces that act upon the musculoskeletal structure and we pay special attention to the interaction between the structure and its environment.

For moving about successfully and efficiently in all kinds of circumstances and for manipulating various objects with purpose and direction, underlying principles inevitably come to light. All motion and all reaction to external forces are governed by principles, whether or not we are aware of them. The keener our awareness, however, and the better our understanding of them, the more skillful our motions and reactions are likely to be, and this means less time wasted on trial and error.

The student who fully grasps the mechanical elements of human movement and recognizes the types of motor skills engaged in by man will be well prepared for identifying the specific mechanical factors inherent in different types of skills and for appreciating the significance of the underlying principles. It has been the intent of this chapter to provide the student with the initial steps to the understanding of the mechanical basis of human movement. As he proceeds through Part I he should project beyond the details of mechanical factors and actions and be on the lookout for applications to specific sports and other activities with which he is familiar, especially in the area of physical education and dance. In this way he will be laying the foundation for subjecting all the activities in which he engages to mechanical analysis, for applying his knowledge to improve performance in the activities, and, eventually, for applying both his knowledge and his experience to effective teaching.

SUPPLEMENTARY MATERIAL

Method of Locating the Line of Gravity. It is a fairly simple matter to determine the relation of an individual's line of gravity to his base of support under experimental conditions. The student will find that it will repay him to do this because it will convince him better than words of the way the body automatically compensates for external loads and for segmental disalignment. It is revealing to see how the body compensates for the sideward raising of an arm, for the forward bending of the trunk, for a briefcase carried in one hand, or a load of books clasped against the chest (Fig. 1–4). No matter what the position, the relation of the line of gravity to the base of support is a remarkably stable one. Its relation to the body segments, however, shifts with every change in position. The segments automatically adjust themselves to maintain a balanced position—a position in which the center of gravity remains approximately over the center of the base of support.

DIRECTIONS FOR DETERMINING THE POSITION OF THE LINE OF GRAVITY

Apparatus (Fig. 1–5.)

1. Scales: preferably either the Toledo or the spring balance type.

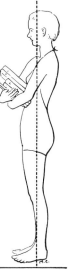

Figure 1–4. Compensatory adjustment of the body for an anterior load. Note that the line of gravity falls close to the center of the base of support.

2. A stool or block the same height as the platform of the scales.

3. A board about 40 cm. wide and a little over 100 or 200 cm. long—the latter if it is to be used for horizontal work. A knife edge should be attached to the underside of each end in such a way that when the board is placed in a horizontal position it will rest on the knife edges. For simplifying the calculations the distance from knife edge to knife edge should measure exactly 100 or 200 cm. The front edge of the board should be marked in centimeters. The board should be tested for accuracy. To do this, the experimenter should see whether it will balance exactly at the center.

Directions

1. Find the subject's total weight.

2. Put the board in place, with one knife edge on the scales platform and the other on the stool or block. Note the reading on the scales. This is the partial weight of the board *(B)*.

3. Have the subject stand approximately in the center of the board, facing the scales and with the heels even. Note the reading on the scales. This is the partial weight of the subject and board together *(S & B)*.

4. Use the following formula to solve for "*d*," this being the distance from the rear knife edge to the frontal plane in which the subject's center of gravity is situated:

$$d = \frac{(\text{Partial wt. of } S \& B) - (\text{Partial wt. of } B)}{\text{Total weight of } S} \times \frac{\text{Length of } B \text{ (from knife}}{\text{edge to knife edge)}}$$

5. Measure the distance "*d*" from the rear knife edge toward the end of the board resting on the scales. A perpendicular erected at this point represents the anteroposterior position of the subject's line of gravity. If desired, a mark may be made on the subject's foot to

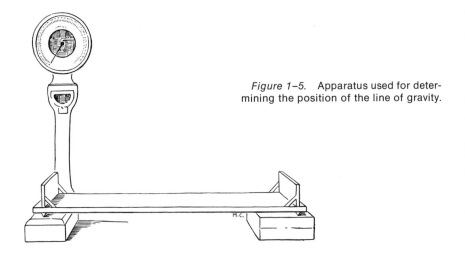

Figure 1–5. Apparatus used for determining the position of the line of gravity.

indicate the location of the line of gravity with reference to the anteroposterior aspect of the base of support. (*Note:* This is not a fixed point.
It moves forward and backward as the subject sways forward and
backward.)

6. The frontal or lateral position of the line of gravity may be
found in the same manner by having the subject stand with his side
toward the scales. In this case "*d*" represents the distance from the
rear knife edge to the sagittal plane in which the subject's center of
gravity is located.

7. If it is desired to find the single point representing the spot
where the line of gravity intersects the base of support, a piece of
paper should be placed under the subject's feet for the side-view
measurement. The outline of the feet should be traced on the paper.
When the first "*d*" is found, the distance should be measured and
marked on both the left and right sides of the paper. The paper should
then be removed and the two points connected by a straight line. When
the subject faces forward for the second measurement, the paper
should be placed on the board so that the subject's feet will fit in the
foot prints. When the second "*d*" is found, the distance should be
measured and marked on both edges of the paper and the two points
connected by a straight line. The point at which the two lines intersect represents the approximate position of the point where the line of
gravity strikes the base of support. This is a crude method of locating
this point and is not strictly accurate, since the subject may not be
standing in exactly the same posture for both measurements. Furthermore, the element of swaying always introduces a source of error. A
more accurate method for determining the position of the line of gravity has been described by Hellebrandt.

DIRECTIONS FOR DETERMINING THE HEIGHT OF THE CENTER OF
GRAVITY. The same equipment is used as for determining the
position of the line of gravity, except that the longer board must be

used for this. Also there should be a perpendicular foot rest at each end of the board, directly over each knife edge. These must not destroy the balance of the board. The subject lies on the back with the head toward the scales and the feet at right angles against the foot rest at the other end. The foot rest should be high enough to support the feet in the proper position. The position the subject assumes should be as much like the standing position as possible. The measurements and calculations are made as before. In this case "*d*" represents the distance from the foot rest to the horizontal plane in which the subject's center of gravity is situated. This is comparable to the distance from the center of gravity to the ground, when the subject is in the standing position. The center of gravity itself is located at the point where the line of gravity intersects this horizontal plane.

PHOTOGRAPHIC METHOD.   This method of determining the position of the line of gravity may easily be adapted to use with photographs. This has several advantages. Photographs of the subject in several positions can be taken in succession and the computations and measurements be made later. Several prints of the same photograph can be made and used for the entire class. The subject can assume positions it would be difficult to hold long enough for the computations and measurements to be made directly. In adapting this method to photographs the length measurements (i.e., total length of board and distance "*d*") are made on the photograph instead of on the board itself. This means that the photographed length of the board must be substituted for the actual length in the formula. Computations will be made easier if the distance of the camera from the board is adjusted so that the photographed length of the board will be a round number, such as 5 or 10 cm. It is possible to do this by taking the back off the camera and looking through a piece of ground glass held behind the camera. The dimensions of the image on the glass will be the same as those on the film.

Center of Gravity Experimentation.   A number of experiments relating to the center of gravity were made by Hellebrandt at the University of Wisconsin. She found the height of the center of gravity in women to be 55 per cent of their standing height. She studied the way in which the body sways when a person attempts to stand still and observed that although the center of gravity of the body as a whole shifts constantly during relaxed and effortless standing, the patterns formed by a trajectory of the shifting center of weight and the mean position of the vertical projection of this theoretical point (i.e., the line of gravity) are relatively constant. She found that the average area of maximal sway for a group of men and women was only 4.09 sq. cm. and that the differences between the men and the women were not statistically significant. It was noted that although the line of gravity intersected the base of support close to its center, in the majority of subjects it was slightly to the left and behind the exact center. In a study on the influence of shoes on the position of the center of gravity Hellebrandt found that shoes of low and of moderate heels had a negligible effect upon postural stability and the position of the line of gravity, but that high heeled shoes tended to cause a forward shifting of the line of gravity and to increase the amount of swaying, apparently indicating a decrease in stability.

In a series of studies on the relation of age to the height of the center of gravity, Palmer found that the latter maintained a fairly constant ratio to the height of the individual at all ages, ranging from 55 to 59 per cent. From the age of 6 fetal months to 70 years the center of gravity was found to descend gradually from the level of the seventh thoracic vertebra to the level of the first sacral segment.

In 1922 Croskey, Dawson, Luessen, Marohn and Wright reviewed methods of determining the position of the center of gravity and then used an improved seesaw method in their own experiment. Using fifty men and fifty women as their subjects, they found the center of gravity in men to be 56.18 per cent of their height, and in women 55.44 per cent. They also found that the height of the center of gravity was considerably more variable in women than in men. They found no correlation between the height of the center of gravity and body weight or height.

A few investigators have been interested in the possibility of a relationship between the line of gravity and standing posture. In their historical survey of this subject Cureton and Wickens noted that no quantitative studies have been found which related the center of gravity to the area of the base as a diagnostic test for posture. Using the Reynolds and Lovett technique for determining the position of the line of gravity and their own method of analyzing anteroposterior posture, they made a number of correlation studies. They concluded that there was a definite relationship between the position of the line of gravity and posture, strength, physical fitness and athletic ability. The coefficient of correlation between their measure of kyphosis and the line of gravity measurement was .256. The relationship between body lean and the line of gravity was indicated by a coefficient of .864. This denotes a high degree of positive relationship, but on the other hand, body lean *is* the position of the body which is associated with the anteroposterior shifting of the line of gravity. They are one and the same thing. In fact, one wonders why the relationship was only .864 instead of 1.0. In correlating body lean with kyphosis, Cureton and Wickens obtained a coefficient of .363. They interpreted this as an indication of a trend for men who habitually stood with their weight more forward to have straighter upper backs. The authors apparently did not investigate the relationship between the anteroposterior position of the line of gravity and the alignment of body segments.

Crowley and Johnston in two separate studies could find no relationship between the anteroposterior position of the line of gravity and total anteroposterior posture as measured by the MacEwan-Howe objective method.[5, 8]

Likewise, Hellebrandt and her co-workers, using this method on a larger number of subjects, could find no relationship between the objective posture score and the anteroposterior shifting of the line of gravity. They suggested that this surprising failure to find a relationship between the two might indicate that the posture criterion in common use is based on an esthetic concept of posture rather than on a physiologic one.

DEMONSTRATIONS AND LABORATORY EXERCISES

1. Construct a simple device to illustrate the planes and axes.

2. Working with a partner, take turns performing simple movements of the head, trunk, upper extremity and lower extremity, and identifying the planes and axes concerned.

3. Determine the anteroposterior position of the line of gravity for three different subjects standing in their natural posture.

4. Determine the position of the line of gravity for a subject in the following positions:

   a. Facing the scales and leaning as far forward as possible with the body in a straight line from the top of the head to the ankles.

   b. Facing the scales and leaning as far backward as possible with the body in a straight line.

5. Determine the lateral aspect (front or back view) of the line of gravity for a subject who is standing with weight balanced evenly on both feet.

6. Determine the lateral aspect of the line of gravity for a subject who is standing on one foot.

7. Determine the height of the center of gravity in a subject (*a*) with the arms against the sides, and (*b*) with the arms extended overhead.

8. Do several original center of gravity experiments.

REFERENCES

1. Croskey, M. I., Dawson, P. M., Luessen, A. C., Marohn, I. E., and Wright, H. E.: The height of the center of gravity in man. Am. J. Physiol., *61*:171–185, 1922.
2. Cureton, T. K., and Wickens, J. S.: The center of gravity of the human body in the antero-posterior plane and its relation to posture. Res. Quart. Am. Assn. Health & Phys. Ed. (Suppl.), 6:93–105, 1935.
3. Hellebrandt, F. A., Riddle, K. S., Larsen, E. M., and Fries, E. C.: Gravitational influences on postural alignment. Physiother. Rev., 22:143–149, 1942.
4. Hellebrandt, F. A., and Franseen, E. B.: Physiological study of vertical stance of man. Physiol. Rev., 23:220–225, 1943.
5. MacEwan, C. G., and Howe, E. C.: An objective method for grading posture. Res. Quart. Am. Assn. Health & Phys. Ed., 3:144–157, 1932.
6. Palmer, C. E.: Studies of the center of gravity in the human body. Child Develop. *15*:99–180, 1944.
7. Reynolds, E., and Lovett, R. W.: Method of determining the position of the center of gravity in its relation to certain bony landmarks in the erect position. Am. J. Physiol., *24*:286–293, 1909.
8. Wellesley College Studies in Hygiene and Physical Education: Factors in antero-posterior posture. Res. Quart. Am. Assn. Health & Phys. Ed. (Suppl.), 9:89–96, 1938.

CHAPTER 2

The Mechanics of Joint Action

The student of kinesiology will have a clearer understanding of human motion if he has acquired the ability of visualizing the action of the joints in each movement he observes. This ability will stand him in good stead not only in the analysis of specific movement skills, but also in the understanding of joint injuries and of abnormalities in joint motion. Such an understanding can be based only on a sound foundation in the structure and function of each joint in the body. Although there are many joints in the skeletal framework, there are relatively few *types* of joints. By first studying the classification of joints one finds the study of individual joints greatly simplified.

Nature has shown an amazing versatility in designing joints to meet a variety of purposes. There are hinge joints, pivot joints and ball-and-socket joints, to name a few. Within these categories there are modifications in the shapes of the articulating bony surfaces, the thickness of cartilaginous plates and disks, and the arrangement of ligaments.

Too often the student thinks of kinesiology primarily as a study of muscular action and he tends to overlook, or at least to underrate, the importance of studying the joints. Consequently, he has such a hazy conception of the mechanics of joint function that he is seriously handicapped later in his profession. He will not understand the exact nature of the strain caused by certain activities, nor the nature of injuries after they have occurred. It is for this reason that the structure and function of the joints are treated in considerable detail in this text. If the student will approach the study of this section in the spirit of the youngster who takes the mechanical toy apart to see how it works, or in the spirit of the youth who, for the same reason, tinkers with the engine of his car, his investigation will be equally rewarding.

Classification. Joints may be classified according to their structure, more specifically according to the way in which the bones (or cartilages) are united. The classifications in two well-known anatomy texts[1, 2] are based on the presence or absence of a joint cavity, i.e., a space between the articulating surfaces of the bones. Each type of joint is further subdivided either according to shape or according to

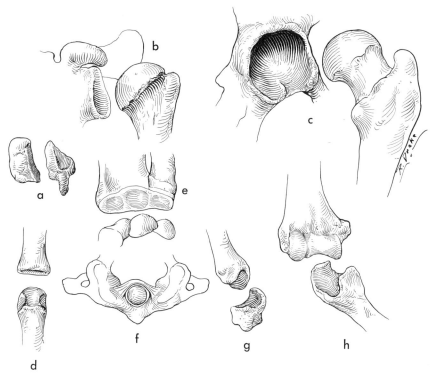

Figure 2–1. Major types of diarthrodial joints. *a,* Plane; *b,* ball-and-socket (shoulder); *c,* ball-and-socket (hip); *d,* condyloid (metacarpophalangeal); *e,* condyloid (radiocarpal); *f,* pivot (atlantoaxial); *g,* saddle (thumb or carpometacarpal); *h,* hinge (elbow or humero-ulnar). (From Hollinshead, W. H.: Functional Anatomy of the Limbs and Back, 3rd ed. Philadelphia, W. B. Saunders Company, 1969.)

the nature of the tissues which connect the bones. These classifications, with their subdivisions, may be grasped more readily if presented in outline form.

    I. Diarthrosis (from the Greek, meaning a joint in which there is a separation, or articular cavity) (Figs. 2–1, 2–2 and 2–3.)

        A. Characteristics

            1. An articular cavity is present.

            2. The joint is encased within a sleevelike ligamentous capsule.

            3. The capsule is lined with synovial membrane which secretes synovial fluid for lubricating the joint.

            4. The articular surfaces are smooth.

            5. The articular surfaces are covered with cartilage, usually hyaline, but occasionally fibrocartilage.

        B. Classification*

            1. Irregular (arthrodial; plane). The joint surfaces are

---

*This classification is based on the one in *Morris' Human Anatomy.*

Fig. 2-2

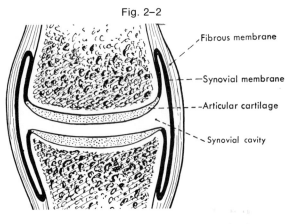

Fibrous membrane

Synovial membrane

Articular cartilage

Synovial cavity

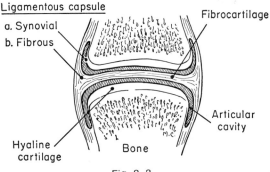

Ligamentous capsule

Fibrocartilage

a. Synovial

b. Fibrous

Articular cavity

Hyaline cartilage

Bone

Fig. 2-3

Figure 2-2.   Frontal section of a diarthrodial joint. (From Hollinshead.)
Figure 2-3.   Frontal section of a diarthrodial joint having fibrocartilage.

irregularly shaped, usually flat or slightly curved. The only movement permitted is of a gliding nature, hence it is nonaxial. Example: the carpal joints (Fig. 14–1).

2. Hinge (ginglymus). One surface is spool-like; the other is concave. The concave surface fits over the spool-like process and glides partially around it in a hinge type of movement. This constitutes movement in one plane about a single axis of motion, hence it is uniaxial. As it is a frontal horizontal axis the movements that occur are flexion and extension. Example: elbow joint (Fig. 13–1).

3. Pivot (trochoid; screw). This kind of joint may be characterized by a peglike pivot, as in the joint between atlas and axis, or by two long bones fitting against each other near each end in such a way that one bone can roll around the other one, as do the radius and ulna of the forearm. In the latter type a small concave notch on one bone fits against the rounded surface of the other. The rounded surface may either be the edge of a disk

(like the head of the radius), or it may be a rounded knob (like the head of the ulna). The only movement permitted in either kind of pivot joint is rotation. It is a movement in one plane about a single vertical axis, hence the joint is uniaxial. Examples: atlantoaxial and radioulnar joints (Figs. 18–10 and 13–1).

4. Condyloid (ovoid; ellipsoidal). An oval or egg-shaped convex surface fits into a reciprocally shaped concave surface. Movement can occur in two planes, forward and backward, and from side to side. The former movement is flexion and extension, and the latter abduction and adduction, or lateral flexion. The joint is biaxial, the axes being frontal horizontal and sagittal horizontal. When these movements are performed sequentially, they constitute circumduction. Example: wrist joint (Fig. 14–1).

5. Saddle (sellar; reciprocal reception). This may be thought of as a modification of a condyloid joint. Both ends of the convex surface are tipped up, making the surface concave in the other direction, like a western saddle. Fitting over this is a reciprocally concave-convex surface. Like the condyloid joint, this is a biaxial joint, permitting flexion and extension, abduction and adduction, and circumduction. The difference between the two is that the saddle joint has greater freedom of motion. Example: carpometacarpal joint of thumb (Fig. 14–4).

6. Ball-and-socket (spheroidal; enarthrodial). In this type of joint the spherical head of one bone fits into the cup or saucerlike cavity of the other bone (Figs. 12–1 and 15–1). It is very like the swivel joint on top of a camera tripod. It permits flexion and extension, abduction and adduction, circumduction (the sequential combination of the preceding), and rotation. It is a triaxial joint, as it permits movement about three axes, namely, frontal horizontal, sagittal horizontal and vertical.

C. Summary classification of diarthrodial joints

Number of Axes:	*0*	*1*	*2*	*3*
	Nonaxial	*Uniaxial*	*Biaxial*	*Triaxial*
Classification:	Irregular	Hinge Pivot	Condyloid Saddle	Ball-and-socket

See Appendix B for a more complete chart of Diarthrodial Joints and their Motions.

II. Synarthrosis (from the Greek, meaning literally "with joint," or according to our usage, a joint in which there is no separation or articular cavity)
   A. Characteristics
      1. In two of the types (cartilaginous and fibrous) the two bones are united by means of an intervening substance, such as cartilage or fibrous tissue, which is continuous with the joint surfaces.
      2. The third type (ligamentous) is not a true joint, but is a ligamentous connection between two bones which may or may not be contiguous.
      3. There is no articular cavity, hence no capsule, synovial membrane or synovial fluid.
   B. Classification
      1. Cartilaginous (synchondrosis; from the Greek, meaning "with cartilage")
         Only the joints which are united by fibrocartilage permit motion of a bending and twisting nature. Those united by hyaline cartilage permit only a slight compression. Example of hyaline type: epiphysial unions. Example of fibrocartilaginous type: articulations between the bodies of the vertebrae (Fig. 18–2).*
      2. Fibrous (suture; from the Latin word for "seam"). The edges of bone are united by means of a thin layer of fibrous tissue which is continuous with the periosteum. No movements are permitted. Only example: the sutures of the skull.
      3. Ligamentous (syndesmosis; from the Greek, meaning "with ligament"). Two bones, which may be adjacent or which may be quite widely separated, are tied together by one or more ligaments. These ligaments may be in the form of cords, bands or flat sheets. The movement that occurs is usually limited and of no specific type. Examples: coracoacromial union (Fig. 12–3); midunion of radius and ulna (Figs. 13–2 and 13–3).
   C. Summary
      The synarthrodial joints of greatest concern to the kinesiologist are those of the vertebral bodies. Owing to the thickness of the intervertebral disks, these permit a moderate amount of motion simulating that of ball-and-socket joints. The movements are flexion and extension, lateral flexion, circumduction and rotation.

Structure and Function of the Joints. As Steindler points out, the shape of a joint is the chief factor in determining its function. Just as the railroad track determines the route available to the train, so the shape and contours of the articulating surfaces determine the

---

*In some anatomy texts these are classified in a separate major category as amphiarthrodial joints.

movement pathways available to the bones.[4] These pathways are further influenced by ligaments, cartilages and tendons which frequently serve as restraining factors.

Steindler names four factors which are responsible for the cohesion of the joints: the joint ligaments such as the lateral ligaments of hinge joints, muscle tension (see stabilizing components of muscular force), fascia and atmospheric pressure. The latter is particularly effective at the hip joint.

In the preceding section joints were classified according to the number of axes about which their movements take place. It was shown that this corresponds to the number of planes in which the segment moves. Thus the movements of the forearm at the elbow joint occur in only one plane because the elbow is a hinge joint and a hinge joint is a uniaxial joint. The femur, on the other hand, can move in three planes because the hip joint is a ball and socket or triaxial joint. Steindler uses the term "degrees of freedom." According to this terminology, the hinge and pivot joints each have one degree of freedom of motion; the condyloid (ovoid), or biaxial joints, two degrees of freedom of motion; and the ball-and-socket, or triaxial joints, three degrees of freedom of motion.

Suggestions for Studying the Joints. In order to understand thoroughly the structure of a joint, and especially the relation of structure to function, the student should supplement his book study with first-hand study of a skeleton or of the disarticulated bones which enter into the formation of each joint. Following this preliminary study, the student will find it extremely helpful to "construct" a joint by taking the disarticulated bones and fastening them together with pieces of adhesive tape, carefully placed to represent the specific ligaments of the joint. Pieces of felt, cut in the proper shape, may be used to represent the fibrocartilage. This technique is particularly helpful for studying the knee, hip, and shoulder joints.

The movements of each joint should be studied both on the skeleton and on the living subject. When using the latter method, the student should take into consideration all the joints involved in the movement being studied. For instance, in studying the movements of the elbow, the articulation between the humerus and the radius must not be overlooked. The close relationship that exists between certain joints should be noted, as for instance the relationship between the elbow joint and the proximal radioulnar articulation. The tilting of the pelvis which accompanies many movements of the lower extremity should be recognized; likewise the movements of the shoulder girdle which accompany those of the shoulder joint. There is a particular pitfall awaiting those who study the movements of the shoulder joint only by observing the living subject. If not forewarned, they are likely to overlook the part played by the shoulder girdle in movements of the arm on the body. The action of the shoulder girdle may easily be detected if the student will palpate the scapula and the clavicle in all movements of the upper arm. He can follow the movements of the scapula by placing his thumb at the inferior angle, one finger on the root of the scapular spine, and another on the acromion process, and by keeping them firmly in contact with these points as the scapula moves.

The x-ray also affords a valuable method of studying the structure and function of the joints. Of even greater value will be the x-ray motion picture when it is made readily available for such purposes.

SUPPLEMENTARY MATERIAL

Method of Measuring Joint Motion. The literature on the measurement of joint motion reveals a notable lack of uniformity in technique and a corresponding disagreement regarding the normal range of motion. In many instances the norms quoted appear to be set up arbitrarily, rather than as the result of experimentation. While much has been achieved in standardizing the techniques of measurement, there is still a need for tables of norms for both sexes and for a complete age range, based on actual measurement. Attention is called to the two excellent reviews of literature on flexibility listed on page 33.

Students should become familiar with the different types of instruments that are used for measuring the range of motion. The simple double armed goniometer is the tool that is universally applicable to all joints (Fig. 2–4). The Leighton Flexometer,[9] designed by a physical educator, is a highly accurate 360 degree gravity type goniometer, which is strapped to the moving segment of the body (Fig. 2–5). A promising electronic instrument for the continuous recording of the movements of body segments is the electrogoniometer, or "elgon," developed by Karpovich (Figs. 2–6 and 2–7).[5] This is receiving increasing attention not only in physical education laboratories but also in orthopedic treatment centers.

1. COMPARISON OF SHOULDER FLEXIBILITY BEFORE AND AFTER CORRECTIVE EXERCISES. In a class in corrective physical education the author made several pertinent measurements at the beginning and end of the season of instruction. Among these was the measurement of forward elevation of the arm on the body. This involves, chiefly, flexion at the shoulder joint, but also includes some movement of the scapula, especially upward rotation. Individuals with resistant

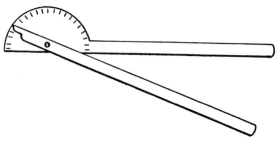

Figure 2–4. Double armed goniometer.

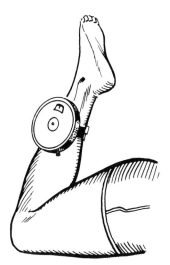

Figure 2–5. Measuring knee flexion with a Leighton Flexometer.

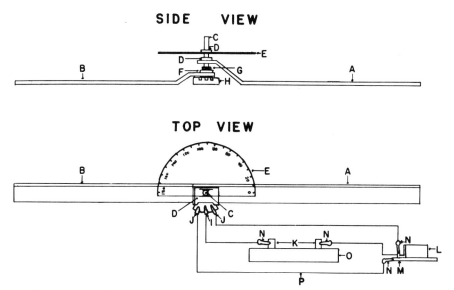

Figure 2–6. Laboratory elgon with protractor, meter and battery. (From Adrian, M.: An introduction to electrogoniometry. *In* Kinesiology Review 1968. Washington, D.C., Am. Assn. Health, Phys. Ed. & Recrn., 1968.)

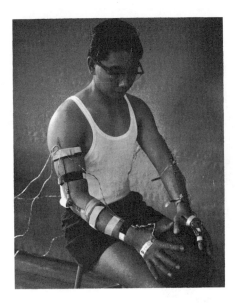

Figure 2–7. Elbow and wrist el-gons on right arm; index finger and forearm elgons on left arm. (From Adrian, M.: An introduction to electro-goniometry. *In* Kinesiology Review 1968. Washington, D.C., Am. Assn. Health, Phys. Ed. and Recrn., 1968.)

forward shoulders have limited motion in the shoulder joint. It is particularly difficult for them to raise their arms to the vertical or beyond when the arms are held just shoulder distance apart. The measurements were made on thirty girls, aged 16 to 18, in the following manner. The subject presented her left side to the examiner and raised both arms forward, upward and backward as far as possible without bending the elbows. Using a large semicircular protractor with a movable arm, the examiner held the protractor with its center opposite the center of motion at the shoulder joint and with the base line parallel with the axis of the subject's upper trunk. She then moved the arm of the protractor until it was in line with the subject's arm and read the anterior angle between the subject's arm and trunk. The results of the two sets of measurements were as follows:

	Range	*Median*
Measurements made in November 1948	129° –170°	142.5°
Measurements made in March 1949	141.5°–175°	162.5°

2. COMPARISON OF MEASUREMENTS OF FORWARD ELEVATION OF THE ARM MADE BY DIFFERENT INVESTIGATORS. A comparison of measurements of a selected joint movement may be of interest to the reader. It should be noted, however, that the techniques used were not standardized and that the measurements were based on relatively small samples, not selected at random. Forward elevation of the arm is the movement selected. The techniques of the three investigators were different, but had this in common: they used either the

vertical or the horizontal as a point of reference rather than the long axis of the trunk.

a. Experimenter: Van Horn[10]

Number, age and sex of subjects: 165 women, aged 16 to 18 inclusive.

Technique. The subject lay on a narrow board with the knees drawn up and the back kept in contact with the board. The angle between the horizontal surface of the board and the subject's arm was measured with a protractor.

Measurements

	Range	*Median*
R:	159°–196°	178°
L:	155°–198°	177°

b. Experimenters: Glanville and Kreezer[7]

Number, age and sex of subjects: ten men, aged 20 to 40 inclusive.

Technique. The subject lay on his back on a table with the shoulder over the edge of the table. The measurement was made with an arthrometer having a circular scale and a weighted metal pendulum type of indicator. This instrument was strapped to the lateral surface of the subject's arm, just proximal to the elbow.

Measurements

	Range	*Mean*
R:	164°–191°	179°
L:	165°–187°	180°

c. Experimenter: Wells

Number, age and sex of subjects: 24 young women, aged 17 to 20.

Technique. The subject sat on a gymnasium bench with the head and back braced against the edge of an open door and raised both arms forward-upward as far as possible, keeping them shoulder distance apart with the palms facing and the elbows fully extended. The anterior angle between the upper arm and the plumb line was measured with a plumb line protractor.

Measurements

	Range	*Median*
L:	161°–186°	172.5°

It is interesting to see that, despite the small number of subjects and in spite of the differences in techniques, the results are fairly consistent. It is also interesting to note the contrast between the results of these three investigations and the one made by the author on the students in the corrective class.

There are doubtless two factors that account for the appreciably lower scores made by the latter group. The first is the fact that the group was selected on the basis of poor posture. The second is the fact that the subject's own trunk was taken as the point of reference. This ruled out the influence of hyperextension of the spine on the position of the arm. Although the latter technique requires the use of subjective judgment in aligning the protractor with the subject's trunk, it is probably a more valid measure of the range of joint motion. This is the technique described by Kraus and Weber.[8]

DEMONSTRATIONS AND LABORATORY EXERCISES

1. Dissect a joint obtained from the butcher and identify the following types of tissue: tendon, ligament, fibrocartilage, hyaline cartilage and synovial membrane. Identify the type of joint and name its movements.
2. By studying a skeleton and observing a living subject, classify the following joints without referring to a textbook: hip, elbow, knee, ankle, wrist, radioulnar, metacarpophalangeal joint of finger, shoulder joint. (Do not confuse the motion at the elbow or wrist joints with that at the radioulnar joints.)
3. From a disarticulated skeleton select the necessary bones to illustrate each type of joint.
4. Using whatever joint-measuring instruments are available, measure the range of motion in the same joint movements that were described in the supplementary section of this chapter.

REFERENCES

Joint Structure and Function
1. Goss, C. M.: Gray's Anatomy of the Human Body, 28th ed. Philadelphia, Lea & Febiger, 1966.
2. Schaeffer, J. P.: Morris' Human Anatomy, 11th ed. New York, McGraw-Hill, Inc., 1953.
3. Sobotta, J.: Atlas of Human Anatomy, trans. by E. Uhlenhuth. New York, Hafner Publishing Co., 1967.
4. Steindler, A.: Kinesiology of the Human Body. Springfield, Ill., Charles C Thomas, Publisher, 1955, pp. 58–63.

Range of Joint Motion and its Measurement
5. Adrian, M. J.: An introduction to electrogoniometry. In Kinesiology Review 1968. Washington, D. C., Am. Assn. Health, Phys. Ed., and Recrn., 1968.
6. American Academy of Orthopedic Surgeons: Measuring and Recording of Joint Motion. Chicago, The Academy, 1963.
7. Glanville, A. D., and Kreezer, G.: Maximum amplitude and velocity of joint movements in normal male human adults. Hum. Biol., 9:197–211, 1937.

8. Kraus, H., and Eisenmenger-Weber, S.: Evaluation of posture based on structural and functional measurements. Physiother. Rev., 25:267–271, 1945.
9. Leighton, J. R.: An instrument and technic for the measurement of range of joint motion. Arch. Phys. Med., 36:571–578, 1955.
10. Van Horn, E. C.: Preliminary work toward the development of a table of norms of the range of motion in the shoulder joint. Unpublished seminar study, Wellesley College, 1947.

RECOMMENDED READINGS

Harris, M. L.: Flexibility (Review of the Literature). J. Am. Phys. Ther. Assn., *49*: 591–601, 1969.
Holland, G. J.: The physiology of flexibility; a review of the literature. *In* Kinesiology Review 1968. Washington, D. C., Am. Assn. Health, Phys. Ed., and Recrn., 1968.

CHAPTER 3

The Mechanics of Muscular Action

The skeletal muscles supply the force for moving the body segments. They do this by virtue of three factors: (1) the unique ability of muscular tissue to contract; (2) the attachments of the muscle to the bones; and (3) the relation of the muscle's line of pull to the joint or joints which it spans.

Properties of Muscular Tissue. In his study of anatomy the student learned that the properties of striated muscle tissue are *extensibility, elasticity* and *contractility.* The first two of these enable a muscle to be stretched like an elastic band and, when the stretching force is discontinued, to return again to its normal resting length. Tendons also possess these properties, being merely continuations of the muscle's connective tissue. The peculiar property of contractility is possessed by muscle tissue alone. Experimenters have found that the average muscle fiber can shorten to approximately one-half its resting length. It can also be stretched until it is approximately one-half again as long as its resting length.[1,10] The range between the maximal and minimal lengths of a muscle fiber is known as the amplitude of its action. The elongation varies proportionately with the length of the fiber, and inversely with its cross section.

When the muscle fibers contract, the muscle as a whole contracts. The degree of its total shortening depends upon its internal structure as well as upon the length of its individual fibers. Only those muscles whose fibers run longitudinally will shorten as a whole in proportion to the shortening of their individual fibers. Penniform and other muscles whose fibers are arranged obliquely will shorten somewhat less, depending upon the length of the fibers and their degree of slant.

Structural Classification of Muscles. The arrangement of the fibers and the method of attachment vary considerably among the different muscles. These structural variations form the basis for a classification of the skeletal muscles.

LONGITUDINAL. This is a long straplike muscle whose fibers lie parallel to its long axis. Two examples are the rectus abdominis on the front of the abdomen and the sartorius, which slants across the front of the thigh.

QUADRATE OR QUADRILATERAL. (Fig. 3–1, *E* and *F*.) Muscles of this type are foursided and are usually flat. They consist of parallel fibers. Examples include the pronator quadratus on the front of the wrist and the rhomboid muscle between the spine and the scapula.

TRIANGULAR OR FAN-SHAPED. (Fig. 3–1, *D*.) This is a relatively flat type of muscle whose fibers radiate from a narrow attachment at one end to a broad attachment at the other. The pectoralis major on the front of the chest is an excellent example.

FUSIFORM OR SPINDLE-SHAPED. (Fig. 3–1, *A*.) This is usually a rounded muscle which tapers at either end. It may be long or short, large or small. Good examples are the brachialis and the brachioradialis muscles of the arm.

PENNIFORM OR FEATHER-LIKE. (Fig. 3–1, *B*.) In this type of muscle a series of short parallel fibers extends diagonally from the side of a long tendon, giving the muscle as a whole the appearance of a wing feather. Examples: extensor digitorum longus and tibialis posterior muscles of the leg.

BIPENNIFORM. (Fig. 3–1, *C*.) This is a double penniform muscle. It is characterized by a long central tendon with the fibers extending diagonally in pairs from either side of the tendon. It resembles a symmetrical tail feather. Examples: flexor hallucis longus and rectus femoris.

MULTIPENNIFORM. In this type of muscle there are several tendons present, with the muscle fibers running diagonally between them. The middle portion of the deltoid muscle is an example of a multipenniform muscle.

Muscular Attachments. Muscles are attached to bone by means of their connective tissue which continues beyond the muscle belly in the form either of a tendon (a round cord or a flat band) or of an aponeurosis (a fibrous sheet). It has been customary to designate the

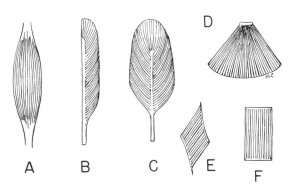

Figure 3–1. Examples of muscles of different shapes and internal structure. *A,* Fusiform or spindle; *B,* penniform; *C,* bipenniform; *D,* triangular or fan-shaped; *E,* rhomboidal; *F,* rectangular.

attachments of the two ends of a muscle as "origin" and "insertion." The origin is usually characterized by stability and by closeness of the muscle fibers to the bone. It is usually the more proximal of the two attachments. The insertion, on the other hand, is usually the distal attachment; it frequently involves a relatively long tendon and the bone into which the muscle's tendon is inserted is ordinarily the one that moves. It should be understood, however, that the muscle does not pull in one direction or the other. When it contracts it exerts equal force on its two attachments and attempts to pull them toward each other. Which bone is to remain stationary and which one is to move depends upon the purpose of the movement. A muscle spanning the inside of a hinge type joint, for instance, tends to draw both bones toward one another. But most precision movements require that the proximal bone be stabilized while the distal bone performs the movement. The stabilization of the proximal bone is achieved by the action of other muscles. Sometimes the greater weight or the more limited mobility of the proximal structure is sufficient to stabilize it against the pull of the contracting muscles.

It has been the author's experience that students tend to have the erroneous impression that there is some physiologic reason for a muscle pulling in a single direction. They fail to grasp the fact that a muscle merely contracts; it does not pull in a predetermined direction. This misconception makes it difficult for them to understand seeming exceptions. Actually there are many movements in which the insertion, or distal attachment of the muscle, is stationary and the origin, or proximal attachment, is the one that moves. Such is the case in the familiar act of chinning oneself. The movement at the elbow joint is flexion, but it is the upper arm that moves toward the forearm, just the reverse of the situation when one lifts a book from a table. The grasp of the hands on the bar serves to immobilize the forearm and thus provide a stable base for the contracting muscles.

In order to avoid the erroneous idea of a muscle always moving its insertion toward its origin, other terms have been substituted for these, terms which it is hoped will have no connotation for the reader regarding direction of pull. These are presented in the introduction to Part II.

Relation of the Muscle's Line of Pull to the Joint. Whether a muscle will cause a joint to become flexed, extended, abducted, adducted or rotated is determined by the relation of its line of pull, or action line, to the joint's axis of motion (Fig. 3–2). For instance, the contraction of a muscle whose line of pull is directly anterior to the knee joint will cause the joint to extend, whereas a muscle whose line of pull is anterior to the elbow joint will cause this joint to flex. The possible axes of motion are of course determined by the structure of the joint itself. It will be recalled that hinge joints have only a frontal horizontal axis; condyloid (ovoid) joints, both a frontal horizontal and a sagittal horizontal axis; ball-and-socket joints, three axes – frontal and sagittal horizontal, and vertical; and pivot joints, a vertical axis only. A muscle whose line of pull is lateral to the hip joint is a potential abductor of the thigh, but muscles whose lines of pull are lateral to

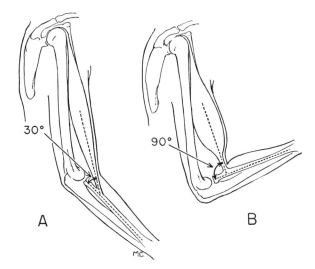

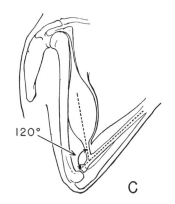

Figure 3-2. Angles of muscle pull. A, An angle less than 45 degrees; B, an angle of 90 degrees; C, an angle greater than 90 degrees.

the elbow joint cannot cause abduction of the forearm because the construction of the elbow joint is such that no provision is made for ab- or adduction. Being a hinge joint, its only axis of motion is a frontal horizontal one and the only movements possible are flexion and extension.

The importance of the relation of a muscle's action line to the joint's axis of motion is seen especially in some of the muscles that act on triaxial joints. Occasionally it happens that a muscle's line of pull for one of its secondary movements shifts from one side of the joint's center of motion to the other during the course of the movement. For instance, the clavicular portion of the pectoralis major is primarily a flexor, but it also adducts the humerus. When the arm is elevated sideward to a position slightly above shoulder level, however, the line of pull of some of the fibers of the clavicular portion shifts from below to above the sagittal horizontal axis of the shoulder joint (Fig. 3-3). Contraction of these fibers in this position contributes to *abduction* of the humerus, rather than to adduction. Similarly, several

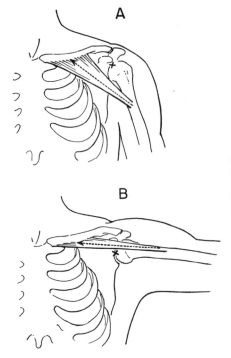

Figure 3–3. The clavicular portion of the pectoralis major muscle reversing its customary function. *A,* The line of pull is below the center of the shoulder joint. *B,* The line of pull is above the center of the shoulder joint.

muscles or parts of muscles of the hip joint appear to reverse their customary function. Steindler pointed out that as the adductor longus adducts the hip joint it also flexes it until the flexion exceeds 70 degrees. Beyond this point the adductor longus helps to extend the hip.

Functional Classification of Muscles. From the point of view of primary function, a useful classification of muscles is one that corresponds to the structural classification of joints.

Diarthrodial Axial Joints	*Muscles*
Uniaxial	
Hinge	Flexors and extensors
Pivot..	Rotators
Biaxial	
Condyloid (ovoid)	Flexors; extensors; abductors; adductors
Saddle	Same as for condyloid joints
Triaxial*	
Ball-and-socket	Flexors; extensors; abductors; adductors; rotators

*Although the joints between the bodies of the vertebrae are cartilaginous synarthrodial joints, and those between the articular processes of the vertebrae are non-axial diarthrodial joints, the movements of the spinal column resemble those of triaxial joints. This is because of the ball-and-socket nature of the nucleus pulposus in the intervertebral disks.

TYPES OF CONTRACTION

The classification of muscular contraction into types is based upon whether the muscle shortens, lengthens, or remains the same length when it contracts. There are three sets of terms for the different types of contraction in which muscles can engage. These are (1) concentric (shortening), eccentric (lengthening) and static; (2) isometric and isotonic; and (3) phasic and tonic.

Concentric, Eccentric and Static Contraction

CONCENTRIC OR SHORTENING CONTRACTION. The muscle actually shortens, and when one end is stabilized the other pulls the bone to which it is attached and turns it about the joint axis. The bone thus serves as a lever and the joint as its fulcrum. This is the usual type of contraction seen in physical activities.

ECCENTRIC OR LENGTHENING CONTRACTION. This is a gradual releasing of the contraction, as when one lowers a weight slowly or gives in to an external force which is stronger than that of the contracting muscle. The term "lengthening" is misleading, as in most instances the muscle does not actually lengthen. It merely returns from its shortened condition to its normal resting length.

STATIC CONTRACTION. The muscle remains in partial or complete contraction without changing its length. There are two different conditions under which this type of contraction is likely to occur.

1. Muscles which are antagonistic to each other contract with equal strength, thus balancing or counteracting each other. The part affected is held tensely in place without moving. Tensing the biceps to show it off is an example of this.

2. A muscle is held in either partial or maximal contraction against another force such as the pull of gravity or an external mechanical or muscular force. Examples of this are holding a book with outstretched arm, a tug of war between two equally matched opponents, and attempting to move an object which is too heavy to move.

Isotonic and Isometric Contraction.

These terms come from the Greek and mean respectively "equal tension" and "equal length."

ISOTONIC CONTRACTION. This is a contraction in which *the tension remains constant* as the muscle shortens. It is commonly, although erroneously, used as a synonym for concentric contraction. The latter term, however, does not indicate the degree of tension; it merely indicates a decrease in length.

ISOMETRIC CONTRACTION. This is contraction *without any appreciable change in length.* According to this definition the term would seem to be synonymous with "static contraction," but according to current usage the muscle is *unable* to shorten because of the magnitude of the resistance. This is very different from merely counter-balancing the pull of gravity. The terms are synonymous only when the static contraction involves maximal contraction.

PHASIC AND TONIC CONTRACTION. These terms are used less now than formerly. They appear to have been replaced by *isotonic* and *isometric* although they are not exactly comparable. In general, the term "phasic" appears to be used for shortening contraction, but there are instances in the literature in which it seems to mean any change in length, either shortening or lengthening. The term "tonic contraction" appears to have exactly the same meaning as "static contraction." Inasmuch as the use of these terms seems to be waning, the student need not be too concerned about their exact meanings.

THE COORDINATION OF THE MUSCULAR SYSTEM

An effective, purposeful movement of the body or any of its parts involves considerable muscular activity in addition to that of the muscles which are directly responsible for the movement itself. To begin with, the muscles causing the movement must have a stable base. This means that the bone (or bones) not engaged in the movement but providing attachment for one end of such muscles must be stabilized by other muscles. In some movements, such as those in which the hands are used at a high level, the upper arms may need to be maintained in an elevated position. This necessitates contraction of the shoulder muscles to support the weight of the arms. Many muscles, especially those of biaxial and triaxial joints, can cause movements involving more than one axis, yet it may be that only one of their actions is needed for the movement in question. A similar situation exists in regard to the muscles of the scapula. A muscle cannot voluntarily choose to effect one of its movements and not another; it must depend upon other muscles to contract and prevent the unwanted movement.

Thus even a simple movement like threading a needle or hammering a nail may require the cooperative action of a relatively large number of muscles, each performing its own particular task in producing a single well-coordinated movement. It is seen then that muscles have various roles, and that what their particular role is in a given movement depends upon the requirements of that movement. In summary, these roles are designated as movers, stabilizers, supporting muscles and neutralizers. Furthermore, if one concedes that the negative function of remaining relaxed can be looked upon as a role, then the muscles that are antagonistic to the movers may also be included as participants in the total cooperative effort. The definitions of these roles are as follows:

Movers. A mover is a muscle which is directly responsible for effecting a movement. In the majority of movements there are several movers, some of them of greater importance than others. These are the principal movers. The muscles which help to perform the movement, but which seem to be of less importance, or which contract only under certain circumstances, are the assistant movers. Muscles which help only when an extra amount of force is needed, as when a movement is performed against resistance, are sometimes called emergency muscles. This distinction between the various muscles which contribute to a movement is an arbitrary one. There may well be some difference of opinion as to whether a muscle is a principal or an assistant mover in a given movement.

Fixator, Stabilizing and Supporting Muscles. This group includes the muscles which contract statically to steady or to support some part of the body against the pull of the contracting muscles, against the pull of gravity, or against the effect of momentum and recoil in certain vigorous movements. One of the most common functions of these muscles is steadying or fixating the bone to which a contracting muscle is attached. It is only by the stabilizing of one of its attachments that the muscle is able to cause an effective movement of the bone at which it has its other attachment (Fig. 3–4). The term "supporting" is used when a limb or the trunk must be supported against the pull of gravity while a distal segment, such as the hand, foot or head, is engaging in the essential movement.

Neutralizers. A neutralizer is a muscle which acts to prevent an undesired action of one of the movers. Thus if a muscle both flexes and abducts, but only flexion is desired in the movement, an adductor contracts to neutralize the abductory action of the mover.

Occasionally two of the movers have one action in common, but second actions which are antagonistic to each other. For instance, one

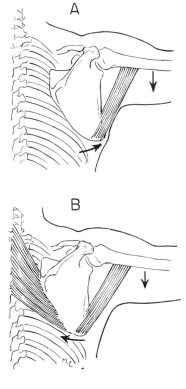

Figure 3–4. If the scapula were not stabilized, the teres major would increase the upward rotation of the scapula as it adducted the humerus. This dual action on the humerus and scapula is shown in A. In B, the scapula is stabilized by the scapular adductors and downward rotators. This permits the teres major to concentrate its force on the adduction of the humerus.

muscle may upward rotate and adduct, the other may downward rotate and adduct. When they contract together to cause adduction, their rotatory functions counteract each other (Fig. 3–5). Muscles which behave this way in a movement are mutual neutralizers as well as movers. Some writers use the term "synergist" for muscles which have this neutralizing function.[12] The term is used by others for muscles that stabilize bones; and by still others for any muscles that work together to contribute to a movement, regardless of the specific function of each.[10] Because of this confusion, the use of the term has purposely been avoided in this text.

Antagonists. An antagonist is a muscle which causes the opposite movement from that of the muscle acting as a mover. Thus in a movement of flexion, the flexors are the movers and the extensors are the antagonists. In accordance with the physiologic principle known as reciprocal innervation, when a muscle contracts, its antagonist automatically relaxes (see p. 175).

Having stated the general rule, it is now necessary to describe what may at first appear to be a contradiction. If a movement performed with great force and rapidity is not checked, it will subject the ligamentous reinforcements of the joint to sudden strain. The tissues would probably be severely damaged. This is particularly true of quick movements of the arm or leg because of the tremendous momentum that can be developed in a long lever. To prevent such injury the muscles that are antagonistic to the movers contract momentarily to check the movement. As they contract, the movers relax, if indeed they have not already relaxed, allowing momentum to complete the movement. The situation is a little like taking the foot off the accelerator in order to put it on the brake. At the moment when the movement is being checked, the so-called antagonistic muscles are not truly antagonistic, but are serving temporarily as movers in eccentric contraction. Thus, in a vigorous movement, the antagonistic muscles may be said to perform two functions. Their first function is to relax in order to permit the movement to be made without hindrance; their second function is to protect the joint by acting as a brake at the completion of the movement.

Ballistic Movement. The concept of ballistic movement was originally described by experimental psychologists.[5, 6, 11] They classified movements first into slow and rapid movements. The slow movements were said to be "moving fixations," because they involve the contraction of opposing muscle fibers. Rapid movements, they said, could be performed either ballistically or as moving fixations. Rapid movements are skillfully executed only when they are performed ballistically. By this they meant that the movement is initiated by muscular contraction, but that the muscles then relax and permit momentum to complete the movement. This type of movement is characteristic of throwing, striking and kicking. On a smaller scale it is represented by typewriting and piano playing. When these activities are performed nonballistically, that is, with a constant muscular contraction, they are uneconomical, hence not skillful. They are then tension movements. This characterizes the way in which begin-

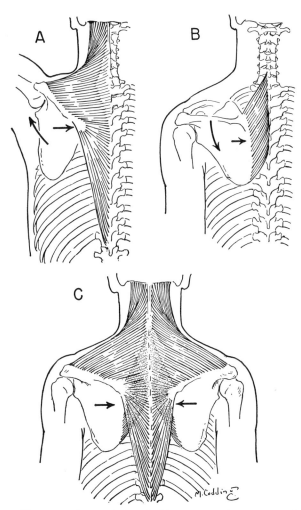

Figure 3–5. The trapezius and rhomboids as mutual movers and neutralizers. *A,* The trapezius alone adducts the scapula and rotates it upward. *B,* The rhomboids alone adduct the scapula and rotate it downward. *C,* Together the trapezius and rhomboids adduct the scapula without rotating it either upward or downward.

ners and young children frequently attempt new coordinations, especially when they are concentrating on accuracy of aim rather than on ease of motion. The psychologists recommend emphasizing form at the expense of accuracy in learning new skills. Otherwise, they say, bad habits of tensing the muscles are likely to be established.

Ballistic movements may be terminated by one of three methods: (1) by contracting antagonistic muscles, as in the forehand drive in tennis; (2) by allowing the moving part to reach the limit of motion, in which case it will be stopped by the passive resistance of ligaments or muscles, as in the case of a high kick; or (3) by the interference of an obstacle, as when chopping wood.

In many movements found both in sports and in skilled labor, three types of muscular action cooperate to produce a single act. This kind of cooperation is seen especially in striking activities which require the use of an implement, such as a tennis racket, golf club or ax. Movements such as these involve (1) fixation to support the moving part and to maintain the necessary position; (2) ballistic movement of the active limb; and (3) fixation in the fingers as they grasp the implement. Hartson suggested that the purpose of the "follow through" in throwing and striking movements in sports is to assure a ballistic type of movement.[5] It would seem that there may be some sport movements which cannot be categorized as either tension or ballistic movements. Where maximum speed or force is desired, it would seem necessary to exert muscular effort throughout the movement, yet undesirable to contract the antagonistic muscles. It would also seem that there are more factors in the "follow through" than are suggested by Hartson's hypothesis. Questions such as these await further research by investigators in the field of physical education.

Cocontraction. A number of investigators have stated that muscles which are antagonistic to each other contract concurrently under certain conditions. Some of the examples cited are the action of opposing muscles of the lower extremity in locomotion, with the action of the antagonists diminishing while that of the agonists is increasing; the contraction of antagonistic muscles in slow tension movements as a means of achieving greater precision and accuracy, or helping to regulate the speed; and the contraction of the antagonistic muscles toward the end of a ballistic movement, e.g., throwing, kicking, or an arm flinging exercise, for the purpose of protecting the joint structures.

True cocontraction would seem to be a contradiction of reciprocal innervation. Therefore, until conclusive evidence to the contrary is presented, this text agrees with the views expressed by Basmajian[2] and by O'Connell and Gardner,[8] namely, that cocontraction is an indication of lack of skill (see page 176). The apparent contradictions may be explained in other ways, for instance, the concept of antagonistic muscles being used to check ballistic movements is entirely acceptable, if by this one means the checking of the limb's momentum after the movers (agonists) have relaxed. A slight overlapping of the opposing muscle groups might occur, but this would seem to be only momentary and of slight importance.

In balance type activities and possibly in slow tension movements, it seems likely that opposing muscle groups may contract in alternation and that they may vary between static contraction and slight concentric or slight eccentric contraction, according to the situation.

It also seems likely that the precise role of a muscle might easily be misinterpreted. A muscle might appear to be contracting antagonistically to the movers, whereas actually it might be a two-joint muscle acting primarily on the other joint, or it might be contracting in the capacity of a fixator or a neutralizer, rather than as antagonist. It is difficult to believe that nature is so inefficient as to require muscles to contract in direct opposition to each other. Evidence of genuine cocontraction would appear to indicate unnecessary tension, hence, lack of skill.

The Influence of Gravity and Other External Forces on Muscular Action. It may surprise the student to learn that when he replaces a book on a low table, or a suitcase on the floor, he is using the same muscles that he used for lifting it, not the opposite group as he might have thought. He uses them in a different way, however. When he lifts the book or the suitcase, the lifting muscles contract in the "normal" way. That is, they gradually shorten and their action is called shortening, or concentric, contraction (Fig. 3–6, *C*). When he *slowly* lowers the object, the same muscles are now gradually returning to their resting length. Although the term is paradoxical this action is known as lengthening, or eccentric, contraction (Fig. 3–6, *A*). A similar action is experienced in reverse by the lower extremity muscles when one lowers the body weight by bending the knees to assume a squat, or semi-squat, position, and then returns to the erect position. As he stoops, the extensor muscles of the hips and knees are undergoing eccentric contraction. They are indeed lengthening in this instance, yet their tension is increasing as they assume the burden of the body weight and gradually lower it in a controlled manner. When the joint action is reversed and the body weight is lifted, the extensor muscles are contracting concentrically until the hips and knees are straight and the body is erect. In the normal standing position the weight-bearing joints are stabilized as the result of the relationship between the gravitational force and the center of motion of the joints.

Similar muscular action is seen when one is opposing an external force which proves too strong for him. In a tug of war, for instance, he may pull with all his strength, but if his opponent is stronger than he is, he (the former) will find his elbows being pulled out straight in spite of himself. This is another example of eccentric contraction. When the muscles contract in this manner they are said to perform negative work.

Tendon Action of Two-Joint Muscles.[3, 4, 7, 9, 10] Another type of coordination of the muscular system is seen in the so-called tendon action of the two-joint muscles, that is, the muscles that pass over and

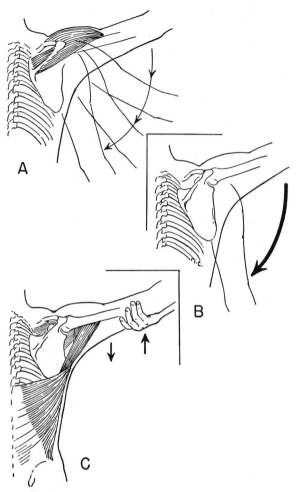

Figure 3–6. Influence of gravitational force on muscular action in sideward depression of the arm (adduction of the humerus). *A,* Eccentric contraction of the abductors in slow lowering of the arm. *B,* Absence of muscular action when the arm is dropped to the side. *C,* Concentric contraction of the adductors when the movement is performed against resistance.

act upon two joints. Examples of these are the hamstrings (semitendinosus, semimembranosus and biceps femoris), which flex the leg at the knee and extend the thigh at the hip; the rectus femoris, which flexes the thigh and extends the leg; the sartorius, which flexes both the thigh and the leg; the gastrocnemius, which helps to flex the leg in addition to its primary function of extending the foot; and the long flexors and extensors of the fingers. The latter are actually multijoint muscles, since they cross the wrist and at least two of the joints of the fingers. A characteristic of all these muscles, whether they act on joints that flex in the same direction, as in the case of the wrist and fingers, or in the opposite direction, as in the case of the knee and hip, is that they are not long enough to permit complete movement in both joints at the same time. This results in the tension of one muscle being transmitted to the other, in much the same manner that a downward pull on a rope which passes through an overhead pulley is transmitted in the form of a pull in the reverse direction to the rope on the other side of the pulley. Thus if the hamstrings contract to help extend the hip, tension is transmitted to the rectus femoris, causing it to extend the knee. Or if the rectus femoris contracts to help flex the hip, tension is transmitted to the hamstrings, causing them to flex the knee. This is a simplified version of what in actuality is a rather complex coordination.

When one-joint muscles contract, their shortening is accompanied by a corresponding loss of tension. In quick movements of the limbs, one-joint muscles lose their tension rapidly. The advantage of two-joint muscles is that they can continue to exert tension without shortening. The two-joint muscles have two different patterns of action. These have been described by Fenn, Steindler and others as concurrent and countercurrent movements.

An example of concurrent movement is seen in simultaneous extension of the hip and knee, also in simultaneous flexion of these joints. As the muscles contract they act on each other in such a way that they do not lose length, and therefore retain their tension. It is as though the pull traveled up one muscle and down the other in a continuous circuit. In simultaneous extension of the hip and knee, for instance, the rectus femoris' loss of tension at the distal or knee end is balanced by a gain in tension at the proximal or hip end. Similarly, the hamstrings, which are losing tension at their proximal end, are gaining it at their distal end.

The countercurrent pattern presents a different picture. In this type of movement, while one of the two-joint muscles shortens rapidly at both joints, its antagonist lengthens correspondingly and thereby gains tension at both ends. An example of this is seen in the rapid loss of tension in the rectus femoris and corresponding gain of tension in the hamstrings, when the hip is flexed and the knee is extended simultaneously. A vigorous kick is a dramatic illustration of this kind of muscle action. The backward swing of the lower extremity preparatory to kicking is a less spectacular but equally valid example. The forward swing in walking is another. In both patterns of movement the one- and two-joint muscles appear to supplement each other, and thus, by their cooperative action, produce smooth, coordinated, efficient movements.

SUPPLEMENTARY MATERIAL

In an article on the mechanics of muscular contraction Fenn described a simple experiment that demonstrates the influence of muscle length on the force which the muscle can exert. The strength of the rectus femoris and of the biceps femoris was tested in two positions by means of the Martin breaking-point test. The rectus femoris is situated on the front of the thigh and attaches to the pelvis just above the hip joint, and, by means of the patellar ligament, exerts its pull on the front of the tibia just below the knee joint. Hence it is a flexor of the hip and an extensor of the knee. The biceps femoris is situated on the back of the thigh and attaches above the hip and below the knee. It therefore is an extensor of the hip and a flexor of the knee.

For the first test the subject lay on his back on a table with his knees at the edge and his legs hanging down. For the second test he sat on the end of the table with his trunk flexed well forward from the hips. Thus the rectus femoris was on a greater stretch in the first position, and the biceps femoris in the second. The results showed that the rectus femoris exerted greater force in the first position than in the second, but the biceps femoris exerted greater force in the second position. These experiments could easily be duplicated in the classroom.[4]

DEMONSTRATIONS AND LABORATORY EXERCISES

1. Referring to a cadaver, a muscle manikin, muscle charts, or samples of meat obtained from a butcher, identify the structural type of several muscles. Also identify some deep fascia.

2. Take two sticks which are joined at one end by a hinge. Attach a single piece of elastic or a long rubber band to the opposite ends of the two sticks.

    a. Separate the ends of the sticks as far as the elastic will permit and then demonstrate the way the elastic will pull both sticks together.

    b. Demonstrate the way the elastic will move only one of the sticks if the other one is stabilized.

    c. Repeat both a and b, using the arm of the skeleton instead of the sticks.

3. Fasten or hold an elastic on a skeleton to represent the line of pull of the clavicular portion of the pectoralis major. Note its relation to the center of motion of the shoulder joint. Now raise the arm sideward above the shoulder level. Again note the relation of the elastic to the center of the joint.

4. Get a subject to hold a heavy dumbbell in his right hand and slowly raise his arm sideward-upward without bending the elbow. Keep your fingers on the clavicular portion of the pectoralis major. Does it contract? If so, at what position of the arm does it begin?

5. Flex the fingers hard. Keep them flexed and flex the hand at the wrist as far as possible. What happens to the fingers? Explain.

6. Extend the fingers, then hyperextend the hand at the wrist as far as possible. What happens to the fingers? Explain.

7. Get a subject to lie on the left side with the hip and knee in a partly flexed position and the right leg fully extended. The right thigh should now be flexed passively by an operator. The subject should attempt to keep the knee straight, but not to the point of interfering

with the hip flexion. What happens? Where does the subject feel discomfort? Explain.

8. With the subject in the same starting position as in 7, have him flex both his right thigh and leg completely. The right thigh should now be passively extended by an operator, the subject attempting to keep the leg flexed at the knee. As the thigh becomes fully extended, what happens to the knee? Where does the subject feel discomfort? Explain. (Caution: Do not use an acrobat or acrobatic dancer as a subject for 7 or 8, or the experiments may not work. Why?)

Note: Laboratory exercises on the action of muscles as movers, stabilizers and neutralizers are not included here because, in order to do them, it is necessary to know the individual muscles. They will be found in the laboratory sections of Chapters 12 through 19.

REFERENCES

1. Arkin, A. M.: Absolute muscle power; internal kinesiology of muscle. Arch. Surg., 42:395–410, 1941.
2. Basmajian, J. V.: Muscles Alive, 2nd ed. Baltimore, The Williams & Wilkins Company, 1967.
3. Brunnstrom, S.: Clinical Kinesiology, 2nd ed. Philadelphia, F. A. Davis Company, 1966.
4. Fenn, W. O.: The mechanics of muscular contraction in man. J. Appl. Physics, 9:165–177, 1938.
5. Hartson, L. D.: Analysis of skilled movements. Personnel J., 11:28–43, 1932.
6. Hartson, L. D.: Contrasting approaches to the analysis of skilled movements. J. Gen. Psychol., 20:263–293, 1939.
7. Lombard, W. P.: The action of two-joint muscles. Am. Phys. Ed. Rev., 8:141–145, 1903.
8. O'Connell, A. L., and Gardner, E. B.: Co-contraction of antagonistic muscles during slow controlled movement. Report presented at Research Section, National Convention of the American Association for Health, Physical Education and Recreation, 1960.
9. Rasch, P. J., and Burke, R. K.: Kinesiology and Applied Anatomy, 3rd ed. Philadelphia, Lea & Febiger, 1967, pp. 280–285.
10. Steindler, A.: Kinesiology of the Human Body. Springfield, Ill., Charles C Thomas, Publisher, 1955.
11. Stetson, R. H., and McDill, J. A.: Mechanism of the different types of movement. Psychol. Monogr., 32(3):18–40, 1923.
12. Wright, W. G.: Muscle Function. New York, Hafner Publishing Co., 1962.

RECOMMENDED READINGS

Craig, A. S.: Elements of kinesiology from the clinician. J. Am. Phys. Ther. Assn., 44:470–473, 1964. A brief but comprehensive article as valuable for physical educators as for physical therapists.
Elftman, H.: The action of muscles in the body. *In* Fenn, W. O. (Ed.): Biological Symposia. Lancaster, Pa., The Jacques Cattell Press, 1941, Vol. 3, pp. 191–209.
Hubbard, A. W.: Homokinetics: muscular function in human movement. *In* Johnson, W. R. (Ed.): Science and Medicine of Exercise and Sports. New York, Harper & Brothers, 1960, Chap. 1.
McCloy, C. H.: Some notes on differential actions of partite muscles. Res. Quart. Am. Assn. Health, Phys. Ed. & Recrn., 17:254–262, 1946.

CHAPTER 4

Simple Machines Found in the Musculoskeletal Structure

If mechanical principles play such an important role in the study of human motion as has been implied, one logical approach to the study of kinesiology would seem to be identification of the machines that are found in the body. Webster's Dictionary and elementary physics texts describe six basic machines, namely the lever, the pulley, the wheel and axle, the inclined plane, the wedge and the screw. The first three of these are represented in the musculoskeletal system. Consideration of some of the tools and implements that we commonly use in the kitchen, garden and workshop will aid in an understanding of their counterparts in the human body.

The Lever. We use levers every day of our lives. In the kitchen the old-fashioned hand can opener, the nut pick, the punch can opener, the bottle opener or lid pry, are all examples of simple levers. In the workshop, or about the house and grounds, the tack lifter, the crowbar, the pinch bar and the wheelbarrow are likewise levers. What do these have in common? Even though their shapes vary and their structures differ in complexity, each of these is a rigid bar. When a force is applied to one of them, it turns about a fixed point known as a fulcrum, and it overcomes a resistance which may, in some cases, be no more than its own weight. All the levers mentioned are for the purpose of using a relatively small force to overcome a relatively large resistance. In levers such as these the range of movement is relatively slight. The tack lifter, for instance, lifts the tack only a fraction of an inch. In other words, the power to overcome a considerable resistance is gained at the expense of range of motion.

The striking implements used in sports are levers that do the opposite of this. The golf club, for instance, is used for gaining range of motion at the expense of force. The length of the shaft enables the club head to travel through a large arc of motion, but it is used to overcome the relatively slight resistance of the weight of the club itself. Tennis and squash rackets, baseball bats, hockey sticks and fencing foils are other examples of levers used for the purpose of gaining distance at the expense of force. These levers do not save the strength of the user, as do the household levers mentioned, but they increase his range and speed of movement. By striking a ball with a racket, for instance, he can impart more speed to it and send it a greater distance than he could by striking it with his hand. This is because the head of the racket travels a greater distance, and therefore at a greater speed, than the hand alone is able to do.

A still different kind of lever is seen in the seesaw on the playground, the scales in the laboratory and the pole used by the Chinese coolie for carrying balanced loads across one shoulder. These levers gain neither force nor distance, but provide for a balancing of weights. If the loads are equal, they will balance each other when they are equidistant from the fulcrum. If they are unequal, they will balance only if the heavier load is placed closer to the fulcrum. There is an exact relationship between the magnitude of the weights and their respective distances from the fulcrum.

This kind of lever may also be used to balance a force and a load. The vagabond carrying a stick on his shoulder, with his bundle tied to one end and his hand holding the other end, is using this kind of a lever. The amount of force exerted by his hand depends upon what portion of the stick is in contact with his shoulder. If it is the midpoint, then the force exerted by his hand must exactly equal the weight of the bundle. The closer the point of contact to the bundle, the less force his hand will need to exert. The slant of the stick is also a factor but for purposes of simplification the horizontal position is the only one considered here.

The Body Segments as Levers. But where in the human body do we have anything even faintly resembling a punch can opener, a hockey stick or a seesaw? The resemblance may not at first be apparent, but when we recognize each of these levers as a rigid bar which turns about a fulcrum when force is applied to it, it is then apparent that nearly every bone in the skeleton can be looked upon as a lever. The bone itself serves as the rigid bar, the joint as the fulcrum and the contracting muscles as the force. A large segment of the body, such as the trunk, the upper extremity or the lower extremity, can likewise act as a single lever if it is used as a rigid unit. When the entire arm is raised sideward, for instance, it is acting as a simple lever. The center of motion in the shoulder joint serves as the fulcrum. The force is supplied mainly by the deltoid muscle and the resistance in this instance is the weight of the arm itself. The point at which the force is applied to the lever is approximately the point at which the deltoid inserts into the humerus and the point at which the resistance is applied is the center of gravity of the extended arm. If a weight is held in the hand the resistance point is then the center of gravity of the arm plus its load and is located closer to the hand than before. If a relatively heavy weight is lifted, for practical purposes the weight of the arm may be disregarded and the resistance point may be assumed to be the center of the object's point of contact with the hand.

An important factor which will be discussed in a later chapter is the angle of application of both the force and the resistance. This refers to the angle between the line, or direction, of force (or of the resistance) and the lever. For the time being only right angle applications will be considered. The student must not fall into the error, however, of assuming that this is the usual situation.

Anatomic levers do not necessarily resemble bars. The skull, the shoulder blade and the vertebrae are notable exceptions to the definition. The resistance point, also, may be difficult to identify, especially in the seesaw type of lever. It is not always easy to tell whether the resistance is the weight of the lever itself, or is the resistance afforded by antagonistic muscles and fasciae which are put on a steadily increasing stretch as the movement progresses. For instance, when the head is turned easily to the left, the resistance point may be regarded as the center of gravity of the head. We can only guess at the approximate location of this. If the turning of the head is resisted by the pressure of someone's hand against the left side of the chin, the resistance point is the midpoint of the contact area. If the head is turned without external resistance, but is forced to the limit of motion, resistance to the movement is afforded by the antagonistic rotators, and possibly by the ligaments and fasciae. The resistance *point* in such a case is the midpoint of the area over which these resisting forces act on the head. As in the first example, the location of this point can only be estimated.

DEFINITION AND CLASSIFICATION OF LEVERS.   It should be clear by now that a lever is any rigid bar which turns about a fulcrum when force is applied to it. In the process of turning, it overcomes resistance. This resistance may be nothing more than the weight of the lever itself, or it may be an external load or a counterforce. In the body internal resistance is an additional factor. This may be caused by friction in the joint, by the tonus of antagonistic muscles or by the tautness of ligaments or fasciae. Whatever the nature of the resistance, its application to the lever can be represented by a single point, that is, the midpoint of the area over which the resistance is applied to the lever.

Thus we see that the lever has three important points: the point about which it turns, the point at which force is applied to it and the point at which the resistance to its movement is applied or concentrated. Since there are three points, there are three possible arrangements of these points. Any one of the three may be situated between the other two. The arrangement of these three points provides the basis for the classification of levers.

1. In a first class lever the fulcrum lies between the force and resistance points (Fig. 4–1, *1*).

2. In a second class lever the resistance point lies between the fulcrum and the force point (Fig. 4–1, *2*).

3. In a third class lever the force point lies between the fulcrum and the resistance point (Fig. 4–1, *3*).

LEVER ARMS.   The portion of the lever between the fulcrum and the force point is known as the force arm of the lever. Similarly,

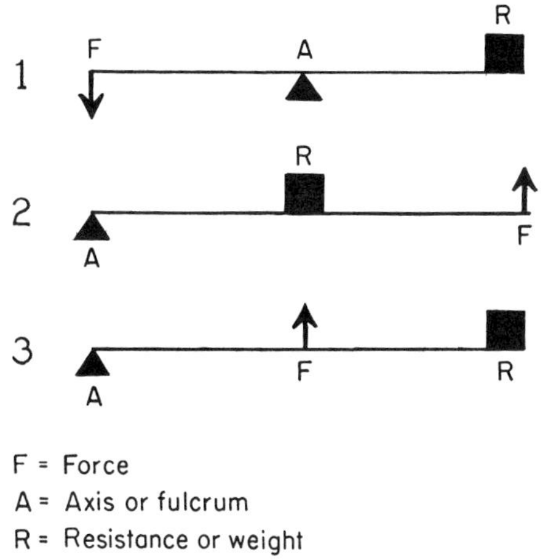

Figure 4-1. Levers. 1. A lever of the first class; 2, a lever of the second class; 3, a lever of the third class.

F = Force
A = Axis or fulcrum
R = Resistance or weight

the portion of the lever between the fulcrum and the resistance point is known as the resistance arm. In the second class lever the force arm coincides with the total lever; hence the force arm is always longer than the resistance arm. In the third class lever the resistance arm coincides with the total lever; hence the resistance arm is always longer than the force arm. In the first class lever, however, the arms may be of equal length, or either the force arm or the resistance arm may be the longer, depending upon the relative position of the fulcrum. The definitions just given, however, presuppose the force and the resistance to be applied at right angles to the lever. A more exact definition of the force arm would be "the perpendicular distance from the fulcrum to the line of force," and of the resistance arm, "the perpendicular distance from the fulcrum to the line of resistance." These definitions are accurate regardless of the direction of the force or of the resistance. They are discussed more fully in the next chapter.

A lever whose force arm is the longer of the two, whether it be a first or second class lever, is said to favor force. Less effort is required to overcome a resistance with this kind of lever than it would take to overcome the same resistance without the aid of the lever. It gains this advantage at the expense of speed and range of movement. Conversely, a lever whose resistance arm is the longer, whether it be a first or a third class lever, is said to favor speed and distance. It lacks force, however. More force is required to move it than would be the case if the relative lengths of the force and resistance arms were reversed. Furthermore, an object of negligible weight can be moved a greater distance and more rapidly by this kind of lever than it could be without the aid of the lever. Regardless of the position of its fulcrum, or of the relative lengths of its two arms, a first class lever is always an arrangement for balance. Examples of these various levers are listed on the following page:

1. First class lever with equal force and resistance arms: seesaw; balance scales.

2. First class lever with relatively long force arm: pump handle; crowbar when one end is placed under a rock, a log is placed under the crowbar, and the opposite end of the crowbar is pushed down.

3. First class lever with relatively long resistance arm: old-fashioned well-sweep; kitchen tongs.

4. Second class lever: wheelbarrow; crowbar when one end is placed under a rock and other end is lifted.

5. Third class lever: screen door with spring supplying the force; fire tongs (hinged at end).

THE PRINCIPLE OF LEVERS. A lever of any class will balance when the product of the force and the force arm equals the product of the resistance and the resistance arm. This is known as the principle of levers. It enables us to calculate the amount of force needed to balance a known resistance by means of a known lever, or to calculate the point at which to place the fulcrum in order to balance a known resistance with a given force. If any three of the four values are known, the remaining one can be calculated by using the following equation:

$$F \times FA = R \times RA$$
(force times force arm equals resistance times resistance arm)

EXAMPLES OF ANATOMIC LEVERS. The head, tipping forward and backward, is a good example of a first class lever in the body (Fig. 4-2). To be sure, it is a sphere rather than a bar, and the axis of motion would seem to be an imaginary one located in the frontal plane approximately between the ears. The force is supplied by the extensors of the head, notably the splenius and upper portions of the semispinalis, and is applied to the head at the base of the skull. The resistance to the movement is furnished by the weight of the head itself, together with the tension of the antagonistic muscles and fasciae, as the limit of motion is approached. The center of concentration of the resistance is difficult to determine. If the head is acting like a seesaw, the resistance would seem to be centered in the front half of the head for hyperextension, and in the rear half for flexion. Additional resistance is provided by the tension of opposing muscles and ligaments, the resistance point being the point at which the various resistant forces are concentrated.

Another first class lever is seen in the foot when it is not being used for weight-bearing, as when the knees are crossed in the sitting position. As the soleus pulls upward on the heel, the foot plantarflexes at the ankle joint where the fulcrum is situated. The resistance seems to be provided by the tonus of the dorsiflexor muscles. The weight of the foot apparently is not a factor here, since the foot has already relaxed into a position of partial plantar flexion. The picture would be changed, however, if the person were lying face down with the leg bent at the knee and the lower leg extended vertically upward.

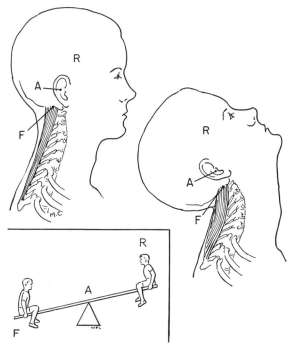

Figure 4-2. The head acting as a first class lever like the seesaw. *A* = The approximate position of the axis or fulcrum; *F* = the point where the force is applied; *R* = the approximate point where the resistance is concentrated.

If the foot were then plantar-flexed, the weight of the foot would be a factor in the resistance.

The forearm is another example of a first class lever when it is being extended by the triceps muscle (Fig. 4-3). The fulcrum is situated at the elbow joint, the force is applied at the olecranon process and the resistance point is located at the forearm's center of gravity when no external resistance is present, and at the hand when the latter is pushing against an external resistance. Internal resistance does not appear to be a factor in this movement. This is a good example of a first class lever in which the force arm is extremely short, relative to the resistance arm. It is therefore similar to a third class lever in that it favors speed and range of movement at the expense of force.

Whether or not there are any second class levers in the body seems to be a controversial matter among anatomists and kinesiologists. Some claim that when the foot is being plantar-flexed in a weight-bearing position, as when rising on the toes, it is a second class lever. The fulcrum is said to be at the point of contact with the ground, the force point at the heel where the tendon of Achilles attaches and the resistance at the ankle joint where the weight of the body is transferred to the foot. Another second class lever might be the forearm if

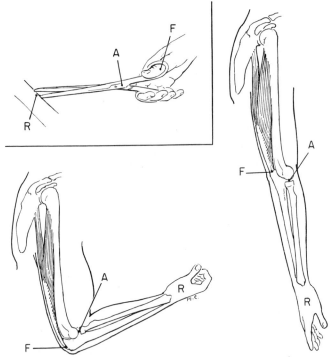

Figure 4–3. The forearm acting as a first class lever with a short force arm and long resistance arm, like a pair of paper shears.

it were being flexed by the brachioradialis alone, but this could occur only if the other flexors were paralyzed.

The forearm is a good example of a third class lever when it is being flexed by the biceps and the brachialis (Fig. 4–4). Another third class lever is seen in the example cited earlier, namely the arm as it is raised sideward-upward by the deltoid muscle (Fig. 4–5).

RELATION OF SPEED TO RANGE IN MOVEMENTS OF LEVERS. The observant reader will have noticed that in the foregoing discussion of levers the terms "speed and range" were usually linked together. There is a reason for this. In angular movements speed and range are interdependent. For instance, if two third class levers of different lengths each move through a 40-degree angle at the same *angular velocity*, the tip of the longer lever will be traveling a greater distance or range than the tip of the shorter lever. Since it covers this distance in the same time that it takes the tip of the shorter lever to travel the shorter distance, the former must be moving faster than the latter. This is easily seen if the shorter lever is superimposed on the longer, as in Figure 4–6. Here the shorter lever, *AB*, has been superimposed on the longer lever, *AC*. The levers are moving from the horizontal position to the diagonal one. Since the point *C* travels to its new position, *C'*, in the same time that it takes *B* to travel to *B'*, point *C* must obviously be moving faster than point *B*.

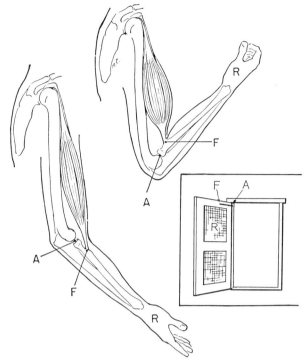

Figure 4-4. The forearm acting as a third class lever with a relatively short force arm, like a screen door.

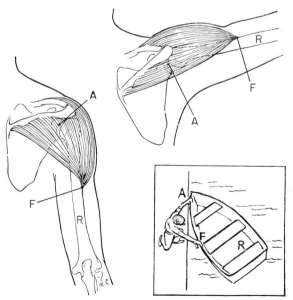

Figure 4-5. The humerus acting as a third class lever with a moderately long force arm, like a boat being pulled alongside the dock.

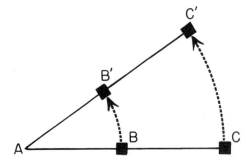

Figure 4–6. Comparison of a long and a short lever turning the same number of degrees. It takes *B* the same amount of time to reach *B'* that it takes *C* to reach *C'*.

CHARACTERISTICS OF ANATOMIC LEVERS.   In skeletal levers the force arm, with few exceptions, is shorter than the resistance arm. Thus anatomic levers tend to favor speed and range of movement at the expense of force. Examples of this are seen in the throwing of a baseball or the kicking of a soccer ball. The hand in the one case, and the foot in the other, travel through a relatively long distance at considerable speed. Both these movements require strong muscular action, in spite of the fact that the balls are relatively light in weight. This type of leverage is the reverse of the kind usually seen in mechanical implements such as the crowbar and the automobile jack, both of which are used to move heavy weights a relatively short distance.

SPORT IMPLEMENTS AS LEVERS.   Sport implements may serve either as levers in themselves or as artificial extensions of the human arm. Frequently the sport implement, the arm and a large part of the rest of the body act together as a system of levers. In batting a baseball, for instance, the trunk forms one lever, the upper arms another, the forearms another and the hands and bat still another. This use of multiple leverage is for the purpose of building up speed at the tip of the bat, for the greater this speed, the greater the force that can be imparted to the ball.

IDENTIFICATION AND ANALYSIS OF LEVERS.   Figures 4–2 to 4–5 depict certain anatomic levers and their mechanical counterparts. These should enable the student to understand the principle of leverage as it applies in the human body and to see how the anatomic levers compare with the levers of everyday life. For each of these levers, and for every lever that the student observes, he should answer these questions: (1) Where are the fulcrum, the force point and the resistance point? (2) What class of lever is this? (3) What are the relative lengths of the force and resistance arms? (4) What kind of movement does this lever favor? After he has studied components of force (p. 92) he should add the questions: (5) At what angle is the force applied to the lever? (6) At what angle is the resistance applied to the lever? (7) What is the true force arm of the lever? and (8) What is the true resistance arm of the lever?

The Wheel and Axle. The wheel and axle device consists of a wheel attached to a central axle about which it revolves. Force may be applied to the wheel either at the rim, as in the case of the steering wheel of the automobile, or to the axle, as in the case of the automobile's rear wheels. The steering wheel is an example of a wheel and axle which magnifies force at the expense of speed and distance. The larger the diameter of the wheel, the greater the magnification of force. Quantitatively, the turning effect of the wheel is the product of the force and the radius. The radius thus corresponds to the force arm of a lever. The doorknob, the water wheel and the helm of the ship are common examples of this kind of wheel and axle. In the helm of the ship the rim of the wheel is absent, but the spokes constitute a wheel nevertheless. In many respects the wheel and axle device is similar to the lever, particularly when the "wheel" consists of a single spoke, as in the case of the meat grinder, the pencil sharpener and the hand-operated clothes wringer. These correspond to a second class lever, in which the fulcrum (actually the center of the axle) is at one end, the force is applied to the other end and the resistance is applied close to the fulcrum.

The type of wheel and axle which is used to gain speed and distance at the expense of force is seen less commonly, perhaps, yet it is present in many of our vehicles. In the automobile the rear wheels are turned by means of force applied to their axles. The same is true of the bicycle, the velocipede and the old-fashioned bicycle, in which the pedals are attached directly to the axle. The Ferris wheel and the merry-go-round are additional examples of this kind of wheel and axle. In each of these the force is applied to the axle and the resistance to the outer circumference of the wheel. More careful inspection of these examples reveals the fact that they are actually combinations of both kinds of wheels and axles. In the velocipede, for instance, the pedal represents the first type of wheel and axle. The force is applied to the outer end of the pedal. This serves to revolve the common axle of the pedal and the front wheel of the velocipede. The front wheel represents the second type of wheel and axle. Force is applied to it at the axle (as the result of the action of the pedal) and resistance, in the form of friction and pressure, is applied to the rim at its point of contact with the ground.

Further consideration of wheels and axles, as seen in common household and industrial devices, shows that they frequently are combined in such a way that a wheel and axle of the first type alternates with one of the second type. There may be several such combinations within one relatively simple mechanism. The common rotary egg beater, for instance, is found to combine four wheel and axle devices, the two types alternating with each other.

Most of the examples of the wheel and axle in the body, like anatomic levers, are arranged for gaining distance and speed at the expense of force. Both kinds are represented, however. A cross section of the upper trunk is a good example. The multifidus, rotatores and semispinalis act on the "axle," that is, the spinal column, and the oblique abdominal muscles and the iliocostalis exert their force on the perimeter of the "wheel" — the ribs in this case (Figs. 4–7 and 4–8). The head and neck also illustrate a wheel and axle mechanism, the force being applied to the perimeter of the "wheel" by the sterno-cleidomastoid and splenius muscles and to the "axle" by the deep spinal muscles.

A cross section of the arm or the thigh likewise presents the characteristics of a wheel and axle. Here the shaft of the long bone serves as the axle, and the peripheral tissues as the wheel. Rotation of the limb about its mechanical long axis constitutes the movement of the wheel and axle, with the force being furnished by the muscles producing the rotation and the resistance by the antagonistic muscles, or by an external resistance, as the case may be. Unlike the usual mechanical wheel and axle, the resistance in an anatomic wheel and axle is frequently applied at the same distance from the center of motion as the force. This is the case when antagonistic muscles provide the only resistance to the movement.

The Pulley. A pulley is usually a spool or wheel with a rope running over it. Although we do not have wheels and ropes in the body, we do have pulleys. In the field of mechanics there are simple pulleys and there are complicated arrangements of block and tackle. Only the fixed single pulley is represented in the musculoskeletal system. It serves the same purpose as the mechanical fixed single pulley, namely, that of changing the direction of a force. This may take the form of giving a muscle a greater angle of pull than it would otherwise have, or of enabling it to produce a totally different movement than it could otherwise produce. For instance, the angle of pull of the gracilis muscle is increased by means of the bulging medial condyles of the knee over which the tendon passes just before it attaches to the tibia

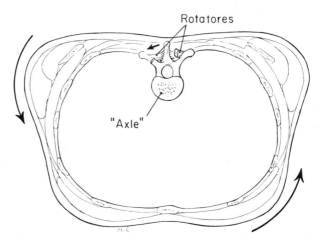

Figure 4–7. A cross section of the trunk representing a "wheel and axle" in which the force of the rotatores muscles is applied to the "axle."

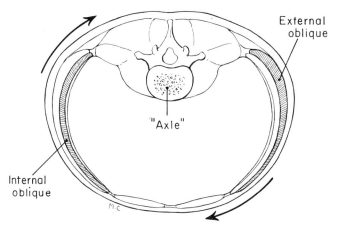

Figure 4–8.   A cross section of the trunk representing a "wheel and axle" in which the force of the oblique abdominal muscles is applied to the "wheel."

(Fig. 4–9). A pulley changing the nature of a movement is illustrated by the peroneus longus muscle, which, by passing behind the lateral malleolus before it turns under the foot to attach to the first cuneiform and base of the first metatarsal bone, plantar-flexes the foot at the ankle (Fig. 4–10). If it passed in front of the malleolus its pull would be shifted in front of the ankle joint and hence it would dorsiflex the foot. In the first example the medial condyles of the femur and tibia are the "fixed single pulley," and in the second example the lateral malleolus serves in this capacity.

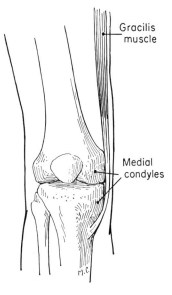

Figure 4–9.   The medial condyles at the knee joint serving as a pulley to increase the angle of pull of the gracilis tendon.

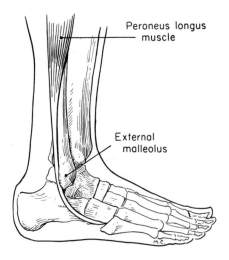

Peroneus longus
muscle

External
malleolus

Figure 4–10. The external malleolus
serving as a pulley for the peroneus
longus tendon.

The function of these machines in the musculoskeletal system,
and their significance in the total movements of the body, will be
discussed at greater length in the chapters that follow.

The Efficiency of Machines.   Machines are judged good if they
are efficient, poor if they are inefficient. How is the efficiency of a
machine measured? Since the machines used in industry and in the
workshop are usually for the purpose of magnifying force, it is customary to measure their efficiency in terms of their *mechanical advantage*, in other words, their ability to magnify force. Another way
of expressing this ability is to state the "output" of the machine relative to its "input." In levers this is the ratio between the force applied
to the lever and the resistance overcome by the lever. It may be expressed in terms of the equation:

Mechanical Advantage = the ratio of the resistance overcome to the

force applied, or simply, $\text{M.A.} = \dfrac{R}{F}$

Since the balanced lever equation (p. 54) may also be expressed

$$\frac{R}{F} = \frac{FA}{RA}$$

it is seen that the mechanical advantage may be expressed in terms of
the ratio of the force arm to the resistance arm. Hence, if

$$\text{M.A.} = \frac{R}{F}$$

it also holds that

$$\text{M.A.} = \frac{FA}{RA}$$

When a muscle is said to have poor leverage it means that it has poor mechanical advantage. In other words, the force arm of the lever upon which it is acting is short compared with the resistance arm.

The mechanical advantage of a wheel and axle is measured in a similar manner, in terms of the ratio of the radius of the wheel (R) to the radius of the axle (r), or

$$\text{M.A.} = \frac{R}{r}$$

We need not concern ourselves with the mechanical advantage of pulleys as the fixed single pulley affects only the direction of a force, not its magnitude.

DEMONSTRATIONS, LABORATORY EXERCISES AND PROBLEMS

1. Place a window pole across the back of a chair, hang a pail or basket containing a 5-pound weight on the hook and hold the other end of the pole. Now adjust the pole so that it becomes increasingly difficult to balance the weight of the pail with one hand. Stop when you reach the point where you are barely able to lift the pail by pushing down on the opposite end of the pole. Have an assistant measure the force arm and the weight arm of the lever. Without shifting the position of your hand, draw the pole toward you until you can easily lift the pail by pushing down on the opposite end of the pole with one finger. Again, have an assistant measure the force and weight arms of the lever. What do you conclude concerning the relative length of the two arms? In which case does the pail move through the greater distance? What do you conclude about the relationship between the force required to move an object by leverage and the distance that the object is moved? This experiment, as you did it, involved a first class lever. Could you perform a similar experiment using a third class lever?

2. Balance a pole across the back of a chair, hanging a 5-pound weight at each end. Let one of these represent the force and the other the weight or resistance. The force arm and the weight arm should be exactly equal if the pole is symmetrical. Now add 5 more pounds to the weight end and adjust the pole until it balances. Measure the force and weight arms. What do you conclude about:

   a. The relationship between the weight and the weight arm; between the force and the force arm?

   b. The relationship between the weight and the weight arm, given a changing weight and a constant force?

Explain the following equation: $F \times FA = W \times WA$.

$$F = \text{force}$$
$$W = \text{weight}$$
$$FA = \text{force arm}$$
$$WA = \text{weight arm}$$

3. Compute the amount of force necessary to lift a weight or resistance of 20 pounds with a 6-foot, first class lever whose fulcrum is located 2 feet from the point at which the weight is attached, and 4 feet from the point at which the force is applied. Assume that both the force and the resistance are applied at right angles to the lever.

4. Where would the fulcrum have to be located in the above-mentioned 6-foot first class lever if there were only 5 pounds of force available to balance the 20-pound weight? Determine this by experiment. Check your answer by the algebraic method.

5. For each of the anatomic levers listed below identify the class of lever represented; identify the fulcrum, the force point and the resistance point; and name the kind of movement favored by this type of lever.

a. Leg being flexed at knee by hamstrings.

b. Leg being extended at knee by quadriceps femoris.

c. Pelvis being tilted to right by left quadratus lumborum.

d. Clavicle being elevated by trapezius I.

e. Lower extremity being abducted by gluteus medius.

f. From supine lying position, lower extremities being raised by hip flexors.

g. From supine lying position, trunk being raised by hip flexors.

6. For each of the following levers in your own body find the force arm and the resistance arm by actual measurement, and calculate the force needed to balance the lever. Work with a partner to get the measurements of lever length and distances of force and resistance points from fulcrum. Although the results will not be mathematically accurate (since the factor of angle of pull is being disregarded), they illustrate the relation between the relative length of the force and resistance arms and the amount of force needed.

a. With the arm extended horizontally sideward, hold a 10-pound weight on the hand. Consider the middle deltoid as the only source of force.

b. With the upper arm extended horizontally sideward, suspend a 10-pound weight from the crotch of the elbow. Consider the middle deltoid as the only source of force.

7. Have a subject raise the arm sideward to the horizontal and, from this position, move it horizontally forward, taking two seconds to perform the horizontal movement. The arm has now moved through 90 degrees. Approximately how many inches did the subject's elbow move? Approximately how many inches did his hand move? Which was moving faster, his elbow or his hand?

8. Identify the "wheel," the "axle" and the place where the force is applied in the example of outward rotation of the humerus by the infraspinatus and teres minor muscles.

9. Using a string to represent the peroneus longus muscle, fasten one end to the proper spot on the leg of a skeleton for its proximal attachment. Making the string pass behind the external malleolus and under the foot, fasten the distal end to the proper point of attachment. Now take another string and fasten it at the same points,

but have it pass in front of the malleolus. Be sure both strings are taut. Study the relationship between each string and the center of motion at the ankle joint. With a protractor measure the angle between the two strings at their distal attachment. Repeat this experiment with the foot in a position of complete dorsiflexion. What effect does the peroneus longus have at the ankle joint that it would not have if it passed in front of the malleolus? What is the mechanical function of the malleolus? (If no skeleton is available, it may be possible to fasten the strings on the skin of a subject's leg.)

10. Find an example of a pulley in the upper extremity.

11. Find the mechanical advantage of the levers in question 6, *a* and *b*.

CHAPTER 5

Stability and Motion

Man is either at rest or in motion. He is therefore constantly governed by mechanical principles: the principles of statics or stability when he is at rest and the principles of dynamics or motion when he is moving. Not infrequently, he is subject to both types of principles at the same time. Animate bodies, unlike inanimate ones, must make quick transitions from one state to the other in order to adjust to the forces acting upon them. They also frequently need to be stable in one part of their body in order to give or receive impetus successfully with another. This in-between state might well be called *balance-in-motion,* or *dynamic balance.*

STABILITY

Because man ordinarily holds himself in an upright position, and because the law of gravity is always in operation on this earth, the problems of stability are ever present. Probably the only time the human body is not adjusting itself in response to gravitational force is when it is in a position of repose. Either consciously or unconsciously, man spends most of his waking hours adjusting his position to the pull of gravity upon his body.

The ability to maintain one's balance under unfavorable circumstances is recognized as one of the basic motor skills. Standing on tiptoes or on one foot without losing one's balance, or maintaining a headstand or a handstand for an appreciable length of time is such a skill. These particular feats are examples of static balance and the mark of skill is to accomplish them with a minimum of motion.

Familiarity with the following factors of stability will enable the student to analyze his balance problems and may suggest to the teacher the means of helping his less skillful students. It should also enable the physical therapist to help the amputees and the victims of paralysis to regain their lost sense of equilibrium.

The Height of the Center of Gravity. Ordinarily man's center of gravity is located approximately at the level of the upper third of the

66

sacrum. Experiments have shown that the height of a man's center of gravity is about 56 per cent of his height,[6] and the height of a woman's is about 55 per cent of her height.[4] These figures hold true only for the normal standing position. If the arms are raised or if a weight is carried above waist level, the center of gravity shifts to a higher position and it becomes more difficult to maintain one's equilibrium. Activities and stunts such as walking on stilts, canoeing and balancing a weight on the head are difficult or dangerous because of the relatively high center of gravity. Lowering the center of gravity will increase the stability of the body (Fig. 5–1). If, for any reason, the equilibrium is too precarious in the standing position, assuming a crouching, kneeling or sitting position will lower the center of gravity and increase stability.

The Size of the Base of Support. It is obvious that a wide base of support adds to the stability of an object. Most of the difficulty experienced in walking on a balance beam, a railroad track or a tightrope, or in ice skating and toe dancing is due to the small base of support. The problem is to keep the center of gravity over the base of support, a requisite for maintaining equilibrium. The wider the base, the easier it is to keep the center of gravity directly above it.

In a man whose weight is supported entirely by his feet, the base of support includes not only his two feet, but also the intervening area (Fig. 5–2). If the feet are separated, the base is widened and the equilibrium improved. An individual on crutches will be more stable if he places the crutches forward, making a triangular base instead of a linear one. (Fig. 5–3 A). There is another factor, however, that must not be overlooked. If one takes a stance that is wider than the breadth of the pelvis, the legs will assume a slanting position. This introduces a lateral component of force. If this is accompanied by insufficient friction between the feet and the supporting surface, as when standing on ice, obviously a widening of the base of support does not make for greater stability. In fact, the wider the stance, the less one can control the sliding of the feet. From this we see that we must observe *all* the

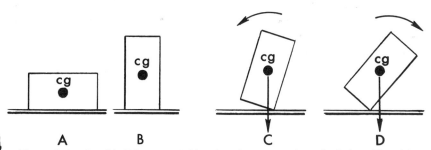

Figure 5–1. An object is most stable when its center of gravity is low. The object in *C* will fall back into place and remain vertical; in *D,* where the center of gravity is not over the base, the object will topple over. (From Williams, M., and Lissner, H. R.: Biomechanics of Human Motion. Philadelphia, W. B. Saunders Company, 1962.)

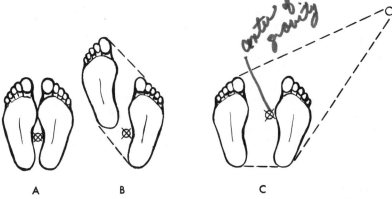

Figure 5-2. The position of the feet determines the size of the supporting area beneath the body. Use of a cane greatly extends the base of support *(C)* and the area over which the body is stable. (From Williams and Lissner.)

principles which apply to a situation. Observance of only one may not bring the results expected.

The Relation of the Line of Gravity to the Base of Support. This factor is closely related to the preceding one. Since an object retains its equilibrium only so long as its line of gravity falls within its base of support, it follows that the nearer the line of gravity to the *center* of the base of support, the greater the stability (Fig. 5-4); conversely, the nearer the line of gravity to the *margin* of the base of support, the more precarious the equilibrium (Fig. 5-5). Once it passes beyond the margin, stability is lost and a new base must be established. It is this factor which constitutes the major problem in some modern dance techniques, in balance stunts, in walking a tightrope and in building pyramids. For developing the neuromuscular control necessary for acquiring such skills as these, there is no substitute for repeated practice. There are, however, a few devices that help one to keep the center of gravity centered over the base of support. One of these we do almost unconsciously. If we carry a heavy weight at one side of the body (e.g., a suitcase or a pail of cement), *this constitutes a unilateral* load which, if uncompensated, would shift the center of gravity to that side, bringing it dangerously close to the margin of the base of support. By raising the opposite arm sideways, by bending or leaning to the opposite side, or by a combination of these, we counterbalance the external load and keep the line of gravity close to the center of the base of support (Figs. 5-6 and 5-7). Another application of the principle of keeping the line of gravity over the center of the base of support is seen in the tightrope walker who carries a balancing pole, or, to a lesser degree, in the gymnast walking on a balance beam with his arms extended sideward. The pole, or the arm, acts as a lever, and the reaction of a lever is in proportion to its length. Even a slight movement at the end of a long first class lever has a considerable reaction at the fulcrum. Hence, if the tightrope walker

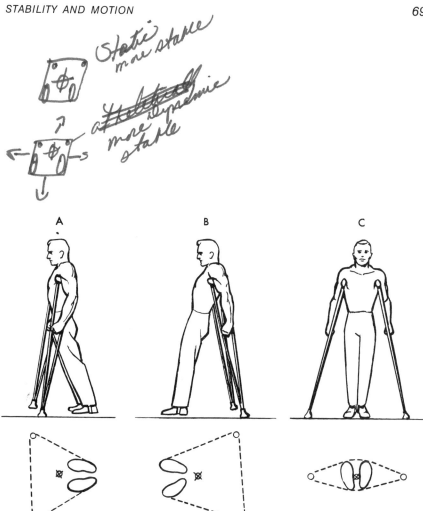

Figure 5-3. Bases of support with varying degrees of stability. Can you rank these from most stable to least stable? The subject in *A* and *B* is secure primarily in the anteroposterior direction; the position in *C* provides greater stability in the frontal plane than in the sagittal plane. (From Williams and Lissner.)

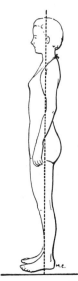

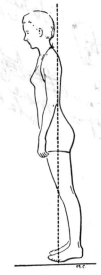

Figure 5–4. Position of the body in which the line of gravity falls approximately through the center of the base of support. This is a stable position.

Figure 5–5. Position of the body in which the line of gravity falls near the anterior margin of the base of support. This position is less stable than the one shown in Figure 5–4.

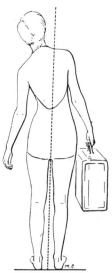

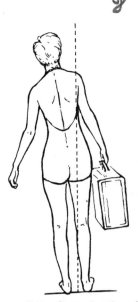

Figure 5–6. Compensating for a unilateral load by bending to opposite side.

Figure 5–7. Compensation for a unilateral load by inclining the entire body to the opposite side.

man + woman = instatic ability

starts to lean too far to the left, an almost imperceptible downward movement of the right end of the pole will be sufficient to help him regain his balance.

The Mass of the Body. The mass or weight of an object is a factor in equilibrium only when motion or an external force is involved. It is a matter of common observation that an empty cardboard carton is more likely to blow down the street than one filled with canned goods. Likewise, a 250-pound linesman is less likely to be brushed aside than is a 130-pound one. In all sports involving physical contact, the heavy, solid individual stands a better chance of keeping his footing than does the lightweight one.

does not affect static stability but does dynamic

Momentum and the Impact of an External Force. Whereas no individual can suddenly increase his weight in order to resist the impact of another individual charging into him at top speed, there are nevertheless two principles, the observance of which makes it possible to withstand this factor of external force. These are (1) inclining the body and (2) widening the base of support *in the direction of the oncoming force.* Leaning into the wind illustrates the first of these (Fig. 5–8); placing the feet in a forward-backward stance when catching a swift ball is an example of the second. When we stand in a bus or a subway train we resist the tendency to be thrown backward when the vehicle starts up either by standing sideways with the feet in a moderately wide stance, or by facing forward and leaning forward. We never face the back of the vehicle from choice, but if we must, we place one foot forward rather than incline the body backward, which would be the alternative. These automatic reactions to external forces are for one purpose only, namely, to enable us to keep our center of gravity over our base of support in spite of the disturbing forces.

(lean forward)

Another form of the effect of external force is seen in the sudden cessation of motion. For instance, if a man is so foolish as to jump off a moving bus, he runs the risk of falling flat on his face. This is because the forward-moving bus has imparted kinetic energy to his body,

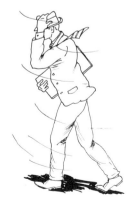

Figure 5–8. Leaning into the wind to balance the effect of its force on the body.

or, as we commonly say, he has received momentum from the moving bus. When he suddenly leaves the bus and ignores the factor of momentum, he loses the kinetic energy suddenly, very suddenly indeed, and finds himself thrown to the ground by an invisible force. He could have avoided this ignominious reaction if, upon jumping from the bus, he had faced forward, leaned backward and taken a few running steps in the same direction as the bus, thus assuring a gradual loss of kinetic energy, instead of an instantaneous one. Better still, he could have waited for the bus to stop.

Friction. Friction as a factor in stability has already been suggested in relation to the size of the base of support. It has even greater influence when the body is in motion or is being acted upon by an external force. Inadequate friction is what makes it difficult to keep one's equilibrium when walking on an icy pavement, particularly if a frisky dog tugs unexpectedly on its leash. When the supporting surface presents insufficient friction, the footgear can make up for it. The person who must walk on icy pavements can wear "creepers" on his shoes; the golfer and the field hockey player can wear cleats; and the gymnast and basketball player can wear rubber-soled shoes.

Segmentation. If, instead of being in one solid piece, an object consists of a series of segments placed one above the other, the problem of retaining its equilibrium is a multiple one. Maximum stability of a segmented body is assured when the centers of gravity of all the weight-bearing segments lie in a vertical line which is centered over the base of support. In a column of blocks, this means that each block must be centered over the block beneath. In a jointed column, as in the human body, one segment cannot slide off another, but it is quite possible for the segments to be united in a zigzag line. Such is all too often the case in man's posture. In fact, the alignment of the body segments is a widely used criterion for judging standing posture. When the segments are aligned in a single vertical line, the posture is not only more pleasing in appearance to most of us, but there is less likelihood of strain to the joints and muscles. When one segment gets out of line, there is usually a compensatory disalignment of another segment in order to maintain a balanced position of the body as a whole. (In other words, for every "zig" there is a "zag.") At every point of angulation between segments there is uneven tension thrown on the ligaments and uneven tonus in opposing muscle groups. This causes fatigue, if not actual strain.

Visual and Psychologic Factors. Factors which belong in this category are less easily explained than the others, but are familiar to everyone. The giddiness that many experience when walking close to an unprotected edge high above the ground, or when crossing a swirling river on a foot bridge, is a real detriment to one's equilibrium. Even if the supporting surface is entirely adequate, the sense of balance may be disturbed. A common means of preserving the balance, both in this type of situation and when walking on a narrow rail, is to fix the eyes on a stationary spot above or beyond the "danger

[handwritten: never make a kid do something he doesn't want to cause he'll get hurt for sure.]

area." This seems to facilitate neuromuscular control by reducing the disturbing stimuli.

Physiologic Factors. Besides the visual and psychologic factors there are also physiologic factors related to the physical mechanism for equilibrium, namely, the semicircular canals. In addition to actual lesions of this mechanism, any disturbance of the general physical condition is likely to affect the sense of balance. Feelings of dizziness accompanying nausea, or any form of debility, reduce one's ability to resist other factors which threaten the equilibrium. These physiologic factors are largely beyond our control. One principle which can be derived from them, however, is that it is better to avoid situations which are likely to threaten the equilibrium when there is a temporary physiologic disturbance.

[handwritten: ear ache will mess up equilibrium (semicircular canals); menstral cycle does not upset equilibrium]

PRINCIPLES OF STABILITY

The principles of stability are stated here as simply and concisely as possible, and brief applications are suggested in each case.

Principle I. Other things being equal, (1) the lower the center of gravity, (2) the larger the base of support, and (3) the more nearly centered the line of gravity with reference to the base of support, the greater will be the body's stability. *[handwritten: stability]*

Applications

a. The easiest and safest pyramids for beginners are those in which the participants are on their hands and knees. This position provides for a lower center of gravity, a larger base of support and greater ease in centering the line of gravity than the kneeling or standing position.

b. In canoeing the kneeling position represents a compromise position which combines the advantages of stability and ease of using the arms for paddling. Kneeling is preferable to sitting on the seat because the lowering of the center of gravity makes the position a more stable one. While it is less stable than sitting on the floor of the canoe, it is a more convenient position for paddling.

c. An external load which is carried anywhere except on the head directly above the body's center of gravity will adversely affect the relation of the line of gravity to the base of support unless the body readjusts its alignment in order to compensate for the load. When carrying a heavy tray, suitcase or bag of cement, for instance, some portion of the body must be shifted in the opposite direction if the center of gravity is to be maintained above the center of the supporting base. If this is not done, the stability of the body will suffer and the muscles on the opposite side of the trunk will become tense in order to brace the body against the pull of the unbalanced load. A unilateral load may be counterbalanced by raising the opposite arm sideways, by bending to the opposite side, or by inclining the entire body to the opposite side, while at the same time keeping the head erect (Figs. 5–6 and 5–7).

Principle II. Other things being equal, the greater the mass of a body, the greater will be its stability.

Application. In sports in which resistance to impact is a factor, heavy, solid individuals are more likely to maintain their equilibrium than lighter ones. This provides one basis for selecting linesmen in football.

Principle III. Other things being equal, the most stable position of a vertical segmented body (such as a column of blocks or the erect human body) is one in which the center of gravity of each weight-bearing segment lies in a vertical line centered over the base of support, or in which deviations in one direction are exactly balanced by deviations in the opposite direction.

Applications

a. This applies to postural adjustments for achieving a pleasing, well balanced alignment of the body segments, both with and without external loads.

b. In pyramid building and other balance stunts in which one person (or group of persons) supports the weight of another person or persons, the chief problem is one of either aligning or balancing the several centers of gravity over the center of the base of support.

Principle IV. Other things being equal, a person has better balance in locomotion under difficult circumstances when he focuses his vision on stationary objects rather than on disturbing stimuli.

Application. Beginners learning to walk on a balance beam or perform balance stunts, and others who for any reason have difficulty in keeping their balance, can minimize disturbing visual stimuli by fixing their eyes on a stationary spot in front of them, either at eye level or somewhat above eye level.

Principle V. There is a positive relationship between one's physical and emotional state and his ability to maintain his balance under difficult circumstances.

Application. Persons should not be permitted to attempt dangerous balance stunts, or activities requiring expert balance ability, when their physical or emotional health is impaired.

DYNAMIC BALANCE (BALANCE IN MOTION)

Dynamic balance, or stability in activity, may seem like a contradiction of terms, yet it is a familiar aspect of many activities. It may be the main feature of the activity, like walking on a balance beam or a tightrope, or it may be incidental to the activity, as when throwing or catching swift balls, taking off for a dive, landing from a vault or jump, and making quick changes of direction in a game situation.

In the giving of impetus, for instance, the magnitude and direction of force and the accuracy of applying the force to the external object are strongly affected by the stability of the performer's stance and the control of his body as a whole. The stance represents the base of support and this is one of the major factors in stability. The principles that deal with the relation of the center of gravity to the base of support apply to bodies in motion just as they do to the balance of static bodies, but the moments of their application are of brief duration.

PRINCIPLES OF DYNAMIC BALANCE

Principle I. In giving and in receiving an impetus with a strong horizontal component, greater stability is obtained if the base of support is widened in the direction of the line of force.

Applications

a. This helps an individual to keep from being thrown off balance when he punches with force, pushes a heavy object or throws a fast ball. It also enables him to "put his weight behind his punch" because with a relatively wide forward-backward stance he can shift his weight from the rear foot to the forward foot as he delivers the impetus.

b. In pushing and pulling heavy furniture he can put his whole body into the act without loss of balance.

c. When catching a fast moving object like a baseball, or a heavy one like a medicine ball, widening the base in line with the direction of the force enables the catcher to "give" as he catches, and in this way to provide a greater distance in which to reduce or stop the motion of the object. It also assures greater accuracy by reducing the likelihood of rebound.

d. Dragging a heavy box forward on a high shelf and then lifting it down is an activity in the home to which this principle applies. Assuming a forward-backward stance for this act gives the individual a wider base for receiving the weight of this forward moving object. This decreases the likelihood of his being thrown off balance when the box suddenly comes free of the shelf. It also enables him to take a step backward which makes it easier for him to lower the box in front of him and to keep control of it. With a sideward stance he would be likely to be thrown off balance as the box comes free. There is also the danger of his exerting so much horizontal force that instead of lowering the box in front of him he swings it back overhead, hyperextending his spine and running the risk of straining his back.

e. Keeping one's balance when standing on a bus or train which is accelerating or decelerating is facilitated by widening the stance in the direction that the vehicle is moving, that is, in a forward-backward direction in relation to the vehicle.

f. Basketball and relay races often require sudden reversals of direction. If the player tries to turn while his feet are close together his momentum is likely to throw him off balance. This can be prevented if he spreads his feet to check his forward motion. He can then quickly pivot to reverse his direction.

Principle II. Other things being equal, the more nearly the weight is centered above the base of support, the more stable the body will be, even though it is in motion and circumstances permit only a limited degree of stability.

Applications

a. Activities which involve a two-foot take-off before the body is launched into the air have what might be called a split-second moment of partial stability. A running front dive is a good example of this. The diver takes his hurdle near the end of the board, comes down on the board on both feet and lets the board toss him into the air. The brief moment between landing on both feet and leaving the board is the moment of dynamic balance. If for any reason the diver comes down with more weight on one foot than on the other, his dive is ruined. His momentary stance affects his take-off, and his take-off determines the pathway his body will take in the air.

(b.) One activity in which it is impossible to widen the base of support is walking on a balance beam. It is a deliberate test of skill, requiring the performer to keep his center of gravity within very narrow limits. Two suggestions have been found helpful in accomplishing this: one, to fix the eyes on a stationary spot straight ahead, either at eye level or somewhat higher; and the other, to use the arms for balance but, in doing so, to keep the movements small and not jerky. A common mistake is to move the arms too suddenly and too far. This invariably causes the performer to lose his balance in the opposite direction.

c. Working on an extension ladder to perform a chore, such as painting the house or cleaning out the gutters, is another example of being limited by a predetermined width for the base of support. The width of the ladder limits the base of support. As this is narrower than the stance frequently chosen for doing the same type of work on the ground, there is likely to be a temptation to lean too far to the side. There is nothing definite that the performer can do to acquire skill in this kind of activity except to develop an awareness of his balance and to familiarize himself with the limitations the ladder imposes on him by starting at a low level and working up gradually.

Principle III. Other things being equal, the greater the friction between the supporting surface and the parts of the body in contact with it, the more stable the body will be.

Application. The wearing of cleats and rubber-soled shoes for sport activities not only aids in locomotion, but also serves to increase one's stability in positions held momentarily between quick or forceful movements, as in basketball, fencing, football, field hockey, lacrosse and other sports.

Principle IV. Regaining equilibrium is based on the same principles as maintaining it.

Applications

(a.) After an unexpected loss of balance, such as when starting to fall or after receiving impetus when "off balance," equilibrium may be more quickly regained if a wide base of support is established and the center of gravity is lowered.

(b.) Upon landing from a downward jump, stability may be more

readily regained if the weight is kept evenly distributed over both feet or over the hands and feet, and if a sufficiently wide base of support is provided.

c. Upon landing from a forward jump, the balance may be more readily regained if one lands with the weight forward and uses the hands if necessary in order to provide support in the direction of motion.

d. Tightrope walkers use a balancing pole to help them regain their balance when they start to lose it. The pole serves as a long first class lever. Since the reaction of a lever is in proportion to its length, even a slight movement of the end of the lever has a considerable reaction at the fulcrum. Hence if the tightrope walker starts to lean too far to the left, an almost imperceptible downward movement of the right end of the pole will be sufficient to help him regain his balance.

From this emphasis on stability it might seem that one should seek maximum stability in all situations. This is not true regarding certain stunts and gymnastic activities that are designed for the purpose of testing and developing body control under difficult circumstances. In many gymnastic vaults, for instance, "good form" stipulates that the performer shall land with the heels close, the knees separated, the arms extended sideward, and the trunk as erect as possible, while he lets his knees bend to assure a light landing. In teaching beginners it would seem wiser to postpone emphasis on form from the point of view of appearance and to stress good mechanics and safety.

MOTION

If we are to understand the movements of the human musculoskeletal system, we need first to turn our thoughts to the concept of motion itself. What causes motion? What kinds of motion are there? What determines the kind of motion that will result when an object — or a part of the human body — is made to move? Under what laws does motion operate and what are the principles that govern its behavior? And finally, how do these generalities about motion apply to the movements of the musculoskeletal system?

Cause of Motion. One cannot easily think of motion without visualizing a specific object in the act of moving. If we did not actually see how it changed from a stationary condition to a moving one, we might wonder what caused it to be set in motion. Did someone pull on it, or push against it, or perhaps blow on it, or even attract it with a magnet? What are these assumed causes of motion? Without exception, they are a form of force. Force, then, is the instigator of movement. If we see an object in motion, we know that it is moving because a force has acted upon it. We know, too, that the force must have been sufficiently great to overcome the object's inertia, for unless a force is greater than the resistance offered by the object, it cannot produce motion. We can push against a stone wall all day without moving it so much as 1 millimeter, but a bulldozer can knock the wall down at the first impact. The magnitude of the force *relative to the magnitude of the resistance* is the determining factor in causing an object to move.

Kinds of Motion. What makes the object move in the way that it moves? Why does the puck sometimes slide across the ice without turning, and why does it sometimes revolve as it slides? Why do arrows, balls and bullets move through the air in a pathway known as a parabola? Why does the hand move in an arc when the forearm turns at the elbow joint and the neighboring joints are held motionless? The student should try to answer these questions for himself before he reads further.

As we note the different ways in which objects move, we are impressed with the almost limitless variety in the patterns of movement. Objects move in straight paths and in curved paths; they roll, slide and fall; they bounce; they swing back and forth like a pendulum; they rotate about a center, either partially or completely; and they frequently rotate at the same time that they move as a whole from one place to another. Although the variety of ways in which objects move appears to be almost limitless, careful consideration of these ways reveals the fact that there are, in actuality, only two major classifications of movement patterns. Either an object turns about a center of motion, or it moves in its entirety from one place to another. Sometimes it does both simultaneously. The former kind of movement is termed *rotatory* or *angular.* This is the kind of motion that is typical of levers and of wheels and axles. A phonograph record is undergoing rotatory motion when it is being played. The partial turning of a sticklike object, or lever, is also rotatory motion. Angular motion is perhaps a more descriptive term to use in the latter case. Rotatory or angular motion is characterized by movement about an axis with all parts of the object moving in an arc, like the movement of a spoke of a wheel or of a paper trimmer (Fig. 5–9). It may be a small arc of motion, or it may be a complete circle.

The second kind of motion is termed *translatory* because the object is translated as a whole from one location to another. Translatory movement may be further classified as *rectilinear* and *curvilinear*

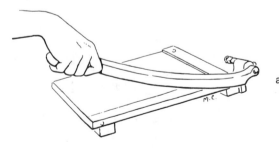

Figure 5–9. An example of angular motion.

Figure 5–10. An example of rectilinear motion.

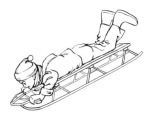

motion. Rectilinear motion, commonly called simply linear motion, is defined as the linear progression of an object as a whole, with all its parts moving the same distance, in the same direction, at a uniform rate of speed (Fig. 5–10). Curvilinear motion refers to all translatory, non-rectilinear movement. The object moves in a curved, but not necessarily circular, pathway.

Not infrequently an object displays a combination of rotatory and translatory movement, the latter often being caused by the former when aided by friction. The bicycle, the automobile and the train move linearly as the result of the rotatory movements of their wheels, provided there is enough friction between the wheels and the supporting surface to keep the former from spinning in place. Likewise man, as he walks or runs down the street, experiences translatory motion because of the angular movement of his lower extremities, aided by friction between his feet and the ground (Fig. 5–11). The angular motions of several segments of the body are frequently coordinated in such a way that a related segment will move linearly. This is true in throwing darts, in putting the shot, and in a lunge in fencing. Because of the angular motions of the forearm and upper arm, the hand is enabled to travel linearly, and thus to impart linear force to the dart and the shot prior to their release, and to the foil (Fig. 5–12).

Motion in a curved path other than a circle or arc is illustrated by the flight of a ball or an arrow—in fact, of any projectile. Although the initial movement of the object through space is rectilinear, the movement path becomes curvilinear as the effect of gravity becomes

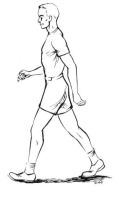

Figure 5–11. An example of linear motion of the body as a whole resulting from the angular motion of some of its parts.

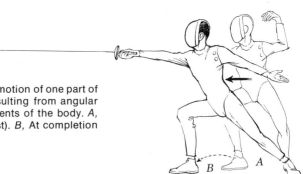

Figure 5–12. Linear motion of one part of the body (the hand) resulting from angular motion of several segments of the body. *A,* Just before lunge (thrust). *B,* At completion of lunge.

apparent. Hence the motion of the projectile is caused by two forces: the impetus imparted to it by the hand, the racket or the bow, and the force of gravity.

Reciprocating motion denotes repetitive movement. The use of the term is ordinarily limited to repetitive translatory movements, as illustrated by a bouncing ball or the repeated blows of a hammer, but technically includes all kinds. The term *oscillation* refers specifically to repetitive angular movements, that is, movements in an arc. Familiar examples of this type of movement are seen in the pendulum, the metronome and the tuning fork.

Kinds of Motion Experienced by the Body. The human body experiences all these kinds of motion (Fig. 5–13). As most of the joints are axial, the body segments must undergo primarily angular motion. A slight amount of translatory motion is seen in the gliding movements of the plane or irregular joints. These movements are negligible in themselves. They occur chiefly in the carpal and tarsal joints and in the joints of the vertebral arches in conjunction with angular movements in neighboring axial joints. The body as a whole experiences rectilinear translatory movement when it is acted upon by the force of gravity, as in coasting (Fig. 5–10) and in the latter part of diving (Fig. 5–15); likewise when acted upon by an external force, as in water skiing (Fig. 5–14). It experiences rotatory motion in forward and backward rolls on the ground, in somersaults in the air and in twirling on

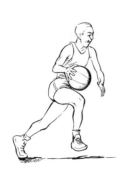

Figure 5–13. An example of movement of the body caused by the body's own muscular action.

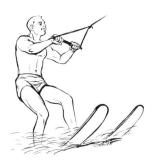

Figure 5–14. An example of movement of the body caused by an external force.

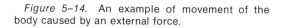ice skates. It experiences curvilinear translatory motion in diving, broad jumping, high jumping and hurdling, and it experiences recipro-cating motion on the trampoline and when swinging back and forth on the rings, trapeze or horizontal bar.

Factors Which Determine the Kind of Motion. Thus far we have considered the cause of motion and the various kinds of motion based on movement patterns or paths. Now we must turn to the question: What determines the kind of motion that will result when an object is made to move? The best way for the student to discover the answer is to produce each kind of motion and then to analyze what he did to obtain the kind of motion he wanted.

In order to make an object move linearly, we discover that either we must apply force uniformly against one entire side of the object, or we must apply it directly in line with the object's center of gravity. The object will move in a straight line provided it does not meet an obstacle or resistance of some sort. If its edge hits against another object, or encounters a rough spot on one side of its pathway, the mov-ing object will turn about its point of contact with the interfering factor. If we attempt to push a tall cabinet across a supporting surface which provides excessive friction such as a cement floor, for instance, the cabinet will tip, even though we place our hands exactly in line with the cabinet's center of gravity and push in a horizontal direction. In

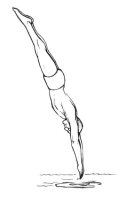

Figure 5–15. An example of movement of the body caused by the force of gravity.

order to move it linearly it will be necessary to apply the push lower than the cabinet's center of gravity to compensate for the friction.

If rotatory motion of a freely movable object is desired, it is necessary to apply force to it "off center" or to provide an "off center" resistance which will interfere with the motion of part of the object. A lever undergoes rotatory motion because, by definition, one portion of it remains in place. If it is desired to move an object in the manner of a lever, it is necessary to provide a fulcrum and to apply force to it at some point other than its point of contact with the fulcrum.

To make an object move in a circular path it is necessary to apply a secondary force or to provide a limited pathway, such as a circular track. When a key is tied to a string and whirled in a circle, the inward pull of the string is the secondary force. This is true of anything which serves to hold the object a uniform distance from the center of motion. An intentional combination of forces, such as consistently longer strides with one leg, or longer strokes with one oar, will also result in circular motion.

Reciprocating motion is caused by a uniform repetition of force applications, and the oscillation of a pendulum is produced by repeated applications of gravitational force to a suspended object which is free to move back and forth and which is in any position other than its resting position.

In summary, it may be said that the kind of motion that will be displayed by a moving object depends first of all upon the kind of motion permitted that particular kind of object. If it is a lever, it is permitted only angular motion; if it is a pendulum, oscillatory motion; and so on. If it is a freely movable object, it is permitted either translatory or rotatory motion, depending upon the circumstances. These circumstances include the point at which force is applied with reference to the object's center of gravity, the environmental pathways of movement available to the object and the presence or absence of additional external factors which modify the motion.

Factors Modifying Motion. Motion is usually modified by a number of external factors, such as friction, air resistance, water resistance and the like. Whether these factors are a help or a hindrance depends upon the circumstances and the nature of the motion. The same factor may facilitate one form of motion, yet hinder another. For instance, friction is a great help to the runner because it enables him to exert maximum effort without danger of slipping, yet on the other hand, friction hinders the rolling of a ball, as in hockey, golf and croquet. Again, wind or air resistance is indispensable to the sail boat's motion, but unless it is a "tail wind" it impedes the runner. Likewise, water resistance is essential for propulsion of the body by means of swimming strokes, and of boats through the use of oars and paddles, yet at the same time it hinders the progress of both the swimmer and the boat, especially if these present a broad surface to the water. It is for this reason that swimmers keep the body level and that boats are streamlined. One of the major problems in sports is to learn how to take advantage of these factors when they contribute to the movement in question, and on the other hand, how to minimize them when they are detrimental to the movement.

There are also anatomic factors which modify the motion of the segments of the body. These include friction in the joints (minimized by synovial fluid), tension of antagonistic muscles, tension of ligaments and fasciae, anomalies of bone and joint structure, atmospheric pressure within the joint capsule, and the presence of interfering soft tissues. Except for the limitations due to fleshiness, these modifying factors come under the heading of "internal resistance."

Laws of Motion. Are there any general truths about motion *question?* that we can count on under all circumstances? Sir Isaac Newton found that there were such truths. As the result of his observations he defined three basic laws of motion. When the effect of modifying factors is discounted, it is seen that these laws hold true for the motion of all objects. The beginner will understand them more easily if he is able to imagine a situation in which extraneous factors such as friction, air resistance and water resistance are eliminated.

LAW OF INERTIA. An object which is at rest will remain so unless acted upon by an external force. An object which is moving will move in a straight line at a uniform speed and will continue to do so unless acted upon by an external force. (It is assumed that the external force is not counteracted by some other external force acting simultaneously.) Thus a ball which is rolling along the ground would continue to roll forever were it not for friction; and a ball sailing horizontally through the air would continue to sail forever, were it not for air resistance and the downward pull of gravity.

LAW OF ACCELERATION. As was stated in the law of inertia, the velocity of a moving object (i.e., the distance traversed per unit of time) will remain constant unless a force acts on the moving object. When such a force does operate, the resulting change in velocity (either increase or decrease) will be directly proportional to the amount of force causing the change, and inversely proportional to the mass of the object. For instance, the amount of force which a horse must use to increase its speed in a race is in direct proportion to its velocity increase. Similarly, it takes more "braking force" to slow a train from 60 to 30 miles per hour than it does to slow the same train from 60 to 50 miles per hour. In both cases the amount of force is directly proportional to the amount of change in velocity.

As an illustration of the effect of variations in mass, the reader might imagine that two balls of equal size are rolling in parallel pathways toward him, an iron ball on the right and a wooden ball on the left. Just as they pass on either side of him he swings both hands, giving each ball a push to help speed it on its way. The speed of the wooden ball will be increased more than that of the iron ball, demonstrating the fact that the change in velocity is inversely proportional to the mass of the object.

LAW OF REACTION. To every action there is an equal and opposite reaction. Another way of stating this law is to say that when a body moves, that is, when it develops momentum, the supporting surface or other object against which it applies its force develops an equal and opposite momentum (Fig. 5–16). To understand this, it is necessary to know that momentum is the product of mass times velocity. When one steps out of a canoe onto the dock, the reaction of the canoe is apparent. This is because the mass of the canoe is so small that the canoe's velocity is great by comparison. When one steps off an ocean liner, on the other hand, the reaction of the boat is imperceptible because its mass is so great that its velocity is infinitesimal by comparison. Nevertheless, in both instances, the mass of the person times his velocity is equal to the mass of the boat (canoe or ocean liner) times its velocity.

When the human body is unsupported in the air, as when diving, it cannot voluntarily alter the pathway of its total movement, that is, it cannot displace its center of gravity. Hence there is no question of action and reaction of the body as a whole. If one part moves, however, such as an arm or a leg, the equal and opposite reaction of the rest of the body is clearly seen. This principle underlies much of the movement in fancy diving and trampolining.

Circular Motion: Centripetal and Centrifugal Force. An object undergoing circular motion is subject to the same laws as an object which is moving in a straight path. That this is not obvious is due to the fact that the object is being restrained in its movement by the centripetal force which is pulling it toward the center of motion. That it is still subject to the Law of Inertia is proved by the fact that it will fly off in a straight line the instant the centripetal force is removed.

The experiment of twirling a string with a key tied to the other end demonstrates this nicely. It is important for the experimenter to understand that the only forces acting on the key are (1) the force causing it to move, provided by the finger, and (2) the inward pull of the string on the key causing its motion to be circular instead of

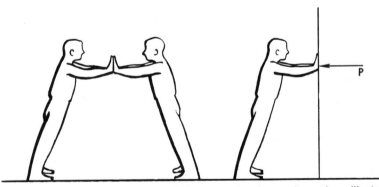

Figure 5–16. A push must be opposed by an equal and opposite push, as illustrated by the two figures. The equal and opposite push of the wall (P) is not as easy to see but it is just as real. (From Williams, M., and Lissner, H. R.: Biomechanics of Human Motion. Philadelphia, W. B. Saunders Company, 1962.)

linear. *Centrifugal force does not act directly on the key.* According to Newton's third Law of Motion, every force has an equal and opposite reaction. Centrifugal force is the equal and opposite reaction to centripetal force, and as such is acting on the finger holding the string, not on the key. When the string is released, there is no longer any centripetal force acting on the key, and therefore no centrifugal counterpull on the finger. The key is now free to travel forward through space in a straight path, which it proceeds to do. Since it is characteristic of centripetal force to act at right angles to an object's normal direction of motion, once this force ceases, the key moves at right angles to the radius of the circle in which it had previously been moving, that is, at a tangent to its former circular pathway. *touches the circle tangent at one point*

Whether an object is moving in a complete circle, as the key on the end of the string, or is moving in a small arc, these same characteristics hold true. Even in the flexing of the forearm centripetal force is present, pulling inward from the fingertips to the elbow joint, and centrifugal force pulling outward from the elbow joint. When a ball is grasped by the fingers, the centripetal force makes it move in the same arc as the hand. When the fingers release it, the ball leaves the hand and starts moving through the air in a straight line at right angles to the forearm. The reason it does not continue to move in a straight line indefinitely is owing to the combined factors of air resistance and the force of gravity.

PRINCIPLES OF MOTION

Principle I (Based on the Law of Inertia). In order to put an object in motion a force must be applied to it—a force which is greater than the force of the resistance.

Principle II (Based on the Law of Inertia). In order to stop the motion of a moving object a force which is greater than the force of the moving object must be applied to it in the opposite direction.

Application. A runner wishing to stop quickly without hurting himself shifts his weight back over the rear foot and reaches well forward with his forward foot. By this means his forward leg is given an appreciable restraining component of force when his foot hits the ground.

Principle III (Based on the Law of Inertia). In order to change the direction of a moving object a force of sufficient magnitude must be applied to it in the desired direction.

Application. Field hockey provides many opportunities for hitting a rolling ball at a slightly different angle to keep it from going out of bounds. It would also be possible to change the ball's direction by letting it hit a stick held firmly at an angle so as to rebound from it. Still another method is used in small puzzles that require the user to roll tiny balls into depressions. Since the balls are under glass the only method available is to tilt the puzzle one way or another, in this way using the force of gravity both to initiate the motion and to change the direction.

Principle IV (Based on the Law of Acceleration). In order to change the velocity of a moving object, a force must be applied to it (1) in the same direction it is moving, if the purpose is to speed it up, or (2) in the opposite direction of its movement, if the purpose is to slow it down.

Application. Rolling a hoop or dribbling in field hockey are good examples of this. In these two instances, however, the acceleration is barely discernible as its purpose is to overcome the slowing down caused by friction.

Principle V (Based on the Law of Action and Reaction). In order to apply an appreciable force effectively, whether to oneself or to an external object, it is usually necessary to have a resistant, non-slippery, stationary surface against which to brace some part of the body.

Application. With every step we take in walking and running or in jumping and hopping, we depend upon a firm, resistant surface against which we can push our feet backward in order to move our bodies forward. Likewise when we attempt to move an external object, especially a heavy or resistant one, by lifting, pushing or pulling, we need a resistant, non-slippery surface against which we can push a foot or other part of the body used for bracing, in order that we may give the necessary impetus to the object. Lifting a heavy weight like a suitcase is a good example for demonstrating the advantage of having a solid surface on which to stand. Assume that we stand with our side to the suitcase, our feet in a forward-backward stance, bend our knees and hips until we can reach the handle with our arm straight down, then rise to an erect position by extending knees and hips. When we lift in this manner we are aware of pressing the feet downward against the ground. If we were standing on thick mud or loose sand we would have difficulty in lifting the suitcase because our feet would sink as we attempted to stand straight with the added weight in our hand. The ineffective action and reaction between feet and supporting surface result in an ineffective lift to the suitcase.

It is important to note that all human motion, whether man is moving only himself or an external object, exemplifies the law of inertia as well as the law of action and reaction. When, for example, one pushes a heavy object along the floor, he must repeatedly overcome the object's inertia by applying sufficient force to cause it to move. The pressure of his hands against the resisting object is *not* an example of action and reaction. Putting an object into motion, by definition, implies exerting a force of sufficient magnitude to exceed the resistance, i.e., the inertia of the object. This illustrates Newton's first law of motion. In order to develop this force he must press his feet backward, as well as downward, against the floor. He may even push one foot against the wall behind him. It is this pressure of the feet, together with the counterpressure of the floor or wall, that illustrates Newton's third law of motion. Note that whereas the push against the object is in the direction one wants it to move, the push of the feet is in the opposite direction.

Principle VI (Based on Characteristics of Circular Motion and on the Laws of Inertia and of Action and Reaction). All circular movements, including those of the human body as a whole and of its individual segments, are characterized by two equal and opposite forces: centripetal—the force pulling inward toward the center, and centrifugal—the force pulling outward from the center, the equal and opposite reaction to centripetal force. The centripetal force holds the object in its circular pathway of motion, apparently nullifying the second part of the law of inertia which states that an object in motion will move in *a straight line.* If the object breaks free from the centripetal force it immediately obeys this law by moving in a straight line at a tangent to the circle. Both of these forces, centripetal and centrifugal, constitute potential hazards.

Application. Rapidly swinging the upper extremity in a circle, either as a flexibility exercise or as a movement preparatory to pitching a baseball, develops considerable centrifugal force. This puts a strain on the ligaments and other structures that surround or cross the shoulder joint and may cause a rupture of the tissues.

A stunt known as "snap-the-whip," performed by ice skaters, constitutes another source of danger. The longer the chain of individuals forming the whip, the faster the outer end moves and the greater the centripetal and centrifugal forces that act on it. In a long "whip" the speed of the end skater can be phenomenal. This puts such a strain on his handclasp with his neighbor that their grip may give way. The end skater then does not continue in a circle but shoots off at a tangent with tremendous speed. If there are obstacles in his pathway before he can get control and change his direction or brake his velocity, a serious accident can occur.

DEMONSTRATIONS AND LABORATORY EXERCISES

1. Continue with the center of gravity experiments from Chapter 1 if you did not complete them.
2. Try to carry a load, first without compensating for it, and then compensating as completely as possible. Check the degree of compensation each time by locating the position of the line of gravity with reference to the center of the base of support. Describe the kinesthetic sensation in the trunk muscles in each case. Do you notice greater tension in one position than in the other?
3. Walk on a low balance beam:
   a. Looking ahead at the wall.
   b. Looking at a person who is in front of the balance beam doing a vigorous exercise such as the jumping jack.
   c. With the eyes closed. What is your reaction in each case? Explain.
4. Walk along with a partner beside you. Without warning, the

partner is to give you a sudden, but not overforceful, sideward push. How do you react? If you did not succeed in "catching your balance," can you explain the reason for your failure?

5. Describe or find references for five pyramids and list them in their order of difficulty. Explain the reasons for the order you have chosen.

6. Do the same for five dual balance stunts.

7. Build two columns of blocks, one with the blocks carefully centered one over the other, the second column with the blocks staggered but balanced. Grasping the lowest block of each column, slide the columns back and forth, changing the speed frequently and suddenly until the blocks tumble. Which column is the first to topple? Why?

8. Take a ruler or a book and make it move in each of the ways listed below. Analyze the cause of each kind of motion produced.

   a. Rectilinear motion.
   b. Curvilinear motion.
   c. Angular motion.
   d. Oscillation.

9. For each of the following activities identify the upper extremity joints at which angular motion occurs and by this motion makes it possible for the hand to move linearly.

   Note: You may identify some principles which are not described in this chapter. If so, discuss them with your classmates and formulate a statement that expresses them clearly.

   a. Drawing a 2-foot straight line on the blackboard at shoulder level.
   b. Putting the shot or throwing a dart.
   c. Drawing the string of an archery bow.
   d. Lunge in fencing.

10. Draw a diagram to represent the path taken by the hand in the sagittal plane in each of the following movements.

   a. Underwater portion of crawl stroke.
   b. Underhand softball pitch (not including the wind-up).
   c. Overhand baseball pitch (not including the wind-up).
   d. Bowling.

11. Place a book on a table and stand a small bottle on top of it. Pull the book toward you with a quick jerk. Which way does the bottle fall? Stand the bottle on the book again and pull the book across the table with a steady pull. Pull it against an obstacle, such as your other hand, so that the movement is stopped abruptly. Which way does the bottle fall now? Explain. Which of the three laws of motion does this experiment illustrate?

12. For this experiment it is necessary to have a smooth surface and a rough surface side by side. A rug partially covering a smooth floor will do nicely. Take two tennis balls and place them on the floor approximately 20 inches apart, one on the rug and the other on the bare floor. Holding a yardstick in a horizontal position, stoop and hit both balls simultaneously, causing them to roll. What causes the

difference in the distance traveled by the two balls? Was there any difference in the force applied to them, or in the resistance offered by them?

13. Roll a ball on a table. Without stopping it, make it turn to the right. How did you change its direction? Is there another way in which you could change the direction of the rolling ball?

14. Attempt to hit a 10-inch target with a tennis ball from a distance of 10 feet in each of the two ways described below. Compare the pathway of the hand's movement in the two methods. Which way is more difficult? Why?

a. Face the target squarely. Keep the upper arm raised in a side-horizontal position and keep the forearm at right angles to it. Throw the ball by moving the forearm in a forward-downward arc. Use as much wrist snap as desired.

b. Throw the ball in the manner that you would normally use if you were playing catch with a friend, or were throwing from one base to another in baseball.

15. In a safe place, swing a weighted rope in a horizontal circle close to the floor and let it go suddenly. Note its pathway in relation to the circle in which it was previously moving.

RECOMMENDED READINGS

Brunnstrom, S.: Clinical Kinesiology, 2nd ed. Philadelphia, F. A. Davis Company, 1966, Chapter 1.
Williams, M., and Lissner, H. R.: Biomechanics of Human Motion. Philadelphia, W. B. Saunders Company, 1962.

CHAPTER 6

Force and Work

FORCE

The human body, like other bodies, both animate and inanimate, is acted upon by various forces. Furthermore, through muscular contraction, the body generates a force of its own which it uses either to balance or to overcome external forces. When opposing forces acting upon a body balance one another or, in the case of the human body, when the external forces acting upon it are balanced by the body's own resisting force, the body remains stationary and is said to be in equilibrium. When there is imbalance between opposing forces, the body moves. The force exerted by muscles on bones obeys the same principles as do all forces applied to external objects, but with this difference: muscles can only pull the bones to which they are attached; they cannot push. The resulting movement of the bony lever, however, can cause either a pull or a push to be applied to the object which resists the lever's movement.

What is force? It can be felt, and its effect can be both seen and measured, but force itself, like the wind, is invisible. Nevertheless it can be described. Force is a push or a pull exerted against something. If we know the strength of the force, the direction in which it is acting and the exact portion of the object on which it is exerting its pull or push, we have the essential information about the force. Hence force can be described in terms of its magnitude, its direction and the point of its application. Since in kinesiology we are particularly interested in muscular force, these three aspects of force will be discussed as they relate to the muscles.

Magnitude. The magnitude of muscular force is in direct proportion to the number and size of the fibers in the muscle which is contracting. If muscles contracted individually it would be a relatively easy matter to measure the force exerted by each one in a given movement. Since they normally act in groups, however, their force or strength is measured collectively. It is customary to measure maximum muscular strength by performing a simple movement against the resistance of a dynamometer, spring balance, or similar instrument.

The instrument thus serves as the resistance to an anatomical lever whose force is provided by a group of muscles which act as a functional team to produce the movement of the lever. Among the muscle groups which are frequently measured by this method are the finger flexors (grip strength), elbow flexors and knee extensors.

Although, to the author's knowledge, there is no way of determining the amount of force exerted by a single muscle in the living body, its potential strength can be calculated from its measurements, its internal structure and the approximate number of pounds (or kilograms) which the average human muscle is known to exert per square inch (or centimeter). The muscle's external measurements and its internal structure form the basis for determining its physiologic cross section, a term which refers to the perpendicular section of all of the muscle's fibers. A study of the internal structure of various muscles reveals a variety of arrangements. In some muscles the fibers are arranged longitudinally; in some, in spindle-like fashion; in some, fanlike; and in some, feather-like (see page 35). Obviously a simple cross section of a penniform or a bipenniform muscle will miss a large number of the fibers; hence a true cross section of the muscle's fibers is one which cuts across every fiber in the muscle. Figure 6–1 illustrates the method of measuring the physiologic cross section of several types of muscles. The cross section does not reveal the actual number of fibers, to be sure, but it corresponds closely enough for us to use this measurement in estimating the muscle's potential force. The physiologic cross section is found by adding the lengths of the lines that cut perpendicularly across the fibers and multiplying their sum by the average thickness of the muscle. Such measurements can, of course, only be made on dissected muscles, but in the living body they can be roughly estimated from the approximate circumference and length of the muscle belly and from a knowledge of the muscle's internal structure. Suppose a penniform muscle is 7 inches long, exclusive of its tendons, and its average thickness is ¾ of an inch.

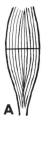
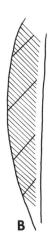
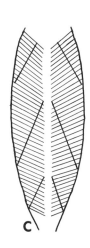

Figure 6–1. Method of measuring the physiologic cross section of three types of muscles. *A,* A fusiform or spindle muscle; *B,* a penniform muscle; *C,* a bipenniform muscle.

A

B

C

Suppose further that it takes three lines, measuring respectively 4, 5 and 3 inches, to cut perpendicularly across the fibers. The physiologic cross section of such a muscle is $\frac{3}{4}(4+5+3) = \frac{3}{4} \times 12 = 9$ sq. in.

The amount of force which the average human muscle can exert has been determined by several experimenters. Fick, one of the early investigators, found that human muscles exerted a force of 6 to 10 kg. per square centimeter of their physiologic cross section.[1,2] This is approximately 85 to 141 pounds per square inch. Recklinghausen, according to Steindler,[4] concluded from his experimentation that human muscles exerted only 3.6 kg. per square centimeter (approximately 51 pounds per square inch) of cross section. It is assumed that these two investigators used male subjects. A more recent investigator, Morris,[3] found that the muscles of male subjects exerted 9.2 kg. per square centimeter (130 lb. per square inch), and of female subjects, 7.1 kg. per square centimeter (101 lb. per square inch). Because of the wide range of figures presented to date further investigation of this matter would seem desirable. A study of the effect of training on muscular force, per unit of cross section, would also be of interest. If 95 lb. per square inch is arbitrarily selected as the force which an average human muscle can exert, the hypothetical muscle described above, having a physiologic cross section of 9 sq. in., would have a potential force of 9×95, or 855 lb.

Point of Application. For practical purposes it may be assumed that the point of application of muscular force is the center of the muscle's attachment to the bony lever. This usually corresponds to the muscle's insertion, or distal attachment. Technically, however, it is the point of intersection between the line of force and the *mechanical axis* of the bone or segment serving as the anatomic lever. This axis does not necessarily pass lengthwise through the shaft of the bony lever. If the bone bends or if the articulating process projects at an angle from the shaft, the greater part of the axis may lie completely outside the shaft, as in the case of the femur. *The mechanical axis of a bone or segment is a straight line which connects the midpoint of the joint at one end with the midpoint of the joint at the other end, or in the case of a terminal segment, with its distal end.*

The position of the point of application, with reference to the fulcrum of the lever and to the point at which the resistance is applied, determines the class of the lever.

Direction. The direction of muscular force is represented by the angle which is bounded by the muscle's line of pull and the portion of the mechanical axis that lies between the point of application and the fulcrum. Figure 6–2 shows a muscle (the biceps) applying its force to a lever (the radius) at an angle of 30 degrees. Figure 3–2 illustrates other angles of pull.

Components of Force. A muscle's angle of pull changes with every degree of joint motion. The size of the angle has a direct bearing on the effectiveness of the muscle's pull in moving the bony lever. Except when the pull is at right angles to the lever, some part of the force exerted by the muscle is not contributing to the lever's movement. The force is then said to consist of two components, a rotatory component (the component that turns the lever) and a non-rotatory component. By definition, these components are at right angles to each other, the rotatory component always being perpendicular to the lever and the non-rotatory component parallel to it. The angle of pull of most muscles in the resting position is less than a right angle and it usually remains so throughout the movement (Fig. 6–2). This means that the non-rotatory component of force is directed toward the fulcrum which gives it a stabilizing effect. By pulling the bone lengthwise toward the joint it helps to maintain the integrity of the joint. Under most circumstances, therefore, muscular force has two simultaneous functions, namely movement and stabilization. In the latter capacity it supplements the ligaments, an excellent example of the body's efficiency, as muscles perform this stabilizing function only during the period when the segment is moving, when the integrity of the joint may be threatened.

Occasionally the angle of pull becomes greater than a right angle which means that the non-rotatory component of force is directed away from the fulcrum and is therefore a dislocating component. This does not happen in many instances, however, and when it does, the muscle is close to the limit of its shortening range and is therefore not exerting much force. (See Fig. 6–3.)

When the angle of pull is 90 degrees the force is completely rotatory. When it is 45 degrees the rotatory and stabilizing components are equal. Since the angle of pull usually remains less than 45 degrees, more of the muscle's force serves to stabilize the joint than to move the lever. In fact, there are some muscles whose angles of pull are always so small that their contribution to motion would seem to be negligible. This appears to be true of the coracobrachialis and the subclavius muscles. It is interesting to note that the upper extremity is frequently called upon to perform violent, powerful movements,

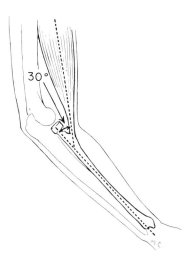

Figure 6–2. The biceps muscle pulling at a 30-degree angle to the mechanical axis of the radius.

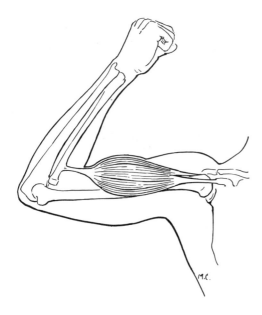

Figure 6–3. The biceps muscle pulling at an angle greater than a right angle. The nonrotatory component is pulling away from the joint.

also to support the body weight in suspension. The joints which bear the brunt of this violence and strain are the shoulder and sterno-clavicular joints. They might well become dislocated more easily than they do were it not for the coracobrachialis and the subclavius muscles which pull the bones lengthwise toward their proximal joints and thus serve to stabilize these joints.

The small angle of pull that most muscles have when in their normal resting position has already been noted. Were it not for ana-tomic devices that serve as fixed single pulleys for increasing such angles, some muscles would probably be unable to effect any move-ment whatsoever. For instance, the condyles both above and below the knee joint serve this purpose for the gracilis muscle (Fig. 4–9); the patella for the quadriceps (Fig. 6–4); and the external malleolus for the peroneus longus (Fig. 4–10). The student should look for additional examples in the body.

Force Applied to External Objects. Force—whether muscular, mechanical or gravitational—when applied to external objects or to other persons, may also consist of more than one component, depend-ing upon the angle of application. If a horizontal push is applied to a piece of furniture, and the push is applied in line with the object's center of gravity, the object will move straight forward in a horizontal direction, provided there is no additional conflicting force or resistance to interfere with the object's motion. This is an example of a force which consists of only one component (Fig. 6–5). On the other hand, if one pushes a low piece of furniture by standing close to it with the arms held at a forward-downward slant, there will be two components, a forward one and a downward one. Only the forward component, in

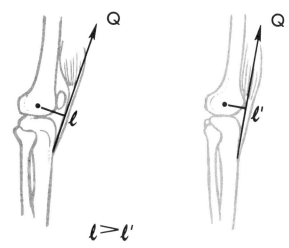

$$\ell > \ell'$$

Figure 6–4. By increasing the angle of pull the patella increases the true force arm of the quadriceps femoris. (From Williams, M., and Lissner, H. R.: Biomechanics of Human Motion. Philadelphia, W. B. Saunders Company, 1962.)

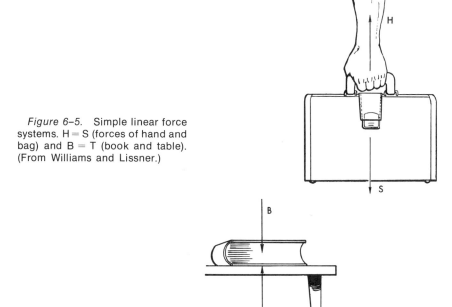

Figure 6–5. Simple linear force systems. H = S (forces of hand and bag) and B = T (book and table). (From Williams and Lissner.)

this case, is effective for producing the desired motion. The downward component merely increases friction.

If a child's cart is drawn by too short a rope, there will be a relatively large lifting component and a small forward-pulling component. Since the purpose is to pull the cart horizontally, it is more efficient to use a long rope because this gives a relatively greater horizontal, or pulling, component.

There are always at least two forces operating on an object that is projected through the air, the propulsive force and the downward force of gravity. The propulsive force frequently consists of two components, a forward and an upward component. If a ball is thrown at an angle of 45 degrees from the horizontal, the upward and forward components of propulsion are equal. The force of gravity, which becomes operative as soon as the ball is released, may not show its effect immediately. The distance traveled by the ball, before the effect of the gravitational force becomes apparent, depends largely upon the magnitude of the propulsive force.

Graphic Representation of Force. It is sometimes desirable to use diagrams to represent muscular force. For this the same method is used as is used in physics. A force may be represented graphically by an arrow. A short linear unit, such as 1/8 inch, is selected to represent a unit of weight, such as 1 pound. A line is then drawn to scale in the direction that the force is applied, and the head of the arrow is placed at the appropriate end of the line to indicate whether the force is a push or a pull. In the case of muscular force it is always a pull. The arrowhead is therefore at the opposite end from the point at which the force is applied. The diagram in Figure 6–6 represents a pulling force of 10 pounds applied to point A in a horizontal direction from left to right. It is customary to indicate the direction of a muscular force in terms of the angle formed between the line of force and the mechanical axis of the bone. Figure 6–2 shows a muscular force pulling on the radius, at an angle of 30 degrees to the bone's mechanical axis.

True Force and Resistance Arms of Lever; Perpendicular Distance. In the discussion of levers in Chapter 4 it was assumed that both the force and the resistance were applied at right angles to the lever. Actually, such is seldom the case. We have seen how the direction, or angle of application, affects the components of force. How does it affect the leverage?

In the earlier examples of leverage, in which the force was applied at right angles to the lever, the force arm was defined as the portion of the lever between the fulcrum and the point at which the force was

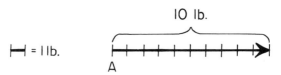

Figure 6–6. A straight line representing a 10-pound pulling force which is applied to point A.

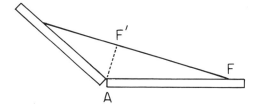

Figure 6-7. The perpendicular distance, AF', represents the true force arm of the lever.

applied. It might equally well have been defined as the perpendicular distance from the line of force to the fulcrum. Likewise, the resistance arm could have been defined as the perpendicular distance from the line, or direction, of the resistance to the fulcrum. These definitions hold true for all levers, regardless of the angle of application of force or the angle of application of the resistance. Whenever these angles are other than right angles, however, the perpendicular distance must be determined by measurement or by calculation, for it is no longer a portion of the lever itself.

The diagram in Figure 6-7 represents a muscle which is pulling at an acute angle to the mechanical axis of the bone. The fulcrum or axis of motion is marked A, and the point where the force is applied is marked F. The portion of the lever, AF, is not the true force arm, however, because the muscle's line of pull is not perpendicular to the mechanical axis of the lever. A line drawn from the fulcrum to the muscle's line of pull, at right angles to the latter, is known as the *perpendicular distance* or *true force arm* of the lever. Thus, in the majority of anatomic levers the true force arm is considerably shorter than one might suppose. Two factors determine this perpendicular distance, namely, (1) the angle of pull and (2) the distance to the point of application of force from the fulcrum. The true resistance arm of a lever is determined in a similar manner.

It should now be apparent that the effectiveness of a muscle in causing movement depends upon both the leverage and the angle of pull, as well as upon the actual force exerted by the muscle. This is because the true force arm of the lever is determined by two factors, namely, the distance from the center of the joint to the muscle's line of pull (which in turn is determined by its angle of pull) and the distance from the center of the joint to the point at which the force is applied, i.e., the point at which the muscle attaches to the moving bone. The product of the force, or tension, and the perpendicular distance (F × F'A) is known as the moment of force, or the torque. It is a measure of the muscle's ability to move the anatomic lever. Hence, if the muscle's force and the true force arm are known, the torque may be determined by multiplying them. Or if, on the other hand, the torque and perpendicular distance are known, the muscle's tension, i.e., force, may be found by dividing the torque by the true force arm of the lever, i.e., the perpendicular distance $\left(F = \dfrac{\text{torque}}{F'A} \right)$. In many instances the shortening of a muscle as it moves an anatomic lever is accompanied by an increase in its angle of pull, and consequently in its perpendicular distance or true force arm. Thus an improvement in mechanical advantage helps to compensate for the diminishing force due to shortening.

The reason for the additional questions about levers, which were suggested on page 58, should now be apparent.

The Composite Effect of Two or More Forces. Frequently two or more nonparallel forces are applied to the same object. For instance, a canoe may be acted upon by both the wind and the paddler, one force tending to send the canoe north and the other, east. In the body it is rarely, if ever, the case that an individual muscle acts by itself to move a segment. For example, there are at least four muscles that flex the forearm, and more than five that contribute to flexion of the leg at the knee joint. It might seem that if we knew the magnitude of each force that contributed to the movement in question, we could assume that the total effect of their combined force would be the sum of their respective forces. This is not the case, however, *unless the several forces are applied to the same point and are acting in identical directions.* Possibly there are two such examples in the body, the gastrocnemius and the soleus acting at the ankle joint, and the psoas and the iliacus acting at the hip joint. In each of these examples it will be noted that the two muscles have a common tendon for their distal attachments. In these cases it seems fair to assume that the total force acting upon the part is the sum of the forces exerted by the two muscles.

This is not true, however, when the forces are applied at different angles, that is, in different directions. In order to determine the composite effect of the forces in such cases it is necessary to use the method of finding the resultant of forces known in physics as the composition of forces. It must be pointed out that the method described here is for determining the resultant of two forces acting at an angle to each other and that it is therefore assumed that they have a common point of application. This is not true of the majority of muscles which act on the same bone. Nevertheless the principle of finding the composite effect of two or more forces, both as to magnitude and direction, is as true for forces acting on body segments as for forces acting on external objects. For purposes of illustration, therefore, let us assume that there are two muscles having a common point of attachment, but different angles of pull. Both the magnitude and the direction of the resultant force can be determined by the construction of a *parallelogram of forces* (see p. 104).

The essential facts for the student of kinesiology to learn from this discussion are summarized as follows:

1. The resultant magnitude of two forces is not their arithmetical sum unless the two forces are acting in exactly the same direction.

2. The resultant direction of two forces is not halfway between them unless the two forces are of equal magnitude.

3. The resultant of two forces depends not only upon the magnitude of each force, but also upon the angle of application, i.e., the direction of each force.

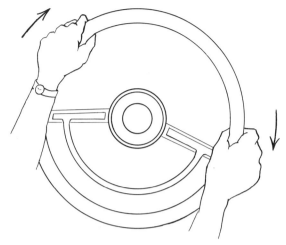

Figure 6–8. When one steers with two hands the hands act as a force couple.

④ The same principles apply to muscular forces acting on body segments as apply to muscular and mechanical forces acting on external objects.

⑤ The multiple muscular action, characteristic of movements of the body segments, is an example of cooperation, not duplication. When several muscles act together to produce a single movement, they act at different points and at different angles. In this way they help to steady and guide the segment throughout its movement.

Figure 6–9. Two force couples acting on the scapula to rotate it upward. (Trapezius II and lower Serratus Anterior are an excellent example. Trapezius II and the lower fibers of IV also tend to act as a force couple although their pulls are not in opposite directions.)

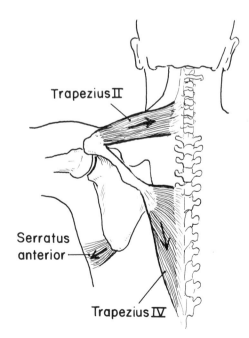

Trapezius II

Serratus anterior

Trapezius IV

A Force Couple. In mechanics the term "couple" or "force couple" refers to a pair of equal parallel forces acting in opposite directions. The effect of such action is rotation. An example of this type of movement is seen in steering a car or a boat when both hands are used on opposite sides of the wheel (Fig. 6–8). There are a number of examples in the human body in which two muscles rotate a bone by acting cooperatively as a force couple; for instance, trapezius II and the lower portion of serratus anterior are a force couple, rotating the scapula upward. Trapezius II and IV, acting on the two extremities of the spine of the scapula, similarly serve as a force couple to help rotate the scapula upward (Fig. 6–9).

WORK

Mechanically speaking, work is the product of the amount of force expended and the distance over which the force is applied. If we let W stand for work, F for force, and d for distance, then we can say that $W = F \times d$, or more simply, $W = Fd$. This equation applies not only to the work of machines, but also to muscular work when the latter is considered from the mechanical, rather than the physiologic, point of view. Suppose, for instance, that there is a rectangular muscle, 4 inches long and $1\frac{1}{2}$ inches wide, that exerts 66 pounds of force as it turns a bony lever. Since the average muscle fiber shortens to one-half of its resting length and the fibers of a small rectangular muscle run the full length of the muscle, the force of the muscle in question is exerted over a distance of two inches (the amount of shortening, equal to one-half the resting length). Therefore, since $F = 66$ lb. and $d = 2$ in. ($\frac{2}{12}$ or $\frac{1}{6}$ of a foot), the muscle is performing 132 inch pounds, or 11 foot pounds, of work. In brief: $W = F(66 \text{ lb.}) \times d(\frac{1}{6} \text{ ft.})$.

If the force of the muscle is not known it is computed from the muscle's cross section. Assuming the muscle in question to be half an inch thick, and the force per square inch of cross section to be 90 lb., the following steps are taken.

1. Find the muscle's cross section.
    Cross section = width × thickness.
    $1\frac{1}{2}$ in. × $\frac{1}{2}$ in. = $\frac{3}{4}$ sq. in. (cross section)
2. Find the amount of force exerted by the muscle.
    Average force = 90 lb. per sq. in.
    Cross section = $\frac{3}{4}$ sq. in.
    $F = 90 \times \frac{3}{4} = \frac{270}{4} = 67\frac{1}{2}$ lb.
3. Find the amount of work performed by this muscle, first in inch pounds, then in foot pounds.
    $W = Fd$
    $W = 67\frac{1}{2}$ lb. × 2 in. = $\frac{135}{2} \times 2 = 135$ in. lb.
    $\frac{135}{12} = 11\frac{1}{4}$ ft. lb.

For purposes of simplification the internal structure of the hypothetical muscle used in these examples was rectangular. This means that a simple geometric cross sectional measure could be used. For penniform and bipenniform muscles, however, it would be essential to determine the physiologic cross section (see page 91). It must also be remembered that "d" in the work equation represents one-half the length of the average fiber in the muscle and that this may or may not coincide with the total length of the fleshy part of the muscle, depending upon its internal structure.

The number of pounds of force per square inch exerted by the average human muscle must be selected arbitrarily, depending upon whose research the student accepts as his source.

A single equation for computing the work performed by a muscle whose average fiber length is known and whose physiologic cross section (PCS) has been determined, would be as follows:

$$W = 90 \times PCS(\text{in sq. in.}) \times \tfrac{1}{2} \text{ the length of the fibers(in inches)}$$

This will give work in terms of inch pounds. Since it is customary to measure work in terms of foot pounds, the result should be divided by 12. The following equation includes this step:

$$W = \frac{90 \ (\text{PCS in sq. in.})(\tfrac{1}{2} \text{ the fiber length in inches})}{12}$$

SUPPLEMENTARY MATERIAL

Methods of Determining the Components of Force. It is a simple matter to find the components of a muscular force when the muscle's total force and angle of pull are known. It can be found either by the use of trigonometry or by constructing a right triangle to scale.

TRIGONOMETRIC METHOD. Although this method requires the use of trigonometry, it is not necessary for the student to have any previous knowledge of this subject. A table of sines and cosines, and a few facts concerning the fixed relationships which exist between the sides and the angles of a right triangle, provide all the necessary information. These facts are as follows:

Definitions (see Fig. 6–10.)

The "side opposite" is the side which faces the angle under consideration.

The hypotenuse is the side which faces the right angle.

The "side adjacent" is the remaining side. It lies between the angle under consideration and the right angle.

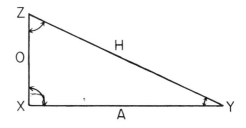

Figure 6–10. A right triangle in which X = the right angle, Y and Z = the two acute angles respectively, H = the hypotenuse, A = the side adjacent (to Y), and O = the side opposite (to Y).

Relationships in a right triangle

The square of the hypotenuse equals the sum of the squares of the other two sides.

The sine of an angle is the ratio of the "side opposite" to the hypotenuse.

The cosine of an angle is the ratio of the "side adjacent" to the hypotenuse.

Hence, in Figure 6–10:

The sine of angle $Y = O/H$

The cosine of angle $Y = A/H$

Applications to muscular force

Problem: The muscle in the diagram (Fig. 6–11) has a force of 150 pounds acting at the distal attachment of the muscle and pulling at an angle of 30 degrees. Find the two components of force.

Method. Construct a right triangle, one angle of which is 30 degrees. This triangle may be superimposed on the original diagram. To do this, a perpendicular should be erected from any point along the long axis of the bone between the joint and the point of attachment. This perpendicular represents the rotatory component of force. The distance along the axis of the bone between the perpendicular and the point of attachment represents the nonrotatory component. The hypotenuse of the triangle, or the portion of the muscle's line of pull between the point of attachment and the perpendicular, represents the total force of the muscle (see Fig. 6–12, A). If desired, instead of superimposing the right triangle on the original diagram, a separate right triangle may be drawn. (Fig. 6–12, B). The size of the triangle is immaterial, provided the proportions are correct.

Referring to a table of sines and cosines, we find that the sine of a 30-degree angle is .5, and the cosine, .866. If the sine of angle $Y = O/H$, then .5 = $O/150$, and O must equal 75. Since O represents the rotatory component, the latter must be 75 pounds.

If the cosine of angle $Y = A/H$, then .866 = $A/150$, and A must equal 129.9, or approximately 130. Hence the nonrotatory component equals approximately 130 pounds.[*]

---

[*] It may surprise the student to discover that the sum of the components is greater than the total force. He should remember the facts concerning a right triangle, however. The square of the hypotenuse equals the sum of the squares of the other two sides.

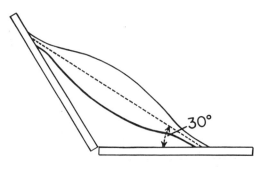

Figure 6–11. A muscle pulling at an angle of 30 degrees.

30°

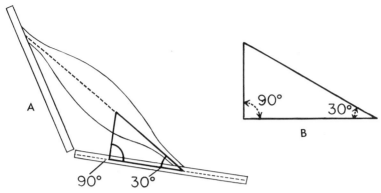

Figure 6–12. Method of constructing a right triangle for the purpose of determining the components of muscular force by the trigonometric method. Note that the hypotenuse coincides with a portion of the muscle's line of pull, and the side adjacent with the mechanical axis of the bone into which the muscle is inserted.

Warning. The angle under consideration is the angle formed by the attachment of the muscle (that is, the muscle's line of pull) to the long axis of the moving bone. One must disregard the angle of the joint between the two bones and the angle between the muscle's line of pull and the stationary bone. Drawing a separate diagram, as in Figure 6–12, *B*, will help the student to avoid this pitfall.

GRAPHIC METHOD. Select a linear unit of measurement to represent a unit of force, such as 1/8 inch to represent 10 pounds of force. Draw a diagonal line to scale, the units of length representing the pounds of total force exerted by the muscle. At one end of this diagonal construct an angle equal to the angle of pull. Continue the side of this angle until it is nearly as long as the original line. From the other end of the diagonal drop a line which will be perpendicular to the second line. Measure the length of each of the two lines drawn from the ends of the diagonal. The line adjacent to the angle of pull represents the nonrotatory component of force, and the line opposite the angle of pull represents the rotatory component of force. This method is simple, but it requires accurate use of the ruler and protractor.

Example (see Fig. 6–13.)
The force of the muscle = 150 pounds
The angle of pull = 30 degrees
Let 1/8 inch = 10 pounds

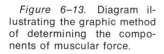

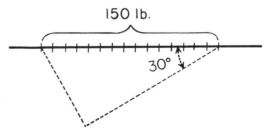

150 lb.

30°

Figure 6–13. Diagram illustrating the graphic method of determining the components of muscular force.

Construct a diagram according to the directions. Measure the lower line. It is found to equal 13 units, that is, 13 × ⅛ inch. Now measure the up-and-down line. It is found to equal 7½ units, or 7½ × ⅛ inch. By computation we find that 13 × 10 = 130 pounds of nonrotatory or stabilizing force, and that 7½ × 10 = 75 pounds of rotatory force.

*Method of Constructing a Parallelogram of Forces for Determining the Composite Effect of Two Forces.** The composite effect of two forces is determined by the construction of a parallelogram, the sides of which are linear representations of the two forces. The first step is to mark a point on a piece of paper. This represents the point at which the two forces are applied. From this point two lines are drawn to scale, with the correct angle between them, that is, the same angle which actually exists between the two forces. By using these two lines as two sides of a parallelogram, the other two sides are constructed by a simple geometric method (Fig. 6–14). The diagonal is then drawn from the point of application to the opposite corner. This diagonal represents, both in magnitude and in direction, the composite effect of the two separate forces. It is known as the resultant of forces.

Note: The student should note that the angle between two muscular forces is the difference between their respective angles of pull.

Measurement of Muscle Strength Relative to Cross Section. In 1948 Morris conducted a study for the purpose of measuring the strength of muscles per square centimeter of cross section. Using twelve college men and twelve college women as her subjects, she computed the areas of the flexor and extensor muscles of the forearm and lower leg by means of a formula based on width, depth and circumference measurements of the upper arm and thigh. These measurements were corrected for fat. To determine the approximate area of each muscle to be tested, she obtained the average proportions of each from two sets of cross section drawings. By means of measure-

---

*When one wishes to determine the resultant of three or more forces, a polygon, rather than a parallelogram, must be constructed. Directions for this procedure may be found in any standard physics text.

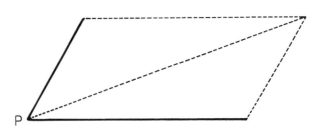

P = Point of application of two forces.

Figure 6–14. A "parallelogram of forces" used for determining the composite effect of two forces applied to the same point.

ments made on x-rays she determined the leverage in which each muscle was involved. The mechanical efficiency of each muscle was computed by the use of the ratio, $\frac{FA}{RA}$. Using the Martin breaking point test, she then tested the forearm flexors, forearm extensors, leg flexors and leg extensors of each subject. From the data so obtained she computed the strength of each muscle per square centimeter of cross section. According to her findings, "the unweighted average of muscle strength was slightly above 9.2 kg./cm.^{2} for men and 7.1 kg./cm.^{2} for women." She concluded that, in general, her findings upheld those of Fick, but not those of Recklinghausen.[3]

DEMONSTRATIONS, LABORATORY EXERCISES AND PROBLEMS

Note: Assume that the muscles can exert a force of 100 pounds per square inch of cross section.

1. How much force can each of the following muscles exert?
   Muscle A, having a cross section of 2 square inches.
   Muscle B, having a cross section of 4 square inches.
   Muscle C, having a cross section of 13 square inches.

2. Find the approximate force of which the muscle shown in Figure 6–15 is capable. Assume that the diagram is drawn to scale, ½ inch being the equivalent of 1 inch. The muscle is 1 inch thick.

3. Estimate the cross section of your own biceps muscle. Approximately how much force should it be able to exert?

4. Approximately how much force should your triceps be able to exert?

5. Measure the width of your gastrocnemius. Assume that it is 1 inch thick. Look at a picture of the muscle to see the slant of the fibers. Estimate the physiologic cross section of your muscle and calculate the amount of force it should be able to exert.

6. On each of the diagrams in Figures 6–16 and 6–17 draw a line to represent the mechanical axis of the bone.

7. In the diagram of the biceps muscle in Figure 6–18, find the size of the angle of pull.

8. Using the data from question 5, draw an arrow (to a scale of your own choosing) which represents the magnitude and direction of the force exerted by your gastrocnemius muscle on the calcaneus bone. Assume that you are standing erect.

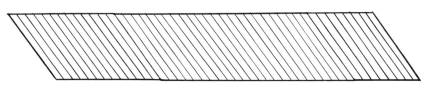

Figure 6–15. What is the approximate force that this muscle can exert? (Scale ½ inch = 1 inch).

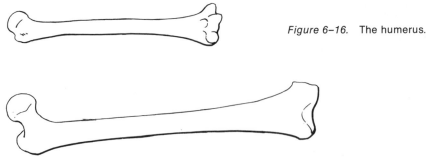

Figure 6-16.   The humerus.

Figure 6-17.   The femur.

9. Using the scale, ⅛ inch = 1 inch, determine the true force arm of the forearm lever in Figure 6–18.

10. For each of the following anatomic levers estimate the approximate length of the true force arm, i.e., the perpendicular distance. Refer to anatomic illustrations or to a muscle manikin to help you estimate the angle of pull of the muscles. Unless otherwise stated, assume that the segments are in their normal resting position. (*Hint:* Use the mechanical axis of the segment for the lever.)

a. The forearm lever with the biceps providing the force.

b. The upper arm lever with the middle deltoid providing the force.

c. The upper arm lever in the side-horizontal position with the entire pectoralis major providing the force. (*Hint:* Which view would show you the angle of pull for this movement, facing the subject or looking down from above?)

d. Same lever as in *c*, with the anterior deltoid providing the force.

11. Referring to the diagrams in Figure 3–2 (p. 37), assume that a weight is suspended from the wrist. Find the true resistance arm of the forearm lever in positions *A*, *B* and *C*. Consider that the scale for these diagrams is 9 inches to the inch.

12. Assume that a muscle having a force of 300 pounds is pulling at an angle of 75 degrees. Find the components of force (*a*) by the trigonometric method; (*b*) by the graphic method.

13. Assuming that the weight used in question 11 is 8 pounds, determine the rotatory and nonrotatory components of the weight (*a*) by the trigonometric method; (*b*) by the graphic method.

14. Determine the amount of work (in foot pounds) performed by each of the following hypothetical muscles:

Muscle A, capable of a total force of 240 pounds and having fibers with an average length of 6 inches.

Muscle B, capable of a total force of 150 pounds and having fibers with an average length of 24 inches.

Muscle C, having a cross section of 4 square inches and fibers with an average length of 12 inches.

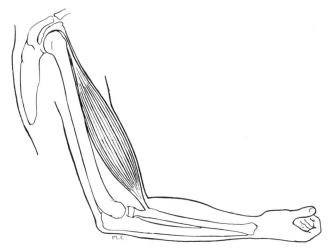

Figure 6–18. The forearm as a lever with the biceps providing the force.

15. In Figure 6–19 muscle *A* has a force of 200 pounds and is pulling on the bone *X-Y* at an angle of 10 degrees. Muscle *B* has a force of 175 pounds and is pulling at an angle of 40 degrees. Find the composite effect of these two muscles in terms of (*a*) the amount of force; and (*b*) the direction, i.e., the angle, of pull.

(*Note:* The angle between two muscular forces, represented by their lines of pull, is the difference between their respective angles of pull. This is not the same as the angle of pull of the resultant.)

16. Referring to Figure 15–15 (p. 267), make a tracing of the femur and the adductor longus muscle. Draw a straight line to represent the mechanical axis of the femur, and another to represent the muscle's line of pull (connecting the midpoints of the proximal and distal attachments).

a. Using a protractor, measure the angle of pull, i.e., the angle facing the hip joint, formed by the intersection of the muscle's line of pull with the bone's mechanical axis.

b. Measure the true force arm of the lever, i.e., the perpendicular distance from the fulcrum (center of hip joint) to the muscle's line of pull. To convert this to a realistic figure use the scale $3/16$ in. = 1 in.

Figure 6–19. Bone *X — Y* with muscles *A* and *B* pulling at indicated angles. Accompanying diagram to Problem 15.

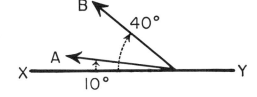

    c. Assuming the muscle's total force to be 250 lb., calculate the moment of force (i.e., the torque) of the lever (see page 97).

    d. Calculate the rotatory and the nonrotatory components of force, using either method.

REFERENCES

1. Fick, R.: Handbuch der Anatomie und Mechanik der Gelenke. Jena, G. Fischer, 1910. Chap. 17.
2. Fick, R.: Review of literature on mechanics of joints and muscles. Z. Orthop. Chir., *51*:320–337, 1929.
3. Morris, C. B.: The measurement of the strength of muscle relative to the cross section. Res. Quart. Am. Assn. Health, Phys. Ed. & Recrn., *19*:295–303, 1948.
4. Steindler, A.: Kinesiology of the Human Body. Springfield, Ill., Charles C Thomas, Publisher, 1955. Lecture V.

RECOMMENDED READING

Williams, M., and Lissner, H. R.: Biomechanics of Human Motion. Philadelphia, W. B. Saunders Company, 1962, Chaps. 5 & 6.

CHAPTER 7

Moving One's Own Body

We walk down the street, we run to catch a bus, we swim, dance, jump and do gymnastic exercises. These are but a few of the many ways in which we move our own bodies. Perhaps we nod to an acquaintance, wave to a friend, rub our hand over our head, shake a foot that has gone to sleep—these are common examples of moving parts of our bodies. There is no movement we perform, no matter how small or inconsequential, that is not governed by specific principles. The basic mechanical principles are derived chiefly from Newton's three laws of motion and from the principles of leverage. These laws apply to all human motion, but the specific behavior of the body in its obedience to these principles may vary according to the environment in which it is moving and to the nature of its support. Before considering these laws, however, it may be well to review briefly the basic principles which apply in all circumstances.

GENERAL PRINCIPLES OF MOVING ONE'S OWN BODY

Principle I (Based on the Law of Inertia). A body will not move until a force is applied to it, a force of sufficient magnitude to overcome the resistance. There must be a constant or regularly repeated application of such force to overcome opposing forces such as the force of gravity, friction, air resistance and water resistance. Whenever possible, momentum should be used in movements that involve continuous motion in order to avoid the necessity of repeatedly overcoming inertia.

Applications

a. In walking, the inertia of the body has to be overcome at each step because of the opposing forces of gravity, air resistance and the restraining push of the forward foot as it makes contact with the ground.

b. In swimming and boating, the chief opposing force is that of water resistance. Strokes must be repeated regularly if movement is to continue. Of the three, the human body, the rowboat and the canoe, the canoe meets the least resistance from the water because it displaces the least water and is the most streamlined in shape. Hence it will glide the farthest before its motion is stopped.

c. When coasting on a sled, once the level ground is reached, the sled soon comes to a standstill because of the opposing force of friction.

d. In activities that require a pull-up followed by a push-up, as in the pole vault and the breast-up on a horizontal bar, there should be no pause between the pull and the push, in order to avoid the necessity of overcoming the body's inertia a second time.

Principle II (Based on the Law of Inertia). Force is needed to change the direction of a moving body.

Application. In walking and running, exaggerated up-and-down movements mean that additional force is being used unnecessarily. The same is true of exaggerated up-and-down movements preparatory to throwing for distance, putting the shot and so on. Elimination of unnecessary changes of direction results in more efficient movement.

Principle III (Based on the Law of Inertia). A body in motion will continue to move until it is acted upon by an external force.

Application. When running, although opposing forces are constantly acting upon the body, an additional force must be introduced in order to make the body lose its momentum in a relatively short space. This is done by inclining the body backward and extending the leg forward at the end of the swinging phase in order to increase the restraining force of the forward leg when the foot strikes the ground.

Principle IV (Based on the Law of Action and Reaction). Every action is accompanied by an equal and opposite reaction.

Applications

a. In walking, running, jumping and so on, the foot is pushed against the ground. The ground pushes back with equal and opposite force, causing the body to move forward or upward, as the case may be. For instance, in walking, running and broad jumping, the foot pushes primarily backward, and because of the counterforce of the ground, the body moves forward. In vertical jumping, the feet push directly downward, and the body moves upward.

b. In attempting to walk on smooth ice, the foot tries to push backward, but is unable to do so because of the absence of friction. Consequently the body does not move forward.

c. In walking on sand or deep snow, although much energy is expended, the feet succeed in exerting only slight backward force against the loose and shifting substance under them, and in return there is a proportionately slight reaction to send the body forward.

d. When the body is not supported by a solid surface, the "equal and opposite reaction" to the action of its parts occurs within the body itself. For instance, a person who has jumped off the high board, or who is floating in the water, will find that when he swings both legs forward from the hips, the trunk will move forward to meet them. Or, when he swings one arm at shoulder level from a sideward to a forward position, the whole body will turn on its longitudinal axis toward the moving arm.

Principle V. When the body as a whole is set in motion, either it will undergo translatory movement as in locomotion, or it will rotate. If it is in contact with the ground, it will either rotate about its own vertical axis, or will rotate about successive points of contact with the ground. In the latter instance this will result in translatory movement of the body as a whole.

Applications

a. Walking and running represent translatory movement of the body as a whole brought about by angular movements of the lower extremities. In the supporting phase of walking, the lower extremity partially rotates about its point of contact with the supporting surface, that is, the point where the foot is in contact with the ground. In a series of cartwheels it rotates about each hand and foot in succession. In a forward roll it rotates about the hands, shoulders, back, buttocks and feet (Fig. 7–1).

b. In fancy dives, such as the one-and-a-half, half or full gainer, the body rotates about its center of gravity at the same time that it is moving through space.

Four Basic Environments or Modes of Body Support

1. The body is supported by the ground or other surface which may be firm, soft or elastic.
2. The body is supported by water. *from something*
3. The body is suspended. – *hanging from something*
4. The body is unsupported, i.e., it is projected or is falling through space. *sky diving*

There may, of course, be various combinations of 1, 2 and 3.

PRINCIPLES OF MOVING ONE'S OWN BODY WHEN IT IS SUPPORTED BY THE GROUND OR SIMILAR SURFACE

Movements of the Body as a Whole. When the body as a whole is set in motion, it is participating either in locomotion by self-propulsion, or in rotation. Locomotion is a form of translatory motion produced by angular motion of the extremities. (For kinesiologic analysis of walking see Chapter 22.) In order for the body to propel itself it must be able to push against a resistant surface. In accord with the Law of Action and Reaction, its action is dependent upon the reaction of the supporting surface. The principles listed below apply specifically to walking. Applications to other forms of locomotion should be made by the student.

Principle I. Since propulsion of the body is effected by the diagonal pressure of the foot against the supporting surface, the efficiency of locomotion depends upon counterpressure and friction.

Principle II. A body at rest will remain at rest unless acted upon by a force. Since walking is produced by a pendulum-like motion of the limbs, the inertia of the body must be overcome at every step.

Principle III. A body in motion will continue in motion unless acted upon by a force. Since motion is imparted to the trunk by the backward thrust of the leg, the trunk has a tendency to continue moving forward, even beyond the base of support. A brief restraining action of the forward limb acts as a check on the momentum of the trunk.

Principle IV. Force applied diagonally consists of two components, horizontal and vertical. The vertical component in walking serves to counteract the downward pull of gravity. The horizontal component serves (1) in the restraining phase, to check forward motion, and (2) in the propulsive phase, to produce forward motion. The horizontal component of force in the propulsive phase must exceed that in the restraining phase if the end result is to be progressive forward motion.

Principle V. The speed of the gait is directly related to the magnitude of the pushing force and to the direction and frequency of its application. This force is provided by the extensor muscles of the hip, knee and ankle joints, and the direction of application is determined by the slant of the lower extremity when the force is being applied.

Principle VI. The economy of the gait is related to its timing with reference to the length of the limbs. The most economical gait is one which is so timed as to permit a pendulum-like motion of the lower extremities in the recovery phase.

Principle VII. Translatory movement of a lever is achieved by the repeated alternation of two rotatory movements, the lever turning first about one end, then about the other.[4]

Principle VIII. Walking has been described as an alternating loss and recovery of balance.[4] This being so, a new base of support must be established at every step.

Principle IX. Stability of the body is directly related to the size of the base of support. In walking, the lateral distance between the feet is a factor in balance.

(*a.*) The absence of lateral distance between the feet, such as occurs when one foot is placed directly in front of the other, increases the difficulty of maintaining balance, since it decreases the width of the base of support.

(*b.*) A wide lateral distance between the feet increases stability, but tends to cause a weaving gait and to make the body sway from side to side.

(*c.*) The optimum position of the feet appears to be one in which the inner borders fall approximately along a single straight line. This gives adequate stability and minimizes lateral motions of the body.

Rotatory Movements of the Body as a Whole. When the body is supported by a solid surface, it can rotate either about its own vertical axis, as when pirouetting on the toes or on skates, or about its successive points of contact with the supporting surface, such as the hands and feet in a cartwheel; the hands, shoulders, back, buttocks and feet, in a forward roll (Fig. 7-1). Two principles which apply specifically to rotatory movements of the body are as follows:

Principle X. Rotatory motion may be accelerated by shortening the radius, and decelerated by lengthening the radius. For instance,

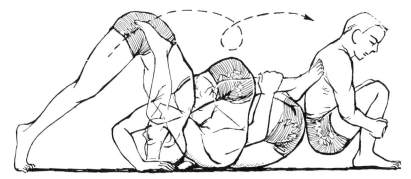

Figure 7–1. The body rotating around its points of contact with the supporting surface. (Redrawn from LaPorte and Renner: The Tumbler's Manual, by courtesy of Prentice-Hall, Inc.)

pulling the arms in close to the body while pirouetting on ice skates will increase the speed, and extending the arms horizontally will decrease it.

Principle XI. A long lever has greater velocity at the end than does a short lever, moving at the same angular velocity (Fig. 4–6). For instance, the hands and feet have greater velocity in a cartwheel than they do in a forward roll.

Movements of Segments of the Body. The following principles apply to movements of bodily segments, movements in which the body as a whole remains in approximately the same location.

Principle XII. Since a long lever has greater velocity at the end than a short lever moving at the same angular velocity, in movements of the arm, the hand has greater velocity when the elbow is kept straight, and in movements of the leg, the foot has greater velocity when the knee is kept straight.

Principle XIII. Centrifugal force is developed in circular movements of bodily segments, as in strenuous arm circling. This should be recognized as a potential source of injury to the shoulder joint, since the centrifugal force creates a dislocating tendency.

Principle XIV. The momentum of any part of a supported body can be transferred to the rest of the body. For instance, if one stands with one arm extended foward and then vigorously flings it horizontally sideward-backward, the whole body will tend to follow the arm. This transfer of momentum could not take place were it not for the reaction of the supporting surface.

PRINCIPLES OF MOVING ONE'S OWN
BODY WHEN IT IS SUPPORTED BY WATER

The problem of moving the body through the water is fundamentally not so different from that of moving it on land. As in walking, it is necessary to push against something in order to move the body

[handwritten margin notes: Blacks bones & muscles are denser so they sink as compared to white; less adipose tissue too; adipose tissue greater in men than women; Water is 4 times greater in resistance than air; Air for the runner]

from one place to another. The chief differences between locomotion in the water and locomotion on land are that (1) in the water the body is concerned with buoyancy rather than with the force of gravity; (2) the substance against which it pushes affords less resistance to the push; (3) the medium through which it moves affords more resistance to the body; and (4) as a means of getting the greatest benefit from the buoyancy and of reducing the resistance afforded by the water, it is customary to maintain a horizontal, rather than a vertical, position. (For kinesiologic analysis of the crawl stroke see Chapter 23.)

Buoyancy differs with individuals and, on the whole, is greater in women than in men. The average person has sufficient buoyancy to float close to the surface of the water. The buoyancy of a body is indicated by the amount of water it displaces. Corresponding to the center of gravity on land, immersed bodies have a center of buoyancy. This is a center of balance in the water. A human body so lacking in buoyancy that it sinks to the bottom is a rarity. The practical problem in swimming is not to keep from sinking, as beginners are inclined to think, but to get the mouth out of the water at rhythmic intervals in order to permit regular breathing. This is a matter of coordination, not buoyancy.

In swimming, as in all motion, the initial mechanical problem is to overcome the inertia of the body. Once the body is in motion, the problem is to overcome the forces which tend to hinder it. In terrestrial locomotion the body exerts its force against the supporting surface, that is the ground, in order to overcome inertia. The forces resisting the progress of the body are the force of gravity and air resistance. In aquatic locomotion the water is both the supporting medium and the source of resistance. In swimming, the hands and feet depend upon the counter pressure of the water in order that the force may be transmitted to the body. Yet, at the same time, the body must overcome the resistance afforded by the water.

Thus the major problems in the mechanics of swimming are the minimizing of resistance and the advantageous application of force. The swimmer reduces the resistance by streamlining his body position, by relaxing in the recovery phase of the stroke and by eliminating useless motions and tensions. There are many different strokes in swimming, but they all involve either a pulling or a pushing motion of the arms, and either a pincer or a thrusting action of the legs. In order to get maximum horizontal propulsion from the arm and leg movements it is necessary to eliminate upward, downward and sideward components of force as much as possible. Swimming with ease, power and efficiency requires a precise coordination of arm and leg motions, of breathing and of use of the trunk muscles in maintaining an optimum position.

The major principles which apply to swimming are as follows:

APPLICATION OF FORCE

Principle I. The body will move in the opposite direction from that in which the force is applied. For instance, a backward thrust will send the body forward; downward pressure will lift it; pressure to the right will send it to the left.

Applications

a. In the crawl stroke, too much force at the beginning of the arc will have too great a downward component, thereby tending to lift the body. This increases resistance and is a needless expenditure of energy. In the breast stroke, the two arms balance each other; hence too great an outward force at the beginning of the stroke, or inward force at the end of the stroke, does not produce lateral motion, but results in a waste of energy.

b. In many aquatic stunts and lifesaving techniques the swimmer deliberately pushes himself up or down by pushing his hands and feet against the water in the direction opposite to that in which he wishes to move. No matter how complicated the movement in a synchronized swimming technique, it is brought about by observing the principle that a body moves in the opposite direction from that in which the force is applied.

Principle II. Maximum force is attained by presenting as broad a surface as possible in the propulsive movements of the limbs and by exerting a backward pressure through as great a distance as possible, provided undesirable forces are not inadvertently introduced.

Applications

a. The full surface of the hand should be used.

b. The use of fins increases the force of the leg stroke.

c. The hand should not enter the water so soon that it shortens the stroke unduly. In the crawl stroke care must be taken not to reach too far, however, as this involves lifting the shoulder and is likely to introduce a lateral force acting on the trunk.

REDUCTION OF RESISTANCE

Principle III. A rapidly moving body in the water leaves a low pressure area immediately behind it. This creates a suction effect and tends to pull the body back.

Application. Although this backward pull cannot be entirely eliminated, it can be reduced in the crawl stroke by keeping the feet close together.

Principle IV. The sudden or quick movement of a swimmer's body, or one of its parts, at the surface of the water tends to cause whirls and eddies. These create low pressure areas which have a retarding effect on the swimmer.

Application. The low pressure areas can be reduced by slicing the hand into the water and by eliminating movements which do not contribute to forward progression. In the flutter kick, movement of the feet in the air does not contribute to the propulsion of the body; hence the feet and legs should be kept just below the surface of the water.

Principle V. The more streamlined the body, the less the resistance to progress through the water. The streamlining of the body in the crawl stroke is accomplished by four actions.

Applications

a. Carrying the head so that the water level is somewhere between the hairline and just below the eyes, depending upon the buoyancy and speed of the swimmer;

b. Carrying the body parallel with the surface of the water;

c. Carrying the buttocks just below the surface of the water;

d. Keeping the legs, ankles and feet close together.

to increase speed in water

Application to Boating and Canoeing.[*] On the whole, the principles which apply to swimming apply also to boating and canoeing. This is particularly obvious in canoeing, for the paddle is used in much the same way as are the arms in swimming. The use of the oars in rowing is more limited, since they must be kept in the oarlocks at all times. In paddling, as in the arm movement of the crawl stroke, too much force at the beginning of the stroke has too great a downward component, and hence too great a lifting effect. Conversely, too much force at the end of the stroke has too great an upward component, and hence a depressing effect on the canoe. In order to make the canoe move smoothly in a horizontal direction, without unnecessary bobbing up and down, it is essential to reduce these two components to a minimum and to emphasize the backward movement of the blade.

The techniques of steering the canoe are based on this same principle. Assuming that there is only one paddler and that he is paddling from the center of the canoe, if he wished to move the canoe broadside to his paddling side he would put his paddle in the water, blade parallel to the keel, directly opposite the center of the canoe, as far out as he could conveniently and safely reach, and then draw the blade squarely toward him at right angles to the keel of the canoe. If he wished to move broadside away from his paddling side, he would slice the blade into the water opposite the center of the canoe and close to it, with the blade parallel to the keel, and then push it directly away from him at right angles to the keel. In order to turn the canoe, he would have to reach either forward or backward and press the blade toward or away from the canoe at a point as far from the canoe's center of buoyancy as he could conveniently reach. A drawing stroke nearer the bow would make the canoe turn toward the paddling side; a drawing stroke nearer the stern would make the canoe turn away from the paddling side. (The direction taken by the canoe as a whole is stated in terms of the bow. As the stern of the canoe moves toward the paddling side, the bow moves away from it.) Steering a canoe is logical and simple when one remembers the principle that movement occurs in the direction opposite to that in which the force is applied, and, at

---

[*]Although it might seem that these activities should be classified with those of giving impetus to an external object, like bicycling they are forms of locomotion by self-propulsion. The primary purpose of boating and canoeing is locomotion of the self on the water, and the locomotion of the craft is of secondary importance. An additional reason for including the discussion of rowing and paddling in this chapter is that the principles of locomotion in the water are the same, regardless of whether the locomotion is caused by movement of the hands and feet or of oars and paddles.

the same time, remembers that a canoe tends to rotate about its center of buoyancy when force is applied at any point other than one in line with this center.

PRINCIPLES OF MOVING ONE'S OWN BODY WHEN IT IS SUSPENDED

Climbing, hanging, swinging and other suspension activities were more commonly engaged in by our early ancestors than by members of recent generations. For primitive man and his forebears they were a common form of locomotion. The modern version of these brachial activities is seen in the trapeze activities of the aerial artist at the circus and in exercises and stunts on the flying rings, traveling rings, horizontal bar, high boom, stall bars, ropes and various forms of hanging ladders in the gymnasium and on the playground (Fig. 7–2). Ladder climbing and brachial locomotion without swinging are modifications of locomotion on the ground. All swinging movements of a suspended body are governed by the principles of the pendulum and of circular motion.

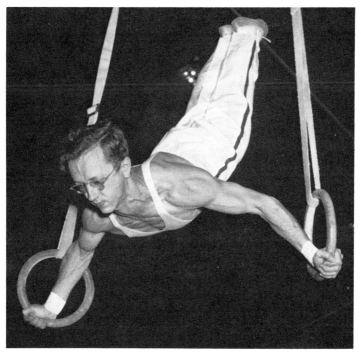

Figure 7–2. Movement of body in suspension. This illustrates need for good muscular development in arms and shoulders. (Courtesy of Springfield College.)

PRINCIPLES RELATING TO THE MOVEMENTS OF A PENDULUM

Principle I.   The movement of a pendulum is produced by the force of gravity. This presupposes a starting position in which potential energy is present. In other words, the pendulum must be moved from its resting position before the force of gravity can make it swing downward.

Principle II.   The upward movement of a pendulum is effected by the momentum developed in the downward movement.

Principle III.   The amplitude of a pendulum, i.e., the range of its swing, depends upon the height from which its movement is initiated. The amplitude may be increased by the application of external force to the pendulum, but at the moment of such application the pendulum is temporarily not being allowed to act as a pendulum.

Principle IV.   The time taken by the pendulum to make a single round trip excursion (known as its *period*) is related to the length of the pendulum. The longer the pendulum, the more slowly it swings. Specifically, the period of the pendulum is proportional to the square root of its length.

Principle V.   The period of the pendulum is not influenced by its weight. A heavy body will swing no faster than a lighter one, or vice versa. This is consistent with the behavior of freely falling bodies.

Principle VI.   As the pendulum swings downward, its speed increases; as it swings upward, its speed diminishes until the zero point is reached. Hence the pendulum's speed is greatest at the bottom of the arc, and least (zero) at each end of the arc.

Principle VII.   The swinging body moves through an arc, first in one direction, then in the reverse direction. Thus it undergoes partial rotation about a center of motion. Since this rotation takes place in a vertical plane, the influence of gravitational pull must be taken into consideration. Whereas the force of gravity *produces* the downward swing, it *opposes* the upward swing. Nevertheless it is indirectly responsible for the latter, inasmuch as the upward swing is caused by the momentum which was built up in the preceding downward swing.

Applications

a. Rotation of a body in the vertical plane can be accelerated by shortening the radius (i.e., distance between the body's center of gravity and the center of rotation) on the up-swing, and lengthening it on the down-swing. Since, in the movement of a pendulum, speed is greatest at the bottom of the arc, shortening the radius at this point accelerates its speed (i.e., its angular velocity) more than in any other position.

b. Observation of this principle provides the means for attaining greater height in swinging on the flying rings or trapeze. As the body passes under the point of support (i.e., the center of rotation) on its forward swing, the knees should be brought up in front of the body. Toward the end of the up-swing the legs should be extended as high as possible. On the entire back-swing, and on the forward down-swing, the body should be relaxed in the extended position.

Principle VIII. When a pendulum reaches the end of its arc, just before it reverses its direction, it reaches a zero point in velocity. At this precise moment the force of gravity is momentarily neutralized by the upward momentum. Also centrifugal and centripetal force neutralize each other at this moment.

Application. The performer can take advantage of this situation by using this moment to perform "trick" movements such as reversing the grasp and facing in the opposite direction, performing cut-offs on the traveling rings, and so forth.

Principle IX. Since the movement of a pendulum is circular, the characteristics of circular motion apply. The grasp of the hands must constantly combat the tendency of centrifugal force to pull the body off the apparatus. If the body does break loose, it will fly off at a tangent to the arc of its swing, and there is danger of injury.

Additional Applications of the Principles Which Pertain to the Movements of a Pendulum

1. The initial problem of the child on the swing and of the gymnast on the flying rings is that of being given potential energy. Without the help of an accomplice, he must find a way of putting himself into a position in which he will have potential energy. He does this usually in one of three ways. He may move the apparatus to some position other than its normal position of rest before he suspends himself from it (i.e., he pulls the rings or swing as far back as he can reach before getting on); his feet may be able to reach the supporting surface when he is on the apparatus, in which case he can push his feet against the floor or take little running steps; or he may use a pumping action to get started. For the man swinging on the rings, this involves bending the legs up in front of the body and then extending them as high as possible. This puts them in a position in which gravity will act on them and the downward movement of the legs builds up momentum. This momentum in turn is then transferred to the rest of the body. The range of the arc of motion may be increased by the repetition of this procedure on the forward-upward phase of the swing. The child in the swing accomplishes the same result by inclining the trunk backward and raising the feet forward. He can start the swing even more effectively if he can pull the ropes toward his body and, at the same time, press forward against the seat.

2. Initiating a pendulum swing on the traveling rings is achieved by flexing each arm alternately. Because of the wide distance between the traveling rings, this procedure moves the body a considerable distance from its resting position, and thus puts it in favorable position for the force of gravity to act on it.

3. Progression on the traveling rings is achieved by releasing the "rear" hand at the "rear" end of the arc, flinging the extended arm sideward-downward slightly in front of the body, and then forcefully upward in a continuous arc of motion. The momentum developed by the arm turns the body toward the other arm, and, as the hand reaches for its new point of suspension, the body has made a half-turn and is facing in the opposite direction. This process is repeated first with one

arm, and then with the other, and with the body turning first one way and then the other, but always as it is moving in the direction of the ultimate goal. Unless sufficient momentum is developed, the performer will have difficulty in reaching the new point of suspension with his free hand.

This activity depends for its success upon the development of adequate potential energy, or energy of position, to assure sufficient kinetic energy to enable the body to rise to the same height at which it started. When the body is suspended by one hand, the only force producing the swing is the force of gravity. Attempts to use muscular force to increase the height of the swing result in jerky, unproductive movements which interfere with the smooth, pendulum-like motion of the body. For effective hand traveling, the principle of the pendulum needs to be kept in mind, namely, that the motion of a pendulum depends upon the force of gravity.

4. The timing of such activities as the cut-off on the traveling rings, uprises on the horizontal bar, changing hands and turning the body around on the flying rings or trapeze, is governed by the fact that the force of gravity and the upward momentum of the body momentarily neutralize each other at the moment when the pendulum reaches the end of its arc, just before it reverses its direction.

5. If it is desirable to control the speed of swinging for any reason, the supporting ropes should be lengthened for a slower swing and shortened for a faster swing.

6. Centrifugal force increases the difficulty of maintaining one's grasp on the rings or trapeze. If the performer loses his grasp, his body obeys Newton's first law of motion and flies off at a tangent to its previous arc of motion. For this reason great care must be taken with beginners and children. The instructor should watch their hands for indications of slipping and should teach them to dismount on the forward swing, preferably just before the base of the arc is reached. The experienced performer, however, will find it more desirable to dismount toward the end of the forward swing, once he has learned how to receive the impact of his own body by losing his kinetic energy gradually (see p. 140).

PRINCIPLES OTHER THAN THOSE RELATING TO THE MOVEMENTS OF A PENDULUM

In hand traveling without swinging, the body is not moving like a pendulum. Locomotion by this means is similar to locomotion on the ground or in the water in that it depends upon the principle of action and reaction. As in walking, force applied against a supporting surface in one direction will cause the body to move in the opposite direction. Hand traveling without swinging on a boom or along the side of a horizontal ladder is achieved by alternately moving one hand away from the other hand, and then moving the second hand toward the first. As the first hand moves, the second hand pushes laterally against the apparatus. Both hands share the weight equally for a moment; then the second hand is released and brought toward the first hand, while at the same time the first hand is pulling laterally on the apparatus. This process is repeated.

PRINCIPLES OF MOVING ONE'S OWN BODY WHEN IT IS IN THE AIR, FREE OF SUPPORT

The unsupported body is eventually drawn to the earth by the force of gravity. Its initial movement through space, however, may be one of projection, the direction usually being horizontally forward, vertically upward, or somewhere between the two (Figs. 7–3 and 7–4). In diving and in high jumping the projection is essentially in an upward direction; in broad jumping and in dismounting from a moving vehicle, it is more nearly horizontal. There are two essential principles which apply to moving the body when it is unsupported. They are of particular importance in their application to diving and to trampoline activities.

Principle I. When the body is unsupported, momentum of the body as a whole cannot be developed. This means that its center of gravity cannot be displaced from its path of motion, this pathway having been determined by the force of gravity and the force of its projection into space (see Figs. 7–5 and 7–6). Once the body is in the air, its center of gravity will follow the same pathway as that of any inanimate object which has been projected at a similar angle by a corresponding force.

Implication. Nothing the diver can do will alter the pathway of his center of gravity, once he has left the diving board.

Principle II. The only total movement which can be initiated in the unsupported body is rotation around its center of gravity. It can be made to rotate around a vertical, frontal-horizontal or sagittal-horizontal axis, or any intermediate axis. Whereas either translatory motion or rotatory motion can be initiated in both the earth-supported and the water-supported body, in the unsupported body there can be no translatory movement other than that caused by gravity and by the initial projection.

Implications

a. The diver must have his center of gravity ahead of the board at the moment of take-off if he is to clear the board when he comes down.

b. The trampoline performer can be confident that no movements he performs in the air can cause him to come down beyond the bed of the trampoline.

DEMONSTRATIONS AND LABORATORY EXERCISES

1. Perform, or observe someone else perform, each of the following, and in each case identify the force that stops the motion of the body:

a. Slide on the ice or slippery floor.

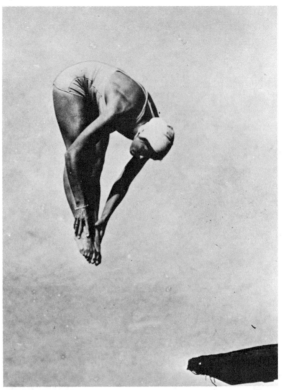

Figure 7–3. Movement of the body in the air free of support. (Anne Ross, Senior National A. A. U. Champion, 1941–1944; Senior National A. A. U. High-board Champion, 1942–1944; Member of All-American Swimming Team, 1941–1944.)

 b. Jump vertically upward.

 c. Plunge for distance in the pool.

 2. Observe someone performing a vertical jump (*a*) with and (*b*) without the help of his arms. Compare the height of the two jumps by noting the level of the top of his head. A chart consisting of numbered horizontal lines should be suspended behind the subject, and the observer should stand on a bench, squarely facing the subject and chart. This experiment should be repeated several times and with several subjects in order to minimize chance variations in the power of the leg action.

 3. *a.* Twirl on the toes (preferably on ice skates) with the arms held close to the body; then extend the arms sideward before the angular momentum is spent. Do the same sitting on a revolving stool.

 b. Repeat this experiment, starting with the arms extended sideward at shoulder level; then pull them in close to the body before the angular momentum is spent.

 What is the effect of extending the arms in *a*, and of pulling them close to the body in *b*? What principle is illustrated?

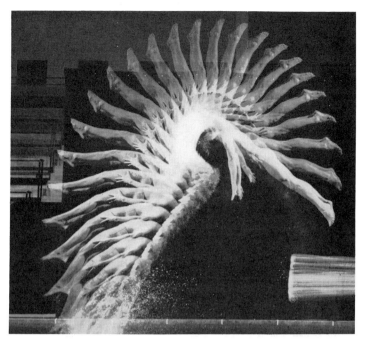

Figure 7–4. Front somersault dive in layout position. An example of rotatory movement of the body as a whole when it is unsupported. (Courtesy of H. E. Edgerton.)

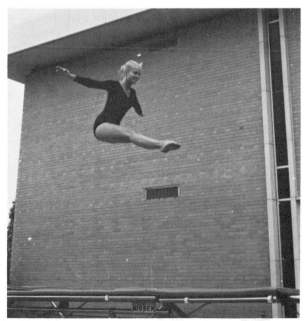

Figure 7–5. Movement of the body in the air, free of support. (Judi Ford, Miss America, 1969; Junior Women's National A. A. U. Trampoline Champion, 1968. Courtesy of Mrs. Virgil Ford.)

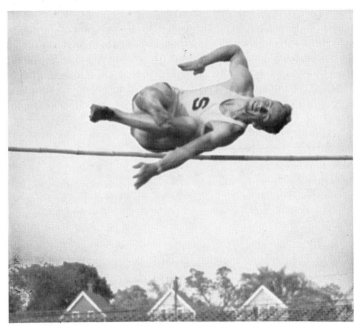

Figure 7-6. An example of flight of body through air as result of strong take-off from ground. (Courtesy of Springfield College.)

4. If you are a reasonably skillful performer, do a backward roll (*a*) starting from a squat position and (*b*) from a standing position. What is the advantage of the latter method, and what are the chief problems? What principles are illustrated?

5. Do the arm movement of the crawl stroke and deliberately press hard with the hand as soon as it enters the water, and, at the end of the stroke, instead of taking the hand out of the water at the proper time, continue the movement of the arm until the hand has pressed upward against the water. What is the effect on the body of these two errors in the crawl stroke?

6. Observe or perform the following swimming stunts and analyze them in terms of the direction in which the body is moved and the direction of the application of force:

    a. Dolphin
    b. Side sculling
    c. Foot foremost surface dive
    d. Little man in a tub

7. Hang from a pair of flying rings which are high enough to enable you to clear the floor with your feet. Hang motionless for a moment, and then start swinging without help from anyone else. How did you initiate the swinging movement?

8. Swing on the flying rings. At the end of the forward swing, at the moment when the momentum of the swing and the force of

gravity neutralize each other, reverse the grasp of one hand. The ability to do this easily is an indication that you have timed the movement correctly.

9. Swing on the flying rings or trapeze without attempting to get much height. Practice dismounting from various positions and notice the effect on the body. As a safety precaution be sure that there are no pieces of furniture or apparatus in your way, and have plenty of mats on the floor.

10. Observe or perform a somersault dive in (*a*) the tuck position; (*b*) the pike position; and (*c*) the full layout position. What is the difference in the speed of rotation and the number of turns possible in a given space? What principle is illustrated?

11. Study diagrams or sequence photographs of several different dives and note the position of the pelvis at the instant of take-off in each of these. This provides the basis for a rough estimate of the position of the center of gravity. What do you estimate to be the position of the center of gravity relative to the end of the board?

12. In the same illustrations note the direction of the application of force just prior to the take-off. Is it vertically downward? If not, how does it deviate from the vertically downward direction?

13. Lie on the side in the water and swing both legs forward vigorously, keeping both knees straight. Does the trunk move? If so, how? What principle is illustrated? (Except for the factor of resistance, this movement simulates that of an unsupported body.)

14. Perform the following movements at the height of a jump from a trampoline and note whether there is any movement of the trunk:

a. With the legs together turn both feet to the left.

b. Start with both arms extended sideward at shoulder level and then swing the right arm horizontally forward.

REFERENCES

1. Bunn, J. W.: Scientific Principles of Coaching. Englewood Cliffs, N. J., Prentice-Hall, Inc., 1959.
2. Dyson, G. H. G.: The Mechanics of Athletics, 3rd. ed. London, University of London Press Ltd., 1964.
3. McCloy, C. H.: Mimeographed material and class notes for course in Mechanical Analysis of Motor Skills, State University of Iowa.
4. Steindler, A.: Kinesiology of the Human Body. Springfield, Ill., Charles C Thomas, Publisher, 1955.

CHAPTER 8

Giving Impetus to External Objects

Impetus, in the words of Webster's dictionary, is "the property possessed by a moving body in virtue of its mass and its motions . . . applied commonly to bodies moving suddenly or violently." Thus both the human body itself and the objects it handles may possess impetus. If two men of unequal weight are running at equal speed, the heavier man has greater impetus than the lighter. Conversely, if two men of the same weight are running at different speeds, the faster runner has the greater impetus. These are examples of impetus associated with horizontal motion, particularly that of self-propulsion. Horizontal motion is experienced also by a man riding on a horse, train or other vehicle, even though his body appears to be motionless. The motion of the vehicle is imparted to him, as is seen if he falls off the horse or jumps from the moving train. Added to the impetus of the horizontally moving vehicle is the impetus of the downward motion resulting from the fall or jump. No wonder, then, that broken bones are likely to result from falls off horses and jumps from moving trains.

A man pushes a lawnmower across his lawn, an archer shoots an arrow from his bow, a baseball pitcher throws a baseball across the plate and the batter hits it into center field, a camper paddles his canoe upstream, a school teacher opens the window, a housewife shuts the sliding door of her closet, a porter lifts a suitcase and puts it up onto the rack. As widely diverse as these activities may seem, they have a common denominator. Each involves the giving of impetus to an external object, whether this is done directly by some part of the body, as the hand or the foot, or through the medium of an implement such as a baseball bat. Together with activities of receiving the impetus of external objects, they comprise the group of activities referred to as manipulative skills. With possibly a few exceptions, the activities in this group may be classified into the following three major categories:

1. Activities characterized by the continuous application of force, e.g., pushing, pulling and lifting. (See Fig. 8–3, A, B, C.)

1, 2, +3 - ways man gives impetus to an object.

2. Activities characterized by the development of kinetic energy in a movable object, followed by the release of the object at the moment of maximum velocity. All throwing activities are included in this category, including throwing with an implement as in lacrosse. (See Figs. 8-1, *A* and 8-3, *D.*)

3. Activities characterized by a momentary contact made with an object by a moving part of the body, or by an implement held by or attached to a moving segment of the body. The object itself may be either stationary or moving. This category includes all forms of striking, such as hitting with the hand (as in handball), striking with a club or racket (as in baseball, golf and tennis), kicking and heading (as in soccer). (See Figs. 8-1, *B*, 8-2, and 8-3, *E.*)

The two activities which do not seem to belong specifically to any of the categories described, but which combine the characteristics of two or three of them, are archery and the use of a sling shot. In these activities the body indirectly applies force to a movable object through the use of an elastic structure with which the object is in contact. Potential energy is imparted to the elastic structure by means of a pull. When the elastic structure is suddenly released the potential energy becomes kinetic energy and this is immediately transferred to the movable object.

man provides secondary impetus

In the chapter on force it was seen that a force could be described in terms of its magnitude, its direction and the location of the point

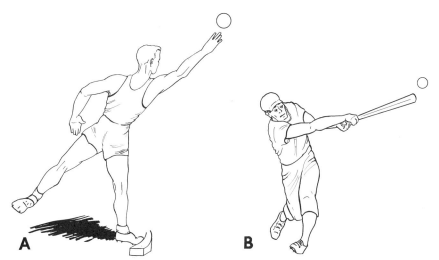

Figure 8-1. Giving impetus to an external object. *A,* Putting the shot; *B,* batting a baseball.

at which the force was applied. These three aspects of force form the basis of most of the principles of giving impetus to external objects. Supplementing these are the factors which relate to the stability of the body at the moment of giving impetus and those which relate to the interaction between the body and the surface which supports it. Unless the body has good stability when it is giving impetus to an object, much of the force is wasted. *(Dynamic stability)*

One should remember that all projected objects, such as balls and arrows, are being acted upon by the force of gravity as well as by the force imparted by the person responsible for projecting them. If one wished to calculate the resultant force acting upon the object, he could do so by the method of constructing a parallelogram of forces, one side of which would represent the force of the impetus and the other side the force of gravity (see p. 104).

The value of a classification such as the one for skills of giving impetus to external objects is that it enables one to see the relationships between activities. This is particularly helpful in the learning of new skills because the principles learned in connection with one skill can be applied to all skills in the same category. One need only recognize the factors common to both the old skill and the new in order to select the principles which apply to the latter. The factors and the principles which pertain to the giving of impetus to external objects are presented below. Anatomic and mechanical principles pertaining to specific forms of these skills are included in some instances.

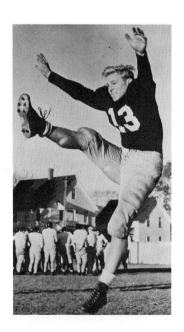

Figure 8–2. An example of giving impetus to an external object. (Courtesy of Springfield College.)

PRINCIPLES OF GIVING IMPETUS TO AN EXTERNAL OBJECT

RELATING TO THE MAGNITUDE OF THE FORCE

Principle I.   The object will move only if the force is of sufficient magnitude to overcome the object's inertia. The force must be great enough to overcome not only the mass of the object, but all restraining forces as well. These include (1) friction between the object and the supporting surface, (2) resistance of the surrounding medium (e.g., wind or water) and (3) the effect of leverage. By the latter is meant the product of the object's weight (or the resistance force) and the weight arm (or resistance arm) of the lever. Other things being equal, the shorter the weight arm of a lever, the less force required to move it.

RELATING TO THE DIRECTION OF FORCE

Principle II.   The direction in which the object moves is determined by the direction of the force applied to it. If the force consists of two or more components, the object will move in the direction of the resultant of those components (see p. 94).

Principle III.   If an object is free to move only along a predetermined pathway (as in the case of a window or sliding door), any component of force not in the direction of this pathway is wasted and serves to increase friction.

RELATING TO THE POINT AT WHICH THE FORCE IS APPLIED

Principle IV.   Force applied in line with an object's center of gravity will result in linear motion of the object, provided the latter is freely movable.

Principle V.   If the force applied to a freely movable object is not in line with the latter's center of gravity, it will result in rotatory motion of the object.

Principle VI.   If the free motion of an object is interfered with by friction or by the presence of an obstacle, rotatory motion may result, even though the force is applied in line with the center of gravity.

RELATING TO THE INTERACTION BETWEEN THE BODY AND THE SUPPORTING SURFACE

Principle VII.   Force exerted by the body will be transferred to an external object in proportion to the effectiveness of the counterforce of the feet (or other parts of the body) against the ground (or other supporting surface). This effectiveness depends upon the

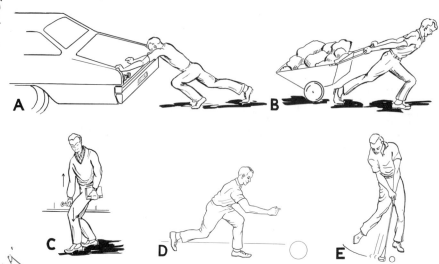

Figure 8–3. Different methods of giving impetus to an external object. *A*, Pushing; *B*, pulling; *C*, lifting; *D*, throwing; *E*, striking.

counterpressure and the friction presented by the supporting surface.

Applications to Pushing, Pulling and Lifting. The chief concern in these activities is economy of effort and avoidance of strain. Economy of effort is assured when the force is applied in line with the object's center of gravity and in the desired direction of motion. If friction tends to impede the movement of the object, this must be taken into consideration also. For instance, suppose one is confronted with the task of pushing a tall cabinet across the room. If the cabinet has casters and if the floor is uncarpeted, the most efficient way to push the cabinet is by placing the hands at the midpoint (assuming the weight of the cabinet to be equally distributed between the top and the bottom) and applying a horizontal push against it. If the floor is carpeted, however, or if the cabinet has no casters, there will be a tendency for the cabinet to tip when the push is applied in line with its center of gravity. In order to assure linear motion, the hands must be placed lower down at a point found by experimentation.

If one's purpose is to cause rotatory rather than linear motion, the effectiveness of the force depends upon the distance of the point of its application from the object's center of motion. In the case of the steering wheel of an automobile or the helm of a ship, the center of motion would be the center of the wheel, and the ideal point for applying force would be at the rim of the wheel or the outer end of a spoke. In the case of a wardrobe trunk which is tipped onto one edge and is being moved by a series of partial pivots on alternating corners, the center of motion is the point of contact with the floor; that is, it is first one corner, then the other. The force is applied at the corresponding upper edge of the trunk, the ideal point for maximum efficiency being the corner diagonally opposite the one serving as the point of contact.

The influence of the resistance arm of the lever is demonstrated when one attempts to open a classroom window by facing it squarely, grasping the handles and lifting it chiefly by means of elbow flexion. At the moment the forearms are in a horizontal position, the magnitude of the resistance may be expressed as the product of the window's weight and the length of each forearm, or half the window's weight and the length of one forearm, provided the arms are sharing the task equally. This, of course, disregards both the restraining factor of friction between the window and its runway and the helpful factor of a mechanism involving counterbalancing window weights. In this method of opening a window the resisting window exerts a rotatory force against the forearm levers. This is especially apparent when the forearms are horizontal. When the forearms are in a position other than horizontal, the magnitude of the resistance may be expressed as the product of the window's weight and the perpendicular distance from the fulcrum (elbow joint) to a vertical line erected through the point of contact between the hand and the window (times two, because both arms are used). (See discussion of true resistance arm of lever on page 96.) If the resisting force of friction is to be considered, this should be added to the weight of the window.

A more efficient way of opening the window, which minimizes or completely eliminates rotatory force against the forearm, is as follows: stand close with the side to the window and the knees bent, the near arm bent close to the body, forearm in a vertical position and heel of hand pushing upward against one of the cross pieces; then extend the knees. This method makes use of the strong hip and knee extensor muscles for applying the force; the arm muscles are used only for stabilizing the arm in the correct position.

The principle of minimizing the resistance or weight arm in order to reduce the amount of force required is also seen in lifting a weight from the floor. For instance, it takes less force to lift and hold a heavy package close to the body than it does to lift and hold it at arm's length. Likewise it takes less force to lift a package by stooping than it does by bending at the waist with the knees straight. In stooping, the weight arm is the horizontal distance from the center of the knee joint to the body's line of gravity; in bending from the waist the weight arm is the horizontal distance from the center of the hip joint to the body's line of gravity. There are other factors involved here, too, but the relative length of the weight arm is an important one. Also, because of the shorter weight arm, it takes less force to lift by stooping with the trunk inclined slightly forward than with the trunk held vertically. Although it is true that more force is required to lift the weight of the body itself from a full stoop than from a bend at the waist, the latter method endangers the joints and muscles of the lower back. These matters are discussed more fully in Chapter 24.

An example of applying the force at an angle to the direction of motion is seen in drawing a low cart by a rope. If the body is erect, the rope will slant upward from the cart to the hand. The pull on the cart therefore consists of two components, forward and upward. Since the purpose is to draw the cart horizontally forward, this upward component of force is wasted. While stooping in order to keep the rope horizontal would assure a single horizontal force, this can hardly be recommended because of the inconvenience and discomfort of maintaining such an unnatural position. A better solution is to use a longer rope. Although this does not eliminate the upward component of force, it serves to make it relatively smaller and the horizontal component relatively greater.

The importance of a solid supporting surface and of the presence of friction between the feet and the supporting surface is readily seen in all the pushing, pulling and lifting activities. One need only imagine attempting a tug-of-war on a muddy field or pushing a car on an icy road to appreciate this.

Applications to Throwing. The efficiency of imparting force to a ball is judged in terms of the speed, distance and direction of the ball after its release. The purpose of the throw determines which of these is given the greater emphasis. Both the speed and the distance of the thrown ball are directly related to the magnitude of the force used in throwing it and to the speed of the hand at the moment of the release. The speed the hand can acquire depends upon the distance through which it moves in the preparatory part of the act (Fig. 8–4, A and B). Hence the longer the preparatory backswing, and the

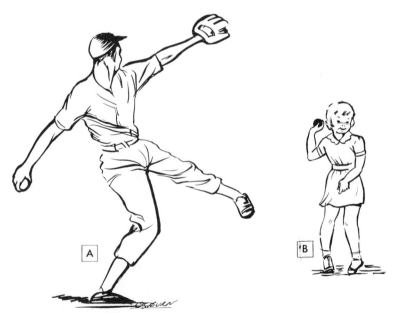

Figure 8–4. Contrasting styles of throwing. *A,* With a long lever and a long backswing. *B,* With a short lever and a short backswing.

greater the distance that can be added by means of rotating the body, shifting the weight, and perhaps even taking a step, the greater the opportunity for accelerating. These preparatory movements, in order to be effective, must be coordinated. Each one must be added to the preceding movement at just the right moment in order for them to contribute to maximum speed.

Greater speed and distance can be attained if internal resistance is reduced. This is accomplished partly by a warm-up immediately preceding the throwing event, and partly by a gradual increase of the range of motion in the joints involved, achieved by preliminary training.

The distance the ball will travel depends upon the angle of elevation as well as the magnitude of the force applied to it. When pushing an object, the force is more effective if applied in a horizontal direction. In throwing a ball for distance, however, the effect of gravity must be considered. As soon as the ball is released, gravitational force starts to operate on it. The effect of this becomes noticeable as soon as the speed of the ball is materially reduced (because of air resistance). Hence greater distance can be obtained if the propulsive force contains an upward as well as a horizontal component. This serves to keep the ball in the air longer and permits longer horizontal travel before the ball hits the ground. Too much elevation is not desired, however, because the upward and the horizontal components of force are in inverse proportion to one another. The optimum angle of elevation for distance throwing is approximately 45 degrees.

It might seem that for maximum distance all the force should be applied in line with the ball's center of gravity. This is not the case, however. If a slight rotatory force is imparted in such a way that a back spin (Fig. 8–5, *B*) results, the ball will travel farther, provided the rotatory force is not sufficient to cut the propulsive force materially. The explanation is that the lower part of the ball meets more air

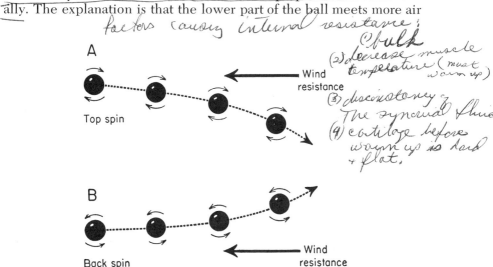

Figure 8–5. The effect of spin on a thrown or struck ball. *A*, Top spin; *B*, back spin.

resistance than the upper when it is spinning backward. This tends to push the ball up and keep it in the air longer. Conversely, top spin (Fig. 8–5, A) decreases the distance the ball travels. When back spin is used, the ball may be released at an angle slightly less than 45 degrees from the horizontal.

While not directly related to the imparting of force, there are three qualities of the ball itself which influence the distance it will travel when thrown. These are the mass and size of the ball and the nature of its surface. A heavy ball will travel farther than a light one of the same size and thrown at the same speed because it is less affected by air resistance. Likewise, a small ball or a smooth-surfaced ball will travel farther than a large or rough-surfaced one because it meets with less air resistance.

The direction taken by a thrown ball depends primarily upon the direction of the force applied to it. If a lateral rotatory force is applied, some lateral spin will result. A clockwise spin (as seen from above) makes the ball go somewhat to the thrower's right; a counterclockwise spin makes it go to his left. Wind also influences the direction of the ball. It imposes an additional force; hence the direction of the ball will be the resultant of the propulsive force and the force imparted by the wind.

Applications to Striking, Hitting, Kicking and the Like. As in the case of throwing, the effectiveness of striking, hitting and kicking is judged in terms of the speed, distance and direction of the struck ball. All the factors that apply to these aspects of a thrown ball apply similarly to a struck ball. There appear to be six major factors which apply to the speed of a struck ball. These are (1) the speed of the oncoming ball, (2) the mass of the ball, (3) the speed of the striking implement at the moment of contact, (4) the mass of the striking implement, (5) the coefficient of restitution (i.e., the elasticity) of the ball and (6) the coefficient of restitution of the striking implement. At least two of these factors, namely, the speed of the approaching ball and the speed of the striking implement, may be further analyzed into secondary factors. For instance, the speed of the striking implement is determined by the magnitude of the force exerted; and the magnitude of the force is dependent upon the distance of the preparatory backswing and upon the speed of muscular contraction. The distance of the preparatory backswing is further dependent upon the range of motion in the joints and upon the timing of the swing. Furthermore, the effectiveness of the force exerted by the body is completely dependent upon a strong grip and a firm wrist for transmission of the force from the body to the striking implement.

PRINCIPLES RELATING TO THE SPEED, DISTANCE AND DIRECTION OF A STRUCK BALL

Principle I. The greater the velocity of the approaching ball, the greater the velocity of the ball in the opposite direction after it is struck, other things being equal. If at first this seems contradictory to the reader, he should think of a ball being thrown against a resisting surface such as a wall. The reader will agree that the faster the ball is traveling when it hits the wall, the faster it will travel on the rebound from the wall. Now, if in addition to the element of rebound, the wall itself moves forward to meet the ball, it is providing an additional force. This is in effect what happens when a pitched ball makes contact with a forward-swinging bat.

Principle II. The greater the velocity of the striking implement at the moment of contact, the greater the velocity of the struck ball, other things being equal. Obviously, a full-powered swing will send the ball farther and faster than will a bunt. Increasing the length of the lever will increase the velocity of the striking implement, and this in turn increases the force of impact (Fig. 8–6).

Principle III. The greater the mass of the ball, *up to a point,* the greater its velocity after being struck, other things being equal. A hard baseball will travel farther and faster than a soft ball. Nevertheless an iron ball would offer too much resistance for the average batter using an average bat.

Principle IV. The greater the mass of the striking implement, *up to a point,* the greater the striking force, and hence the greater the speed of the struck ball, other things being equal. A good baseball player usually selects a heavy bat. Too heavy a bat, however, is in-

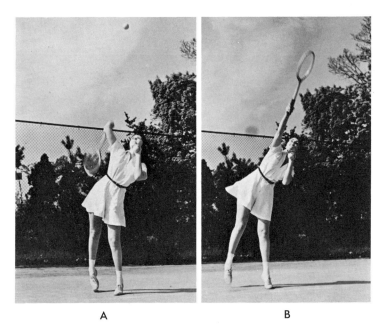

A   B

Figure 8–6. Tennis serve. The entire body acts as a lever to impart maximum force to the ball. (Photo by Loder.)

advisable because of the difficulty of swinging it with sufficient speed and control.

Principle V. The higher the coefficient of restitution (i.e., the elasticity) of the ball and of the striking implement, the greater the speed of the struck ball, other things being equal.

Principle VI. Other things being equal, the greater the ball's speed of departure, the greater the distance of its flight (or roll). As in the case of a thrown ball, the optimum angle of elevation is approximately 45 degrees. This angle is slightly less when back spin is imparted to the ball, and greater when top spin is imparted.

Principle VII. The more skillful the striker, the more successful he will be in sending the ball where he wants it to go. The four factors that influence the direction taken by a struck ball are as follows: (1) the direction of the striking implement at the moment of contact;

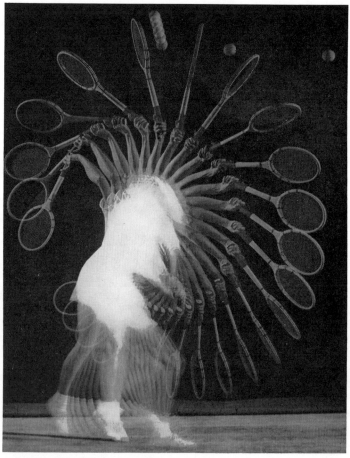

Figure 8–7. Tennis serve. An example of giving impetus to a ball. (Courtesy of H. E. Edgerton.)

(2) the relation of the striking force to the ball's center of gravity (an off-center application of force causes spin, and spin affects direction); (3) degree of firmness of grip and wrist at moment of impact; and (4) the laws governing rebound. According to the last, the angle of rebound equals the angle of incidence, except in the case of a soft ball (that is, a ball which compresses greatly when hit), in which case the angle of rebound is slightly less than the angle of incidence. An understanding of the angle of rebound is of particular importance in the racket games. It forms the basis of one of the essential skills of such games — the accurate placing of the ball (Fig. 8–7).

DEMONSTRATIONS AND LABORATORY EXERCISES

1. Raise a window from the bottom:
   a. Standing at arm's length.
   b. Standing close, facing the window and using both hands.
   c. Standing close, side to the window and pushing it up with one hand with the elbow bent and the forearm in a vertical position.

   Which is the best method for a heavy window or a window that sticks? Explain in terms of components of force and the direction of application of force.

2. Open (or close) a sliding door:
   a. Standing at arm's length.
   b. Standing close, facing the door.
   c. Standing close, facing in the direction that the door is to move, using a pushing motion with the forearm parallel with the door.

   Which is the best method? Explain in terms of direction of application of force, and of components of force.

3. Push a heavy piece of furniture. Experiment to find the most efficient method.
   a. At what point on the object did you apply the force? Explain the underlying principles.
   b. What was the position of your arms? Explain the advantage.
   c. What was the position of your body? Explain the advantage.

4. Throw a tennis ball or baseball for distance:
   a. Standing still, facing in the direction of the throw.
   b. Standing with the left side toward the direction of the throw, with the feet apart and the weight evenly distributed, getting a full arm swing and body twist with the throw.
   c. Same as in b, except with the weight on the right foot to begin with, shifting to the left as the ball is thrown.

   Compare the three methods for distance. Explain in terms of length of backswing, speed at moment of release, and total distance used in applying force to ball before releasing it.

5. If possible, observe a small child or an untrained girl, and then a trained boy or girl, throw a small ball at a target 20 or 30 feet away.

Analyze the motions of each with reference to the pathway of the hand immediately preceding, at the moment of, and following the release. Explain the factors differentiating the good throws from the poor.

6. Observe slow motion films of throwing, striking and other forms of giving impetus. Look for the application of the principles stated in this unit, or for the lack of such application.

RECOMMENDED READINGS

Broer, M. R.: Efficiency of Human Movement, 2nd ed. Philadelphia, W. B. Saunders Company, 1966, Chaps. 16, 17, 18, 19.

Dyson, G.: The Mechanics of Athletics, 3rd ed. London, University of London Press, Ltd., 1964.

CHAPTER 9

Receiving Impetus

Impetus from vertical motion is experienced by anyone who falls through space. Such motion, which occurs subsequent to a downward jump, a dive or an accidental fall, has a rapidly increasing velocity due to the effect of gravitational force. Falling bodies are known to increase their velocity at the rate of 32 feet per second, each second. When the body lands on a supporting surface, its impetus is said to have been received. Likewise, the impetus of a horizontally moving body is received when its motion is stopped as the result of contact with a resisting surface, such as a wall or other obstacle.

Examples of receiving the impetus of external objects are commonly seen in sports. Baseballs are caught or fielded with the hands; hockey balls and pucks are received with a stick; soccer balls are trapped with the feet; and blows from an opponent's fists are received by various parts of the body. Examples of receiving the impetus of external objects are also seen in industry and in daily life. Cartons and tools are tossed from one man to another; red hot rivets are tossed and caught with tongs; victims from a fire are caught in nets.

Problems and Principles. What are the particular problems involved in these diverse forms of receiving impetus, and what are the principles which enable us to solve these problems satisfactorily? Considering first the reception of the body's own impetus, the chief problems would seem to be those of avoiding injury and of regaining equilibrium promptly. It is the abrupt loss of motion resulting from collision with an unyielding surface that is likely to cause an injury. To use more technical terms, and hence more exact ones, all moving bodies have what is known as kinetic energy—the energy of motion. Like impetus, and like momentum, kinetic energy is related both to the mass of the body and to its velocity. (Momentum = mv; kinetic energy = $\frac{1}{2}$ mv^2.) In order to avoid injury from too abrupt a loss of kinetic energy it is necessary to find some means of losing it more gradually. This is achieved only by increasing the distance over which the kinetic energy is lost. The various devices we use for absorbing the shock of impact serve this purpose.

Another factor in injury which should not be overlooked is the relation of the force of impact to the size of the area which bears the brunt of the impact. A force of 100 pounds concentrated on 1 square inch of body surface, for instance, is likely to cause more serious injury than is the same amount of force spread over an area of 36 square inches. The problem here is clearly to increase the size of the area which receives the force of impact. This is especially important when there is limited opportunity for increasing the distance over which the kinetic energy is lost.

The problem of regaining equilibrium is largely a problem in controlling the placement of the limbs in preparation for landing, for equilibrium is regained when an adequate base of support is established. This requires sufficient control to place the feet, or perhaps both the hands and the feet, in a position which will provide a favorable base. The problem of regaining equilibrium is closely related to that of avoiding injury, since establishing an adequate base is dependent upon the integrity of the bones and joints which receive the force of impact.

Various methods of falling are taught in classes in tumbling and modern dance. Perhaps one of the most effective measures for the prevention of injury in accidental falls is this kind of instruction, followed by the practice of a variety of falls until the techniques have been mastered. This helps to establish the right patterns, patterns which will be followed automatically when accidental falls occur.

The problems involved in receiving the impetus of external objects appear to be threefold: namely, avoiding injury, maintaining equilibrium and receiving the object with accuracy and control. As in the case of receiving the impetus of one's own body, avoidance of injury in catching or receiving external forces is achieved by increasing the distance over which the object's kinetic energy is lost. When catching a swift baseball, the experienced player will not hold his hands rigidly in front of him, but will "give" with the ball. By moving his hands toward his body through a distance of 10 to 20 inches as he receives the ball, he is making it possible for the ball's kinetic energy to be lost gradually. This same principle is likewise true for the player who is reaching for a high ball with one hand. The extended arm acts as a lever, the force being applied by the impact of the ball on the palm. The "moment of force" is therefore the product of the force of impact and the perpendicular distance from the shoulder joint to the ball's line of flight at the instant it is caught. If this line of flight is perpendicular to the outstretched arm, the "moment of force" is the product of the force of impact and the length of the arm. Catching a fast ball with the arm extended can put a tremendous strain on the shoulder joint, as well as endanger the bones of the hands. To avoid injury the player should "give" by reaching somewhat forward for the ball and drawing his arm back at the moment of impact, also by rotating his body and by stepping back if the force is sufficiently great.

[handwritten margin note: If doesn't know how to run & fall is screwing — of overstriding]

If he lets the elbow flex slightly, he will shorten the lever of his arm and thus reduce the "moment of force."

Another factor in avoiding injury when catching swift balls is the position of the hands. Beginners often reach with outstretched arms and point their fingers toward the approaching ball. This leads to many a "baseball finger." The fingers should be pointed either down or up, according to whether the ball is below or above waist level. Balls approaching at approximately waist level can be caught above the waist if the player bends his knees.

The second problem in receiving the impetus of external objects, that of maintaining equilibrium, is often neglected. The player should prepare for it in advance, for a swift ball or a sudden blow can easily catch him "off balance" and cause him to lose his equilibrium. There is little advantage to catching a swift ball successfully if, in the process of catching it, the player falls over backward. The stance is of great importance here. The base needs to be widened in the direction of the ball's flight, thus making it possible for the catcher to shift his weight from the forward to the rear foot at the moment of impact. This not only increases his chances of maintaining his equilibrium, but also contributes to the gradual reduction of the ball's motion. Widening the stance in a direction at right angles to the flight of the approaching ball does little to increase the catcher's stability.

The third problem, that is, receiving the ball or other object with accuracy and control, is perhaps the one given the most emphasis in a game situation. As in the attempt to avoid injury, one of the key factors is the gradual loss of the object's kinetic energy. This reduces the danger of the ball's bouncing off the hands. Accurate vision, judgment and positioning of the body are of vital importance. "Keeping the eye on the ball" is essential to judging its speed and direction, and hence to adjusting the position of the body. Thus accurate judgment depends upon accurate vision, and accurate adjustment of the body depends upon both of these, as well as upon agility and smoothness of neuromuscular response. Together, these factors make up what is known as "hand-eye and foot-eye coordination." To a certain extent this is innate, but it is also developed and improved by practice.

In receiving both the impetus of one's body and that of external objects, an important factor to be considered is the subsequent movement one expects to make. It may be the determining factor in deciding on the stance to assume. For instance, if a run is anticipated, a forward-backward stance will be more favorable than a lateral one. Furthermore, it will be desirable to have the weight over the forward foot. If a catch is to be followed immediately by a throw, the movements used for "giving" may be blended into the preparatory movements of the throw. These are fine points which have much to do with the degree of one's skill in an activity.

A summary of the principles to observe in receiving impetus, both that of one's own body and that of external objects, is presented below, together with some representative applications of these principles.

PRINCIPLES OF RECEIVING IMPETUS

PRINCIPLES RELATED TO AVOIDING INJURY

Principle I. The more gradually the kinetic energy of a moving body is lost, the less likely is the loss to cause injury.

Applications to receiving the impetus of one's own body

a. For landing from jumps wear rubber-soled shoes and use landing pit or gymnasium mat.

b. When landing from a fall, attempt to land on the more heavily padded parts of the body.

c. When landing from a jump, attempt to land on the balls of the feet, and immediately let the ankles, knees and hips flex, controlling the action by means of eccentric contraction of the extensor muscles of these joints (see Fig. 9–1).

d. When horizontal motion is terminated by a fall or jump, as in the case of falling off a horse, tripping and falling when running, jumping off a moving vehicle and so on, attempt to diminish the horizontal motion gradually by rolling, somersaulting, taking a few running steps or doing a series of "frog jumps."

e. When landing from a jump, if the suggestions in *c* are not adequate, attempt to transfer the downward motion of the body to horizontal motion by rolling or somersaulting.

f. When landing from a fall following horizontal motion, if the suggestions in *d* are not feasible, attempt to take some of the weight on the hands, letting the arms "give" at the wrists, elbows and shoulders. When falling forward in an extended position, attempt to arch the back as the hands take the weight, turn the face to the side, and rock down on the front of the body. This method is especially applicable to tripping and falling when running. It takes a high degree of skill, however.

Applications to receiving the impetus of external objects

a. Wear a thickly padded glove when catching fast balls. This

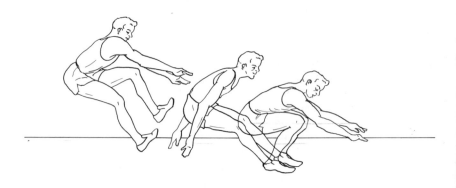

Figure 9–1. Effecting a gradual loss of kinetic energy by bending the knees upon landing from a jump.

reduces the shock of impact by effecting a slightly more gradual reduction of the ball's velocity. The greater the mass of the ball, the thicker the padding needed.

b. When catching a ball with both hands, "give" with the arms by pulling them in toward the body at the moment of impact, and, if necessary, shift the weight backward and take a backward step or two.

c. When catching a high ball with one hand, allow the arm to move horizontally backward and rotate the body in the same direction. By bending at the elbow the likelihood of straining the shoulder will be reduced. By placing oneself in a favorable position in the first place, the need for overreaching will be prevented.

d. The method of reducing kinetic energy gradually when catching a ball may be adapted in such a way that it will serve as the preparatory movement for throwing. In catching a basketball, for instance, swinging the arms down to one side and rotating the body not only assure a gradual loss of the ball's velocity, but also serve to put the hands and ball in a favorable position for throwing. The transition from catching to throwing is thus made with one continuous motion.

e. The principle of "giving" when catching balls applies also to "spotting" and to receiving in apparatus work in the gymnasium. In receiving the weight of another person the "giving" is effected by a lowering and bending of the arms and bending of the knees, or by taking several steps, according to whether the motion is chiefly vertical or horizontal.

Principle II. The larger the area of the body which receives the force of impact, the less will be the force per unit of surface area.

Applications to the act of landing from a fall

a. When falling forward, rocking onto the front of the body serves to increase the area which receives the force of impact, as well as to effect a gradual loss of kinetic energy.

b. When one seems to be in danger of falling on the elbow, a slight twist may make it possible to roll onto the upper arm and shoulder and thus increase the area receiving the force of impact.

c. When one seems to be in danger of falling on one knee, it may be possible to twist onto the side of the leg and rock onto the side of the thigh, perhaps using one arm to help absorb the shock.

PRINCIPLES RELATED TO MAINTAINING AND REGAINING EQUILIBRIUM

Principle III. Other things being equal, the larger the base of support and the better centered the center of gravity above this base, the greater will be the body's equilibrium.

Applications to receiving the impetus of one's own body

a. In any jump or fall the body's equilibrium is temporarily lost. In order to gain prompt control of the body upon landing, a favorable base of support can be established by adjusting the position of the feet *before landing* in such a way that they will provide a base of adequate width when the landing is made.*

b. In connection with the above, the position assumed by the feet should be such that it will facilitate the equal distribution of body weight over them.

c. External aids to making a controlled landing include a smooth landing surface and appropriate footwear. These help to prevent turned ankles and stubbed toes which might spoil an otherwise good landing.

d. When one lands with so much force that it is difficult to estab- lish an adequate base of support with the feet alone, one or both hands should be used to establish a temporary base large enough to assure a quick recovery of equilibrium.

e. In order to provide an adequate base of support for the re- covery of balance following forceful horizontal movements, the larger dimension of the base should be parallel with the direction of the horizontal movement. This will necessitate a forward-backward stance if one is facing in the direction of the horizontal motion. It will necessitate a sideward stance if one lands facing sideward with reference to the direction of motion. This adjustment of stance is particularly applicable to vaulting and tumbling activities. When one trips while running, the body automatically uses this method in its attempt to prevent a fall.

Applications to receiving the impetus of external objects and forces

a. In preparation for catching a swift ball, especially a heavy one such as a medicine ball, assuming a moderately wide stance with the feet separated in the direction of the approaching ball will enable the catcher to keep his balance. It also enables him to increase the dis- tance for stopping the ball's velocity.

b. When standing in a moving train or bus, balance is maintained more readily as the vehicle accelerates and decelerates if one takes a moderately wide stance parallel with the long axis of the vehicle, in other words, with the direction of movement.

c. If the body is subjected to pushes, pulls or blows, it can main- tain and regain balance more readily if the feet are separated in a stance which is parallel with the direction of the force.

PRINCIPLES RELATED TO ACCURACY AND CONTROL IN RECEIVING EXTERNAL OBJECTS

Principle IV. The more gradually the velocity of an external ob- ject is reduced, the less likely is the object to rebound when its impetus is received.

---

*The practice of teaching landing with the feet together when vaulting over gym- nastic apparatus is not in keeping with this principle. This method of landing is not to be condemned for that reason, but it should be recognized as a test of skill. The skillful gymnast can regain his balance in spite of a narrow base of support. Beginners should be permitted to land with their feet separated.

All the methods suggested for avoiding injury when receiving the impetus of external objects also apply to preventing rebound.

Principle V. "Keep the eye on the ball." Whether the object whose impetus is about to be received is a ball, a carton or a fist, keeping the eyes on it will enable one to judge its speed and direction and to respond accordingly. The tendency of some novices to shut the eyes should be corrected at the outset.

Principle VI. Catching an external object with accuracy and control is dependent largely upon the position of the catcher relative to the direction of the approaching object. Putting oneself in the most favorable position possible is an essential objective for accurate catching. This is basic to the prevention of injury and to the maintenance of equilibrium.

DEMONSTRATIONS AND LABORATORY EXERCISES

1. Jump from a low bench to the floor, landing on both feet.

a. Landing with minimum "give," that is, with as little flexion at the ankles, knees and hips as possible.

b. Landing with maximum "give," that is, allowing the ankles, knees and hips to flex to a full squat position. The head should be kept erect.

c. Landing as in *b*, but looking down at the feet.

Which method is preferable? Why?

2. Trip on the edge of a mat and fall forward, landing first on the knees, then on the hands.

a. Keeping the arms rigid, elbows straight.

b. Letting the elbows flex, arching the back, rocking down onto the abdomen and chest, with the head turned sideways.

3. Jump down from a table or gymnasium box, using the parachute landing technique, that is, landing on the toes with the feet together, bending the knees slightly and turning sideward, rolling onto the side of the leg, thigh and hip, then onto the back of the shoulder, keeping the arms close in front of the chest and the head flexed forward.

4. Catch a medicine ball thrown straight toward your chest.

a. With your arms rigidly outstretched.

b. With your hands held close in front of your chest.

c. With your arms outstretched at first, but brought in toward your chest at the moment of impact.

Which method is preferable? Why?

5. Receive a hard drive in field hockey, (*a*) with, and (*b*) without, "giving" with the stick. Compare the results both as to control of the ball and sensation in the hands.

PART TWO

Anatomic and Physiologic Fundamentals of Human Motion

INTRODUCTION TO PART TWO

Parts II opens with a chapter on basic anatomic concepts. Following this is a chapter on neuromuscular structure and function, an area in which great advances have been made in recent years. This is followed by eight chapters on functional regions of the musculoskeletal structure, each chapter presenting information concerning the joints and muscles, especially as it relates to movement.

Much of the information about joints and muscles in the early textbooks of anatomy and kinesiology was based on dissection, and on inspection and palpation of living subjects. The range of motion for each joint has been measured by many investigators and clinicians who use various kinds of protractors and other instruments such as the double armed goniometer and Leighton's Flexometer (Figs. 2-4 and 2-5). In the last century, Duchenne made an important contribution to our knowledge of muscular function by his electrical stimulation of the muscles of living subjects and his careful observation and recording of the resulting movements. In the present century, especially in the third quarter of it, electronic devices have provided more exact methods of investigating the movements of living persons, not merely isolated movements of single segments, but movement patterns occurring in normal activities. Electromyography is a technique which permits investigation of several muscles at a time and can be used for analyzing the muscular actions in skills such as a tennis serve or a golf drive, as well as to analyze dance techniques, walking, stair climbing and movements used commonly in industry and housework. It gives precise information about the timing and intensity of the muscular involvement and provides objective records for future reference and comparison. Such research has been invaluable to students of kinesiology. In this textbook, for instance, in each edition since the first, revisions of muscle actions, brought to light by electromyographic research, have been incorporated.

Somewhat more recently the electrogoniometer has been introduced as a device for making continuous recordings of joint action (Figs. 2-6 and 2-7). Its use makes it possible to determine with great accuracy the precise joint movement occurring during the course of a motor act. Other advances in the study of joint functions include both still and motion photography and radiography which are being used with increasing frequency.

As valuable as these devices are, the best method for studying muscular actions in the undergraduate kinesiology course is undoubtedly that of palpation and inspection in conjunction with book study. Experience proves palpation to be an effective teaching technique and for that reason it is the basis for the laboratory exercises in this section.

The aim of Part II is to prepare the student for analyzing movements. Hence this section should not be looked upon simply as a review of anatomy, but as the very foundation for the analysis of human movement. The student's emphasis in his study should therefore be on the nature of the joints and the movements performed by the muscles, rather than on muscular attachments. Nevertheless, the attachments are important because they indicate the line of pull in relation to the joints they act upon and this is basic to understanding the reason for the movements they cause.

It is not necessary to complete the entire anatomic section before beginning to analyze movements. In fact, attempting to analyze basic movements as soon as possible serves as a stimulus to the study of anatomy. As an example, let us consider flexing the elbow joint or, more specifically, flexing the forearm on (or against) the stabilized upper arm, starting from the anatomic position. Note that we have already defined the starting position and the movement. We could be even more specific and state whether the movement was executed quickly or slowly and whether it was performed against a resistance, as though lifting a weight.

The next step would be to consider the joint itself. The structure of the elbow joint should be reviewed. Since it was stipulated that the movement was made from the anatomic position, it would be advisable to review the radioulnar articulations also, especially the proximal joint because of its close relationship to the elbow joint. It would be helpful to refer to Chapter 2 or Appendix C to check on the types and characteristics of these joints.

The muscles performing the movement should be considered next and an attempt made to answer such questions as the following: What muscles flex the elbow joint? How are they affected by the starting position and the position of the forearm throughout the movement? Try to discover whether there is a clear cut difference in the importance of the participating muscles in this particular movement, but do not overstress this point. Include all of the muscles that unquestionably contribute to flexion in this position without being overly concerned as to whether they are "principal movers" or "assistant movers." Review the section on the coordination of the muscular system (page 58) and try to identify muscles serving in the capacity of stabilizers and of neutralizers.

Following the above procedure throughout the study of Part II will pave the way for later analysis of more complex movements. Procedural steps for analyzing fitness exercises, sport skills, and other physical activities, are presented in Appendix F. For the present, however, it is suggested that the student make simple joint and muscle analyses until he is thoroughly familiar with this process.

REFERENCES

1. Karpovich, P. V., Herden, E. L., Jr., and Asa, M. M.: Electrogoniometric study of joints. U.S. Armed Forces Med. J., *11*:424–450, 1960.
2. Leighton, J. R.: An instrument and technic for the measurement of range of joint motion. Arch. Phys. Med., *36*:571–578, 1955.

RECOMMENDED READINGS

Jokl, E.: G. B. Duchenne's Physiology of Motion. J. Health, Phys. Ed. and Recrn., *38*:67–70, 1967.
Waterland, J. C., and Shambes, G. M.: Electromyography: one link in the experimental chain of kinesiological research. J. Am. Phys. Ther. Assn., *49*:1351–1356, 1969.

CHAPTER 10

Basic Anatomic Concepts

This chapter contains four categories of anatomic information which are basic to the study of kinesiology. These are: (1) a classification of the types of bones in the skeleton; (2) definitions and descriptions of bony contours, projections and depressions; (3) definitions of terms used for positional, directional and surface orientation; and (4) the terminology used in this text for muscle attachments.

Classification of Bones

1. Long Bones. Characterized by a cylindrical shaft and two extremities, usually broader than the shaft. The bones belonging to this group are the bones of the upper arm, forearm, fingers, thigh, leg, toes and the clavicle. (See Figs. 6–16 and 6–17.)

2. Short Bones. Relatively small, chunky, solid bones. They include the bones of the wrist (carpals), of the ankle (tarsals), and the patella. (See Fig. 14–1.)

3. Flat Bones. Broad, flat bones which provide either protection or broad surfaces for muscular attachment. They include the bones of the skull, the scapulae, sternum, ribs and pelvis. (See Figs. 19–2, 12–1 and 15–16.)

4. Irregular Bones. Bones which do not come under any of the above three categories. They include the bones of the spine and some of the facial bones. (See Fig. 19–3.)

Bony Contours, Projections and Depressions

Bones have knobs, ridges and hollows which are frequently used as points of reference by anatomists and kinesiologists. An accurate conception of these is essential for learning muscular and ligamentous attachments.

PROJECTIONS AND EMINENCES

Condyle: A rounded projection or enlargement at the end of a long bone, usually involved in articulation with another bone.

Examples: Lateral condyle at distal end of femur (Fig. 16–2) and lateral condyle at proximal end of tibia with which the former articulates to form the lateral portion of the knee joint; medial condyle at distal end of humerus.

Crest, Ridge or Line: A rough, relatively narrow edge or elevation. Examples: Crest of the ilium (Fig. 15–1); intertrochanteric line on anterior surface of femur between greater and lesser trochanters.

Head: An enlargement at the end of a long bone forming part of the joint. Examples: Head of femur (femoral portion of hip joint); head of radius (radial portion of elbow joint) (Fig. 13–1).

Process: A generic term for any projection. Examples: Transverse process of vertebra; spinous process of vertebra; acromion and coracoid processes of scapula (Fig. 12–2).

Spine: A sharp, slender, usually pointed projection. Examples: Anterior superior and inferior spines of ilium (Fig. 15–16); posterior superior and inferior spines of ilium. (*Note:* The spine of the scapula is an exception to the definition. It is more truly a ridge.)

Styloid process: A long, pointed process, similar to a spine. Examples: Styloid processes at distal end of ulna and radius (Fig. 13–1); styloid process of fibula (proximal end).

Trochanter: Specific term for two protuberances situated below neck of femur (greater and lesser trochanter). (See Fig. 15–1.)

Tubercle: A small tuberosity. (The two terms are sometimes used interchangeably.) Examples: Tubercle of femur, a prominence at the junction of the greater trochanter with the neck; adductor tubercle at summit of medial condyle of femur. (See distal attachment of adductor magnus, Fig. 15–15.)

Tuberosity or protuberance: A broad, usually rounded projection, partially roughened. Examples: Greater tuberosity of humerus on lateral surface of superior (proximal) end; tuberosity of the ischium, the roughened, rounded eminence on the posterior portion of the inferior ramus (arm) of the ischium (lower pelvic bone), popularly known as the "sitting bone"; external protuberance of occipital bone. (See lowest part of pelvis, Figs. 15–4 and 15–18.)

DEPRESSIONS

Fossa: Usually a shallow hollow or concave surface. Examples: Glenoid fossa or cavity, the portion of the scapula that articulates with the head of the humerus to form the shoulder joint; supraspinatus fossa, on the posterior surface of the scapula above the spine of the scapula; infraspinatus fossa, on the posterior surface of the scapula below the spine of the scapula (Fig. 12–17); subscapular fossa, the entire anterior surface of the scapula.

Groove: A furrow. Example: Bicipital (intertubercular) groove, at upper end of humerus, running vertically between greater and lesser tubercles and providing passage for tendon of long head of biceps muscle. (See Fig. 12–3.)

Notch: Name is self-descriptive. Examples: Scapular notch, a small notch on superior aspect of scapula between coracoid process and superior border of glenoid cavity (Fig. 12–3); greater sciatic notch, a large notch on posterior aspect of hip bone between posterior inferior spine and spine of ischium.

FORAMEN

A hole, opening or perforation. Example: Obturator foramen, a large hole in lower portion of hip bone, surrounded by arms (rami) of ischium and pubis and by acetabulum. (See Fig. 15–1.)

Positional, Directional and Surface Orientation

A variety of terms is used in anatomy and kinesiology to indicate the location of musculoskeletal structures and the directions in which body segments move. Familiarity with these will aid the student in his understanding both of this text and of the supplementary literature that he reads.

Anterior: Front aspect of the head, trunk or extremities (i.e., the aspect of the extremities that would be facing forward if the anatomic position were assumed).

Caudad: Toward the feet. (Literally, toward the tail.)

Cephalad: Toward the head; the opposite of caudad.

Distal: Away or farther from the point of attachment, or from the midline of the trunk. Used mostly in connection with the extremities.

Dorsal: Rear or posterior aspect of the head, trunk or extremities, when the anatomic position is assumed.

Inferior: Below or lower than.

Inner: Closer to the sagittal (median) plane of the body. Used commonly both for surfaces of bones and for rotatory movements of body segments.

Inward: Toward the sagittal (median) plane of the body.

Lateral: Side of the body or of an extremity; in a sideward direction away from the sagittal (median) plane of the body.

Lower: When referring to position, same as inferior; when referring to direction, same as caudad.

Medial: Toward or nearer to the sagittal (median) plane of the body. See also "inner" and "inward." The opposite of lateral.

Outer: Farther from the sagittal (median) plane of the body; commonly used both for surfaces of bones and for rotatory movements of body segments; the opposite of inner.

Palmar: Refers to the palm of the hand.

Plantar: Refers to the sole of the foot.

Posterior: Rear aspect of the head, trunk or extremities (i.e., the aspect that would be to the rear if the anatomic position were assumed); the opposite of anterior.

Proximal: Closer to the point of attachment, or to the midline of the trunk; the opposite of distal.

Sideward: Same as lateral or lateralward.

Superior: Above or higher than; the opposite of inferior.

Upper: Same as superior; the opposite of lower when the latter refers to position.

Ventral: Same as anterior; the opposite of dorsal.

Volar: Refers to the flexor surface of the arm and the palmar surface of the hand.

Terminology for Muscle Attachments

For the reasons given on page 36, the following terminology for muscular attachments is used in preference to the terms, "origin" and "insertion."

Attachments of Muscles of the Head, Neck and Trunk

Upper attachment ⎫
                 ⎬ for muscles whose line of pull is more
Lower attachment ⎭   or less vertical

Medial attachment ⎫
                  ⎬ for muscles whose line of pull is
Lateral attachment ⎭   more or less horizontal

Attachments of Muscles of the Extremities
    Proximal attachment
    Distal attachment

Attachments of the Diaphragm
    Peripheral attachment
    Central attachment

Lest these terms confuse students who have become accustomed to "origin" and "insertion" from their study of anatomy, the initials "O" and "I" are inserted parenthetically following the new terms.

CHAPTER 11

The Neuromuscular Basis of Human Movement

The mechanical aspects of muscular action were discussed in Chapter 3; the emphasis in this chapter is on the neurological aspects and on the unique provisions for coordinated movement. In his chapter on neuromuscular integration in the book *Science and Medicine of Exercise and Sports*, Loofbourrow presents this topic so succinctly and vividly that his introductory paragraph is quoted here in full as an introduction to the present chapter.

The forces which move the supporting framework of the body are unleashed within skeletal muscles on receipt of signals by way of their motor nerves. In the absence of such signals, the muscles normally are relaxed. Movement is almost always the result of the combined action of a group of muscles which pull in somewhat different directions, so the control of movement involves a distribution of signals within the central nervous system (CNS) to appropriate motor nerves with precise timing and in appropriate number. In order for movements to be useful in making adjustments to external situations, it is necessary for the central nervous system to be appraised of these situations, which are continually changing. A means of providing this information promptly exists in a variety of receptors sensitive to changes in temperature, light, pressure, etc. These receptors are signal generators which dispatch signals (nerve impulses) to the CNS over afferent nerve fibers. The CNS receives these signals together with identical ones from within the muscles, joints, tendons, and other body structures and is led thereby to generate and distribute in fantastically orderly array myriads of signals to various muscles. This, despite the enormous complexity of the machinery involved, enables the individual to do one main thing at a time. This is integration. It is what Sir Charles Sherrington meant by "the integrative action of the nervous system."[12]

The following discussion does not presume to be an exhaustive treatise on neuromuscular mechanisms. It attempts rather to present as simply as possible those mechanisms which are pertinent to the study of kinesiology. Because of the newer techniques made possible by electronic devices during the past ten to twenty-five years, great strides have been made in acquiring more accurate information concerning the intricacies of muscular function.

SKELETAL MUSCLE: NATURE OF TISSUE AND
CHARACTERISTICS OF ITS BEHAVIOR

The muscles which are responsible for the movement and positioning of the bony segments of the body are known as skeletal muscles. They are constructed of bundles of striated muscle fibers which differ in both structure and function from the highly specialized cardiac muscle and from the smooth muscle of blood vessels, digestive organs, urogenital organs and so forth.

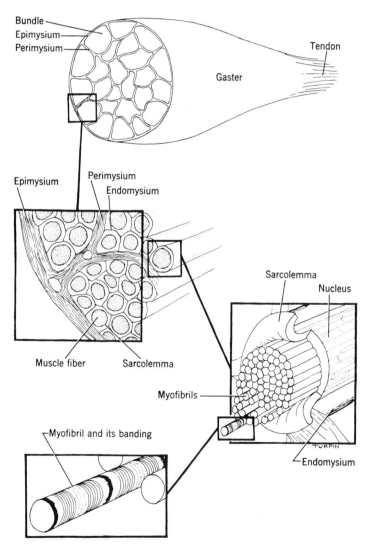

Figure 11–1. The architecture of a skeletal muscle and its fibers. (From Torrey, T. W.: Morphogenesis of the Vertebrates. New York, John Wiley & Sons, 1962.)

A single muscle cell is a threadlike fiber about one to three inches in length. Microscopic examination reveals that the fiber consists of many myofibrils embedded in sarcoplasm and that it is held together by a delicate membrane known as sarcolemma. Each fiber is enclosed within a thin connective tissue sheath called *endomysium.* The microscopic myofibrils, which are arranged in parallel formation within the fiber, are made up of alternating dark and light bands which give the muscle fibers their striated appearance. The electron microscope has revealed the striations to be a repeating pattern of bands and lines due to an interdigitating arrangement of two sets of filaments. It is postulated that these are filaments of the contractile proteins, mainly actin and myosin, and that when stimulated they slide past each other.[10] This is a condensed and highly simplified explanation of contraction, a function which is the unique property of muscle tissue.

The muscle fibers are bound into bundles within bundles (Fig. 11-1). Each individual bundle of muscle fibers is enclosed in a fibrous tissue sheath called *perimysium;* the group of bundles that constitutes a complete muscle is in turn encased within a tougher connective tissue sheath called *epimysium.* In long muscles whose fibers run parallel to the long axis of the muscle, the bundles form "chains" which function as though the individual fibers ran the entire length of the muscle.[11]

On the basis of their muscle hemoglobin (myoglobin) content the fibers of striated muscles are classified as red or white. The two types are roughly comparable to the dark and white meat of chicken. Red muscle fibers, which contain a rich supply of hemoglobin, tend to be more plentiful in the muscles which are responsible for long-continued contractions such as those engaged in by the antigravity muscles, also in muscles like the diaphragm which participate in regularly repeated contractions. White muscle fibers, on the other hand, tend to predominate in the flexor muscles, the muscles which in general are responsible for relatively brief, but often extremely forceful, contractions. In man, however, the distinction between red and white fibers is not nearly so clear-cut as these statements might lead one to think.

THE NERVOUS SYSTEM AND
BASIC NERVE STRUCTURES

It is assumed that the kinesiology student is already familiar with the general plan of the nervous system, hence it will not be described in full here. Only a brief outline of the major divisions is presented below, the purpose being to give the reader an orientation framework for the topics which have been selected for discussion.

   I. Central Nervous System
     A. Brain
     B. Spinal cord
  II. Peripheral Nervous System
     A. Cranial nerves (12 pairs)
     B. Spinal nerves (31 pairs)
 III. Autonomic Nervous System

This is not a distinct system based on structure and geographic location, as are the central and peripheral systems, but rather a functional division which overlaps with those in specific areas. It includes those portions of the brain, spinal cord and peripheral nervous system that supply cardiac muscle, smooth muscle and gland cells.

Neurons. A neuron, which is the structural unit of the nervous system, is a single nerve cell consisting of a cell body and one or more projections. There are two kinds of neurons whose long fibers constitute the peripheral nervous system. These are sensory or afferent, and motor or efferent (Fig. 11–2). In addition to these there are numerous connector (internuncial) neurons within the central nervous system.

The cell bodies of the majority of efferent or motor neurons are situated within the anterior horns of the spinal cord. (There are also some in the brain stem and sympathetic ganglia.) Many short threadlike extensions of the cell body, known as dendrites, make contact, i.e., synapse, with the axons of other cells, the latter being either sensory or connector neurons.

Each motor and connector neuron has a specialized process termed an axon. The axon of the motor neuron emerges from the spinal

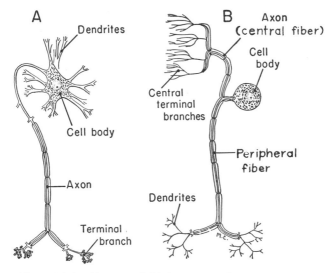

Figure 11–2. Neurons. *A,* Motor neuron; *B,* sensory neuron.

cord in a ventral root. It then travels by way of a peripheral nerve to the muscle that it helps to innervate. There it divides and subdivides into smaller and smaller branches, the most distal being known as the terminal branches. Each terminal branch ends within a single muscle fiber in the structure called the motor end-plate.

The cell body of a spinal afferent or sensory neuron, unlike that of a motor neuron, is situated in a dorsal root ganglion just outside of the spinal cord. (The cell bodies of cranial sensory neurons are in cranial nerve ganglia.) The neuron has a single short process that projects from the cell body and then bifurcates into two branches which go in opposite directions. One, the so-called central fiber, travels in the dorsal root of the nerve to the posterior horn of the spinal cord where it divides into numerous branches. It may terminate in the cord or it may ascend in the cord to the brain and terminate there. The other branch of the afferent neuron is the long peripheral fiber which comes from a receptor. It travels in a nerve trunk to the vicinity of the appropriate dorsal root ganglion where it unites with the cell body via the short stemlike process mentioned above (Fig. 11–2, B).

Authorities differ in their choice of nomenclature for the parts of a sensory neuron. Some apply the term "axon" to the short stemlike process; others apply this term to the central fiber, i.e., the branch that enters the spinal cord. This text adopts the latter use of the term as it is in keeping with a commonly accepted definition, namely that an axon is the fiber over which impulses are conducted *away from* the cell body, as opposed to dendrites which convey impulses *toward* the cell body. When referring to a sensory neuron, the term dendrite is applied not to the long fiber which conveys impulses from peripheral regions to the cell body, but rather to its branches. The long sensory fiber itself is known simply as the peripheral fiber. Some authorities, however, do not designate any part of the sensory neuron as a dendrite, but say merely that the peripheral fiber and its branches *function like dendrites.*

It was noted above that the dendrites of efferent (motor) neurons make contact within the spinal cord either with the terminal branches of afferent (sensory) neurons or with connector neurons. Connector neurons, also known as internuncial neurons, are a third type of nerve cell. They exist completely within the central nervous system and serve as connecting links. They may vary from a single small neuron, connecting a sensory neuron with a motor neuron, to an intricate system of neurons whereby a sensory impulse may be relayed to many motor cell bodies. We know from common experience that a complex motor act may result from a single sensory impulse. For instance, a sudden loud noise may cause us to jump, turn around and tense nearly every muscle in our body. The connector neurons are responsible for this widespread response to the single sensory impulse. Thus there may be only one connector neuron participating in a movement, or there may be an intricate network making possible an almost limitless number of connections with other neurons.

Nerves. Just as an electric cable is an insulated bundle of wires

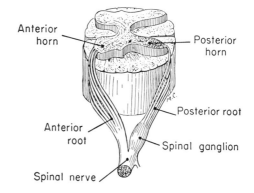

Anterior
horn

Posterior
horn

Figure 11–3. Section of the spinal cord showing the anterior and posterior roots of a spinal nerve.

Posterior root

Anterior
root

Spinal ganglion

Spinal nerve

for the transmission of electric currents, so a nerve is a bundle of fibers, enclosed within a connective tissue sheath, for the transmission of impulses from one part of the body to another. A nerve, or nerve trunk as it is frequently called, may consist entirely of outgoing fibers from the central nervous system to the muscles and other tissues; or it may consist only of incoming fibers from the sensory organs to the central nervous system. The typical spinal nerve, however, is mixed, that is, it contains both outgoing and incoming fibers. Each spinal nerve is attached to the spinal cord by a ventral (motor) root and a dorsal (sensory) root (Fig. 11–3). The dorsal root bears a ganglion and it is just beyond the ganglion that the two roots unite to form the spinal nerve. Once outside the vertebral canal, each spinal nerve divides into an anterior and a posterior branch, each of which contains both motor and sensory fibers. The anterior branches supply the trunk and limbs, the posterior branches the back.

THE MOTOR UNIT

To recapitulate, the structural units of the nervous and motor systems are, respectively, the neuron and the muscle fiber. Functionally, the two systems combine to form the neuromuscular system. The functional unit of the neuromuscular system is the *motor unit* and it consists of a single motor neuron (Fig. 11–2, A) together with all of the muscle fibers that its axon supplies.

Motor units vary widely in the number of muscle fibers supplied by one motor neuron. In some motor units there may be as many as 1000 or more muscle fibers; in others there may be fewer than 100. The number of motor units in a muscle depends in part upon the total number of fibers in the muscle and in part upon the number of fibers in a single motor unit.[6] A muscle which has a large number of motor units in relation to the total number of fibers, that is, a small ratio of muscle fibers to motor neurons, is capable of more precise movements than is the muscle with a small number of motor units for the same number of muscle fibers. Hence the ratio of muscle fibers to motor neurons has a direct bearing on the precision of the movements executed by the muscle. For example, the small muscles of the thumb and index finger are capable of effecting movements of great precision because their motor units have such a low ratio of muscle fibers to motor neurons, or to state it differently, such a large number of motor neurons per muscle. By way of contrast, the gluteus maximus has a relatively small number of motor neurons for its size, hence a large number of muscle fibers per neuron. It does not need to be pointed out that the movements for which the gluteus maximus is responsible can scarcely be described as precise.

RECEPTORS

The sensory nerve terminals whose function is to pick up and transmit sensory stimuli are called receptors. There are several ways of classifying these depending upon the particular aspect in which one is interested. For example, one classification is based on the type of energy required to produce the stimulus. This classification would include such categories as mechanoreceptors, chemoreceptors, thermoreceptors and so forth. Another basis of classification is location. On this basis the receptors may be divided into two major categories, exteroceptors and interoceptors, according to whether the stimuli they receive come from the external environment or from within the body. The former division includes the eyes, ears, tongue, nose and skin; in other words, the receptors of the familiar five senses: sight, hearing, taste, smell and cutaneous sensations (touch, heat, cold, pain and pressure) (Fig. 11–4). The interoceptors may be subdivided into visceroceptors (receptors which receive and transmit impulses from the viscera) and proprioceptors (receptors which receive and transmit impulses from the muscles, tendons and joints) (Fig. 11–5). It is the latter group in which students of movement are particularly interested because these are the receptors that transmit information concerning the positions and movements of the body. They include the labyrinthine receptors, the muscle spindles, the Golgi tendon organs and the Ruffini endings (Fig. 11–6). The pacinian corpuscles, receptors of deep pressure impulses, are also classed by some as proprioceptors, but by others as cutaneous exteroceptors.

Labyrinths. The labyrinths of the inner ear consist of the cochlea, the three semicircular canals, and the utricle and saccule. The cochlea is concerned with hearing, but the rest of the labyrinth is concerned with the sense of balance or equilibrium. Each of the canals contains a membranous tube, and the bony spaces for the maccule and saccule contain membranous sacs correspondingly named. The entire membranous labyrinth is filled with fluid. Certain parts are specialized in that the membrane consists of hair cells which are sensitive to the movement of the fluid as the head moves and which are intimately related to branches of the eighth cranial nerve. Thus,

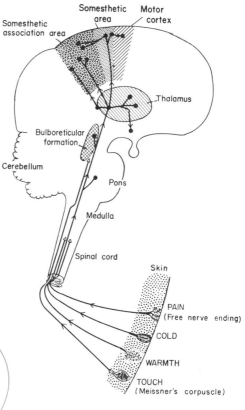

Figure 11–4. Transmission of exteroceptive sensations to the brain, showing the sensory receptors and the nerve pathways into the brain. (From Guyton, A. C.: Function of the Human Body, 2nd ed. Philadelphia, W. B. Saunders Company, 1964.)

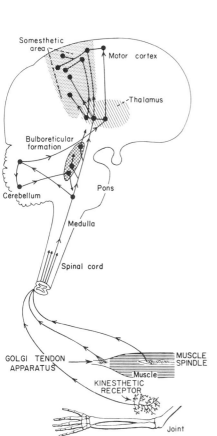

Figure 11–5. Transmission of proprioceptive sensations to the brain, showing the sensory receptors and the nerve pathways for transmitting these sensations into the brain. (From Guyton.)

movement of the head is translated into nerve impulses reaching the brain. The hair cells in the maccule and saccule have, in addition, an overlying gelatinous substance in which otoliths (small carbonate of lime crystals) are embedded. The otoliths accentuate the effects of gravity on the hair cells. The maccule and saccule are thus sensitive to position as well as to movement of the head. The anatomic arrangement of the entire labyrinth is such that some part of it is especially sensitive to any position or direction of movement of the head.*

Muscle Spindles. Muscle spindles are found in most muscles, and are of interest to kinesiologists because of their significance in the production of accurate, well-coordinated movements (Figs. 11–6 and 11–7). A muscle spindle is a tiny capsule (about 1 mm. in length) situated in the fleshy part of the muscle near its junction with the tendon. It lies between the muscle fibers and is parallel with them. It contains one or more special muscle fibers which, because of their location within the capsule, are known as intrafusal fibers. These fibers are unique in that their midsections are not striated and are therefore noncontractile. Each spindle is supplied with one afferent neuron which has a characteristic ending known as the primary or annulospiral ending. This ending is divided into as many branches as there are intrafusal fibers and each little branch is coiled around the noncontractile midsection of the intrafusal fiber. The annulospiral (AS) ending is sensitive to changes in fiber length and by virtue of this sensitivity is credited with being responsible for the stretch reflex.[3, 12]

In addition to the AS ending, most of the muscle spindles also have from one to five sensory endings which, because of their appearance, are given the picturesque name of flower-spray (FS) endings. Each FS ending has its own sensory fiber.[3] The flower-spray endings (also called secondary endings) are found at either end of the noncontractile midsections of the intrafusal fibers. They are believed to register static muscular length, but their precise function is yet to be determined.[3, 12] One theory is that they inhibit further contraction of a muscle if the spindle is being overstretched.[11]

Muscle spindles are also supplied with their own small efferent fibers. To differentiate these from the motor neurons of the "regular" muscle fibers (i.e., not the special intrafusal fibers) these are termed *gamma fibers* in contrast to the "regular" motor neurons whose axons are termed *alpha fibers* (Fig. 11–6). As a group, the gamma fibers form a *gamma fiber system.* Impulses conveyed by gamma fibers (also called gamma efferents) cause the intrafusal muscle fibers to contract. This shortening of the spindle muscle fibers stretches their central noncontractile region where the AS endings are situated and this stimulates them, causing their rate of firing to increase. Hence the effect of the gamma system is to increase the sensitivity of the spindle afferents. As Loofbourrow has noted, the AS endings can be caused to

---

*The author is indebted to Dr. Ernest Gardner for this discussion of the labyrinths.

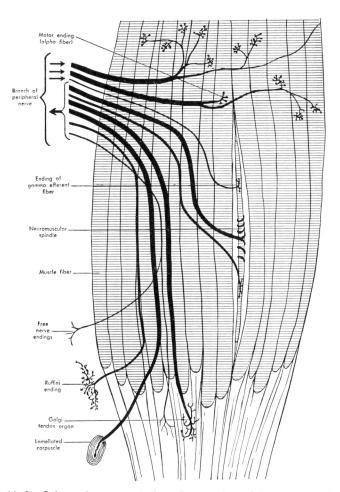

Motor ending
(alpha fiber)

Branch of
peripheral
nerve

Ending of
gamma efferent
fiber

Neuromuscular
spindle

Muscle fiber

Free
nerve
endings

Ruffini
ending

Golgi
tendon organ

Lamellated
corpuscle

Figure 11-6. Schematic representation of a muscle and its nerve supply. Arrows indicate direction of conduction. Each muscle fiber has a motor ending from a large myelinated (*alpha*) fiber. The muscle fibers within a spindle have motor endings from small myelinated (*gamma*) fibers. Muscle nerves have many sensory fibers. Some are large myelinated fibers coming from primary sensory (annulospiral) endings in spindles, from neurotendinous spindles (Golgi tendon organs), and from lamellated corpuscles (pacinian corpuscles) in the connective tissue between muscle fibers or external to the muscle as a whole. Smaller myelinated fibers arise from proprioceptive endings (such as Ruffini endings) in the connective tissue in and around muscle, or in joints. Finally there are small myelinated and nonmyelinated fibers that form free endings (presumably for pain) in the connective tissue in and around muscle. (From Gardner, E.: Fundamentals of Neurology, 4th ed. Philadelphia, W. B. Saunders Company, 1963. Modified after Denny-Brown.)

fire, not only by passive stretch of the muscle as a whole, but also, in the absence of such stretch, by the function of the gamma system.[12] In this way the gamma discharges are said to compensate for the loss of tension on the spindle caused by the muscle's contraction.[12] The practical aspect of this is that the greater the resistance to shortening, due to the magnitude of the load, the more effective the gamma system is in adjusting the length of the spindle to the length of the muscle. In this respect its function has been likened to that of a thermostat.

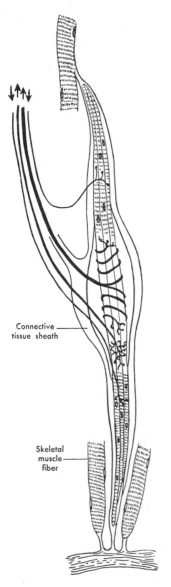

Connective tissue sheath

Skeletal muscle fiber

Figure 11–7. Schematic representation of a neuromuscular spindle. Parts of three skeletal muscle fibers are shown (cross-striated, nuclei at edge). Inside the connective tissue sheath of the spindle are three muscle fibers (thinner than regular skeletal muscle fibers, with central nuclei, and striations minimal or absent in region of sensory endings). Sensory nerve fibers form primary (annulospiral) and secondary (flower-spray) endings, the primary arising from the large fibers. (The form of primary and secondary endings varies according to species. In some, such as rabbit and man, the primary endings of the large fiber may be flower-spray in type, not winding around the muscle fiber). Small nerve fibers (*gamma* efferents) form motor endings at each end of the spindle muscle fibers. Motor discharges over *gamma* efferents cause the spindle muscle fibers to contract at each end, thus stretching the intervening, non-contractile, sensory region and activating the sensory endings. Arrows indicate direction of conduction. (From Gardner, based on Barker, D.: Quart. J. Micr. Sc., vol. 89, 1948.)

Golgi Tendon Organs. The Golgi tendon organ is another special receptor for impulses from muscles (Fig. 11–6). It consists of a mass of nerve endings which are enclosed within a connective tissue capsule and embedded in a muscle tendon. It is situated close to the junction of the tendon with the fleshy part of the muscle in such a way that it has an end-to-end relationship with the muscle fibers. These organs are stimulated by stretch, both the stretch occasioned by the passive stretch of the entire muscle and the stretching of the tendon caused by the muscle's contraction. The threshold for stretch stimulation is higher in the Golgi tendon organs than in the muscle spindles, hence the tendon organs do not respond as readily as do the spindles. They are concerned chiefly with reflex action and their particular function is inhibition. For instance, if sufficient external force is applied to a rigidly extended limb in an attempt to flex it, the extensor muscles will suddenly let go as a result of the inhibiting effect that the Golgi tendon organs have on them.

Ruffini Endings and Pacinian Corpuscles. Ruffini endings are found in the connective tissue around muscles and bones and in the capsules of diarthrodial joints. Some pacinian corpuscles, the receptors that are sensitive to deep pressure, are also present in these tissues. The various endings that are present in the vicinity of joints are concerned with transmitting information about the positions and movements in which the joints are involved.

In short, the significance of the proprioceptors is that as a result of their function a constant flow of information toward the CNS is assured, and because of this feedback system, the muscles can adjust as necessary in order to make the appropriate responses. A very simple illustration of this is seen when one lifts an object whose weight he has misjudged. In a fraction of a second the muscles make their adjustment and lift the object with accuracy and control.

THE SYNAPSE

As was mentioned in the discussion of neurons, the connection between neurons in the central nervous system is known as a synapse. A synapse, and there may be thousands between any two neurons, is a contiguity of the membrane of an axon and the membrane of a dendrite or a cell body. There is no physical union between them. Conduction of impulses takes place in one direction only, namely from the axon of one neuron to the dendrites or cell body of another. The transmission of an impulse across a synapse depends upon the release of a transmitter substance by the axon. This substance diffuses through the membranes and stimulates or inhibits the next cell.*

---

*The author is indebted to Dr. Ernest Gardner for his help in this definition of a synapse.

REFLEX MOVEMENT

A reflex movement is one which occurs without volition and without the need of direction from the cerebrum. The anatomic basis for a reflex act is the reflex arc (Fig. 11–8). This consists of an afferent neuron which comes from a receptor organ, enters the spinal cord, and there makes a synaptic connection either directly with the dendrites and the cell body of an efferent neuron, or indirectly through one or more connector neurons. The axon of the efferent neuron extends from the cord to the muscle where its distal branches terminate in muscle fibers. (It will be recalled that the axon of the efferent neuron together with all of the muscle fibers that it serves constitutes a motor unit.) The point of contact between an axon and a muscle fiber is known as a myoneural junction, also as a motor end-plate. The number of reflex arcs and the number of motor units involved depend both upon the nature of the reflex and upon the extent of muscular activity needed.

As could be inferred from the discussion of receptors, there are two main classes of reflexes related to skeletal movements, namely exteroceptive and proprioceptive. Many of the exteroceptor reflexes exhibited by animals and man are familiar to us. A horse will twitch its skin when flies alight on it; a dog will scratch when its skin is irritated by a flea, or perhaps tickled by a man. A human being jumps when he hears a sudden loud noise. He also blinks when a foreign body strikes his eyeball, or even threatens to strike it. Three exteroceptive reflexes which may be of special interest are the extensor thrust, the flexor and the crossed extensor reflexes.

Extensor Thrust Reflex. Pressure against the sole of the foot stimulates the pacinian corpuscles in the subcutaneous tissue and elicits the reflex contraction of the extensor muscles of the lower extremity. When the weight is supported by the feet the pressure of the floor is sufficient to bring about this reaction. Some authorities classify this reflex as a proprioceptor, rather than an exteroceptor reflex.[7] (See page 162.)

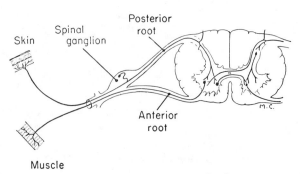

Figure 11–8.   Reflex arc mechanism.

Flexor Reflex. The flexor reflex operates in response to pain and is a device for self-protection. Because of the flexor reflex we quickly withdraw a part of the body the instant it is hurt. If a finger is pricked by a pin or if it inadvertently touches a hot pan, we do not have to decide to remove our hand from the source of pain; we jerk it back even before we realize what has happened to it. Furthermore, all of the necessary muscles for withdrawing it are innervated prompt-ly, not just those in the immediate vicinity of the injury. Although we are all too aware of the pain, this awareness plays no part in the reflex action of withdrawal. The value of the awareness is rather in teaching us to avoid repetition of the act that caused the pain.

Crossed Extensor Reflex. This reflex functions cooperatively with the flexor reflex in response to pain in a weight-bearing limb. For instance, when an animal injures its paw, the flexor reflex causes it to withdraw the paw. Simultaneously, owing to the crossed extensor reflex, the extensor muscles of the opposite limb contract to support the additional weight thrust upon it. Similarly, if a man who is bare-foot happens to step on a tack with his right foot he quickly shifts his weight to his left foot and withdraws his right foot from the floor. As the flexors of his right limb contract to enable him to lift his foot, the extensors of his left limb contract more strongly to support the weight of his entire body.

Guyton also cites the example of a non-weight bearing limb in man responding in like manner.[8] For example, if a pain stimulus is applied to one hand, at the same moment that the hand is withdrawn the opposite arm will extend as though to push the body away. The majority of authorities, however, appear to look upon the crossed extensor reflex as a mechanism for providing support for the body when one foot has been lifted.

Proprioceptive Reflexes. Earlier in this chapter receptors were classified as exteroceptors and interoceptors, the latter being sub-divided into visceral receptors and proprioceptors. Proprioceptive reflexes are generally described as those reflexes which occur in response to stimulation of receptors which are located in the skeletal muscles, the tendons and the joints. According to this interpretation the only proprioceptive reflexes are those related to the effect of stretch on muscles and tendons and the effect of movement on the connective tissues associated with joints.

Many texts use the term *myotatic reflex* synonymously with *stretch reflex* and this would appear to be logical as the word comes from the Greek words for muscle (mys) and stretching (tasis).[6] Other authorities classify stretch reflexes as a special type of myotatic reflex.[5] This should not disturb the student, however, for it is obvious that classifications are man-made devices for facilitating study and re-search. It is not surprising that there should be discrepancies in such classifications and even in the interpretations of the same classification.

Stretch Reflexes. This type of reflex is of particular interest to the physical educator. In its simplest form the stretch reflex is a local response to stretch. For example, a muscle is subjected to stretch.

The muscle spindles pick up the stretch stimulus and transmit it by way of the afferent neuron to the spinal cord. There the central terminal branches of the sensory neuron synapse directly with the dendrites of the motor neuron which innervates the same muscle fibers that were stretched. These fibers then contract. This is the simplest type of reflex arc and is commonly known as a monosynaptic arc. Gardner prefers the term "two-neuron reflex arc" and describes it as involving one "area of synaptic junction." This is more accurate as an arc consisting of a single sensory neuron and a single motor neuron is not restricted to a single synapse. The important characteristic of this type of reflex arc is that it does not make use of connector neurons in the spinal cord. (Many authorities state that *all* stretch reflexes have this characteristic, but some state more cautiously that *most* of them do.[5, 6])

Gardner classifies stretch reflexes as phasic and static types. The phasic type is the kind described above and includes familiar clinical tests like the knee jerk. Reflexes of this type are extremely rapid and the contraction is of brief duration. The word "jerk" gives an accurate picture. While it is true that the cause of the stimulus in this instance is exteroceptive in nature (it being a rubber-headed hammer or the edge of the hand) it is nevertheless classed as a proprioceptive reflex. Another example of a phasic type of stretch reflex is probably present in the violent movement of the arms in certain gymnastic exercises and sport skills. If the stretch is sudden and sufficiently severe the stretched muscle contracts, apparently in an attempt to protect itself from injury.

In the static type of stretch reflex the muscle is stretched slowly which means that several spindles are stimulated, not simultaneously but in succession. This results in a more sustained muscular contraction. Such reflexes may be elicited by stretch due to the contraction of the antagonistic muscles or by stretch due to the tendency of gravity to cause weight bearing joints to flex.[6] Some authorities refer to this type as the antigravity reflex and, in some instances, they include the response of lower extremity and trunk muscles to the involuntary forward-backward swaying that usually occurs when a person stands in one position for a long time.

Ralston and Libet, who have made extensive electromyographic studies of muscular action, apparently do not accept this concept of an antigravity reflex.[15] In 1953 they stated that investigators did not find electrical activity accompanying stretch unless the stretch was of such speed that it invoked the jerk type of reflex. They also stated that the short bursts of activity that accompanied swaying were apparently not simple stretch reflexes in spite of the fact that they were probably initiated by local stretch receptor impulses. As evidence of the latter conclusion they stated that the contraction of the tibialis anterior and the soleus which had been observed in a "standing at ease" position was initiated by a degree of angular motion at the ankle joint that they claimed was far less than that which is required to elicit a stretch reflex. They concluded that the hypothesis that stretch reflex discharge occurs automatically to help maintain a given postural attitude in normal man was not supported by the available evidence. In 1957 Ralston reaffirmed this conclusion.[16] Clearly this matter needs further investigation.

Posture and Locomotor Mechanisms. Whether due to reflex action or to some other mechanism, it seems apparent that there are certain provisions in the human body for remaining more or less erect and for engaging in locomotion, and that these follow the general pattern of reflex behavior. The coordinated efforts of the body to resist the downward pull of gravity include the extensor thrust reflex, the static type of stretch reflex in response to gravitational pull, the muscular action evoked by forward-backward swaying and the various mechanisms for preserving equilibrium, including visual orientation and labyrinthine reflexes.

In regard to locomotion, the action of the legs of a four footed animal has been attributed to reflex action. Some classify this reflex as a division of the crossed extensor reflex;[17] others refer to it simply as a walking reflex.[8] Because the research in this area has been done primarily on dogs and cats it has been suggested that this reflex exists only in quadrupeds. Nevertheless, it is logical to assume that it exists also in man inasmuch as his early forms of locomotion — creeping and crawling — resemble the locomotion of quadrupeds. Even after he assumes the erect position the swing of his arms in opposition to his lower extremities reflects his earlier four-footed gait.

"MUSCLE TONUS"

For many years it was thought that the firmness of muscles in their resting state was the result of the continuously alternating contraction of a small number of motor units. The technique of electromyography, however, has shown this explanation to be erroneous.[15] Muscular contraction, whether of slight or great intensity, is known to be accompanied by electrical activities called action potentials. The presence of action potentials, however slight, can be recorded by electromyography. Repeated experimentation has failed to reveal the presence of action potentials in relaxed muscles, no matter how firm the muscles were when tested. This quality of firmness is now thought to be a manifestation of normal elasticity and turgor of muscle tissue.[1, 15]

de Vries undertook an investigation in 1965 to discover the source of the low level activity that earlier investigators had reported from the use of surface electrodes. Using more sensitive equipment he discovered a high degree of linearity in the relationship between the force of contraction and integrated muscle action potentials at low levels. He concluded that even the smallest potentials recorded with surface electrodes were probably weakened action potentials.[2]

The excessive "firmness" of an obviously hypertense muscle should not be mistaken for the normal firmness of a relaxed, well-developed muscle. Experimentation has shown that the hypertense muscle does show electrical activity, even though no motion is evident.[1] Abnormal muscular tension, such as this, would seem to be a matter of involuntary static contraction resulting from certain emotional states.

VOLITIONAL MOVEMENT

This topic involves such an extensive and complex body of knowledge that only the bare essentials and a few of the newer concepts can be touched upon here. The chief anatomic structures concerned with volitional movement, in addition to those mentioned earlier (skeletal muscle, basic nerve structures, motor units and sensory receptors) are the cerebral cortex, the cerebellum, the brain stem, the corticospinal tracts and the numerous motor pathways, both pyramidal and extrapyramidal.

The portion of the cerebral cortex in which impulses for the majority of volitional acts are thought to arise is the fold situated just in front of the transverse central fissure. Because of its location, this is known as the precentral gyrus; and because it was originally thought to consist entirely of motor cells, it is referred to as the motor area of the cortex (Fig. 11–9). In front of this area is another area having to do with movement. It is called the premotor area and is thought to be responsible for the more complex movement patterns.[7, 8]

Regarding the topography of the motor area, it used to be thought that this area was divided into distinct sub-areas, each of which was solely responsible for the contraction of particular muscles or groups of muscles. Recent studies, however, have revealed that there is considerable overlapping of motor unit territories.[7, 9] This appears

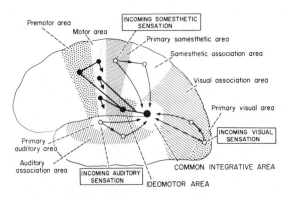

Figure 11–9. Integration of sensory signals from several different sources into a common thought by the common integrative area of the brain, showing also the primary and association areas for vision, for auditory sensations, and for somesthetic sensations. (From Guyton, A. C.: Function of the Human Body, 2nd ed. Philadelphia, W. B. Saunders Company, 1964.)

to be a provision for the performance of complex movement patterns as well as for a variety of movement combinations.

The axons of the motor cells, called Betz's cells, descend through the brain stem and the spinal cord. Together, these axons form the corticospinal tracts. They pass through the anterior portions of the medulla which constitute the pyramids, and it is here that most of the fibers cross to the opposite side. Because of their route through the pyramids the fibers are known collectively as the pyramidal system and their cell bodies as pyramidal cells. The fibers from the premotor area and from other parts of the cortex do not pass through the medulla pyramids; hence they are referred to as the extrapyramidal system.

It was originally thought that the pyramidal system consisted exclusively of Betz cell axons. More recently, however, it has been discovered that the majority of pyramidal fibers actually come from cortical cells outside of the traditional motor area, also that the extrapyramidal system includes many fibers from the motor area.[7] Furthermore, the precentral gyrus is no longer thought to be exclusively a motor area, but rather a sensorimotor area because it is now known to receive some afferent impulses. There is experimental evidence to show that proprioceptive impulses have been received by the motor area after the sensory area in the postcentral gyrus had been removed.[7]

One of the most important of the newer concepts concerning volitional movement is that continued sensory stimulation is essential to motor unit function. There has been ample clinical evidence to show that when sensory innervation is impaired there is a noticeable impairment of volitional movement. It is realized now that for the successful and appropriate execution of volitional acts, sensory stimuli are as indispensable as motor stimuli. This is true throughout all stages of the movement.[7, 9] It is obvious from this that the stimulus-response concept, as formerly interpreted, is no longer adequate for explaining volitional acts.[9]

It has been discovered that the position of a limb is a factor in the intensity of response when a given muscle is made to contract by means of cortical stimulation. For instance, in an electromyographic study of the triceps muscle it was found that the response of the muscle to stimulation of the appropriate cortical area differed according to the size of the angle at the elbow joint. When the joint angle was acute, the response of the triceps to cortical stimulation was stronger than when the joint angle was obtuse. The significance of this experiment is the evidence it presents of the part played by the proprioceptors in relaying information about the position of the joint.[7, 9]

A concept currently receiving wide attention is known as the reafferent or servo-mechanism concept of overt behavior.[4, 9] This mechanism is responsible for feeding back inhibitory impulses to motor neurons and thereby keeping the discharge frequency of the latter under control and safeguarding them against possible convulsive activity.[9, 12]

Many of the structures and mechanisms which influence volitional movement belong to the extrapyramidal system. Among these is the cerebellum which has the important task of controlling the timing and governing the intensity with which the muscles contract (Fig. 11–10). There is also the reticular formation in the brain stem, a mechanism for exerting facilitatory and inhibitory influence on spinal centers, especially the centers for the antigravity muscles,[12] and thus providing for finer coordinations. The thalamus in the brain stem is responsible for receiving sensory impulses and integrating them in coordinated patterns of movement; and the hypothalamus, which responds to emotional stimuli, is responsible for eliciting increased muscle power.[7] These are but a few of the ways in which the pyramidal and the extrapyramidal systems are seen to work together in volitional movement.

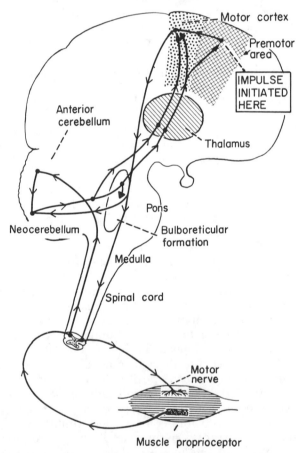

Figure 11–10. Feedback circuits of the cerebellum for damping motor movements. (From Guyton, A. C.: Function of the Human Body, 2nd ed. Philadelphia, W. B. Saunders Company, 1964.)

GRADATIONS IN THE STRENGTH
OF MUSCULAR CONTRACTIONS

Common experience indicates that the same muscles contract with various gradations of strength according to the requirements of the task. The elbow flexors, for example, are able to contract just enough to enable the hand to lift a piece of paper from the desk; they can also contract forcefully enough to lift a fifteen pound briefcase. How do they adjust to such extremes?

There are two major factors in the gradation of contraction. These are (1) the number of motor units which participate in the act, and (2) the frequency of stimulation. If the stimulus is of threshold value, all of the muscle fibers in the motor unit will contract maximally. If the stimulus is subliminal, in other words, below threshold value, none of the muscle fibers in the unit will contract at all. This characteristic is known as the *all-or-none principle of muscular contraction.* It must be emphasized that the principle applies only to individual motor units, not to entire muscles. To reiterate, if the stimulus is of threshold value, each muscle fiber in the participating unit will contract. Hence it follows that, other things being equal, the more motor units that contract, the greater will be the total strength developed.

If stimuli are discharged at low frequency, the muscle fibers will partially relax between impulses, but if the stimuli are discharged at high frequency the fibers will have insufficient time to relax and the result is summation or maximal contraction. If these two factors are combined, that is, if the maximum number of fibers are stimulated with the impulses being discharged at high frequency, the resulting contraction is of maximal strength.

RECIPROCAL INNERVATION AND INHIBITION

One of the mechanisms that provides for economical and coordinated movement is the one known as reciprocal innervation and inhibition, first described by Sherrington. According to this concept, when motor neurons are transmitting impulses to muscles, causing them to contract, the motor neurons that supply their antagonists are simultaneously and reciprocally inhibited. The antagonistic muscles, therefore, remain relaxed and the movers, or agonists, contract without opposition. Reciprocal inhibition operates automatically in movements elicited by the stretch reflex, also in familiar volitional movements. In more complicated and in less familiar coordinations its operation depends upon the degree of skill developed by the performer.

Not all investigators are in agreement with respect to the operation of reciprocal innervation and inhibition in volitional movement. Some believe that muscles that are antagonistic to each other do contract concurrently under certain conditions and they refer to this as cocontraction (see page 44). This text, however, agrees with those who state that simultaneous contraction of antagonistic muscles, when it does occur, is indicative of unskilled performance, and that skillful performance is characterized by the absence of antagonistic action.[1, 13]

REFERENCES

1. Basmajian, J. V.: Muscles Alive. Baltimore, 2nd ed. The Williams & Wilkins Company, 1967.
2. de Vries, H. A.: Muscle tonus in postural muscles. Am. J. Phys. Med., 44:275–291, 1965.
3. Eldred, E.: The dual sensory role of muscle spindles. J. Am. Phys. Ther. Assn., 45:290–313, 1965.
4. Fischer, E.: Physiological basis of volitional movements. Phys. Ther. Rev., 38: 405–412, 1958.
5. Fischer, E.: Neurophysiology a physical therapist should know. Phys. Ther. Rev., 38:741–748, 1958.
6. Gardner, E.: Fundamentals of Neurology, 5th ed. Philadelphia, W. B. Saunders Company, 1968.
7. Gellhorn, E.: The physiology of the supraspinal mechanism. In Johnson, W. R. (Ed.): Science and Medicine of Exercise and Sports. New York, Harper & Brothers, 1960, Chap. 7.
8. Guyton, A. C.: Function of the Human Body, 3rd ed. Philadelphia, W. B. Saunders Company, 1969.
9. Harrison, V. F.: Review of the neuromuscular bases for motor learning. Res. Quart. Am. Assn. Health, Phys. Ed. & Recrn., 33:59–69, 1962.
10. Huxley, H. E.: The contraction of muscle. Sci. Am., Nov. 1958 (offprint).
11. Karpovich, P. V.: Physiology of Muscular Activity, 6th ed. Philadelphia, W. B. Saunders Company, 1965.
12. Loofbourrow, G. N.: Neuromuscular integration. In Johnson, W. R. (Ed.): Science and Medicine of Exercise and Sports. New York, Harper & Brothers, 1960, Chap. 6.
13. O'Connell, A. L., and Gardner, E. B.: Co-contraction of antagonistic muscles during slow controlled movement. Report presented at Research Section, National Convention of the American Association for Health, Physical Education, and Recreation, 1960.
14. Ralston, H. J.: Mechanics of voluntary muscle. Am. J. Phys. Med., 32:166–184, 1953.
15. Ralston, H. J., and Libet, B.: The question of tonus in skeletal muscle. Am. J. Phys. Med., 32:85–92, 1953.
16. Ralston, H. J.: Recent advances in neuromuscular physiology. Am. J. Phys. Med., 36:94–120, 1957.
17. Ruch, T. C., and Patton, H. D.: Medical Physiology and Biophysics, 19th ed. Philadelphia, W. B. Saunders Company, 1965.

CHAPTER 12

The Upper Extremity: The Shoulder Region

Nowhere in the body is anatomic cooperation more beautifully illustrated than in the movements of the arm on the trunk. The arm travels through a wide range of movements. In each of these the scapula contributes to the movement by placing the glenoid fossa in the most favorable position for the head of the humerus. For instance, when the arm is elevated sideward, the scapula rotates upward; when the arm is elevated forward, the scapula not only rotates upward, but also tends to move away from the spinal column and to slide partially around the rib cage. There are some circumstances in which this latter movement is deliberately inhibited, as for instance in the arm placings and flingings of formal gymnastics. In all natural movements, however, the scapula shares with the humerus in the movements of the arm on the trunk.

These movements of the scapula occur not in one joint, but in two. The scapula articulates with the clavicle, and the clavicle, in turn, articulates with the sternum (Fig. 12–1). All movements of the scapula involve motion in both these joints. Thus, just as the scapula cooperates with the humerus, so the clavicle cooperates with the scapula. This is but one of the many illustrations of teamwork found in the human mechanism.

In order to understand the movements of the arm as a whole, each joint which participates in these movements should be studied separately.

THE SHOULDER JOINT (GLENOHUMERAL ARTICULATION)

Structure. The shoulder joint is formed by the articulation of the spherical head of the humerus with the small, shallow, somewhat pear-shaped glenoid fossa of the scapula (Fig. 12–1). It is a ball-and-socket joint. The structure of the joint and the looseness of the capsule (permitting between 1 and 2 inches of separation between the two bones) account for the remarkable mobility of the shoulder joint.

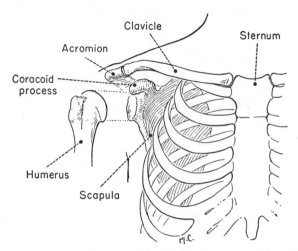

Figure 12–1. Anterior view of shoulder joint and shoulder girdle.

Both the humeral head and the glenoid fossa are covered with hyaline cartilage. The cartilage on the head is thicker at the center; that which lines the cavity is thicker around the circumference. The glenoid fossa is further protected by a flat rim of white fibrocartilage, likewise thicker around the circumference. This cartilage, called the glenoid labrum, serves both to deepen the fossa and to cushion it against the impact of the humeral head in forceful movements (Fig. 12–2).

The joint is completely enveloped in a loose sleevelike articular capsule which is attached proximally to the circumference of the glenoid cavity, and distally to the anatomic neck of the humerus. The capsule is reinforced both by ligaments and by muscle tendons. The latter are particularly important in preserving the stability of the joint. Apparently they do not prevent downward dislocation, however. Two electromyographic investigations have thrown light on the role of certain structures in stabilizing the shoulder joint and, in particular, preventing downward dislocation. In their extensive study of the shoulder region in 1944, Inman, Saunders and Abbott noted the stabilizing function of the four muscles that constitute the "rotator cuff" — the supraspinatus, infraspinatus, teres minor and subscapularis.[8] In 1959 Basmajian and Bazant investigated the muscles whose fibers cross the shoulder joint vertically, as compared with those whose fibers cross it horizontally. To their surprise they discovered that it was the horizontal fibers, not the vertical, that were active in preventing downward dislocation of the humerus. After doing a dissection of the shoulder joint they agreed that the slope of the glenoid fossa was an important factor. Because of this slope, the head of the humerus was forced laterally as it was pulled downward, and it took the horizontally directed muscle fibers to check this lateral movement which, in turn, stopped the downward movement. They concluded that

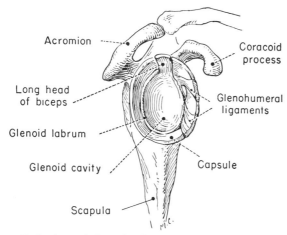

Figure 12–2. Lateral view of right scapula showing glenoid cavity.

downward dislocation of the humerus was prevented primarily by three factors, namely, (1) the slope of the glenoid fossa, (2) the tightening of the upper part of the capsule and of the coracohumeral ligament, and (3) the activity of the supraspinatus muscle and, to a lesser extent, of the posterior fibers of the deltoid.[1]

LIGAMENTOUS REINFORCEMENTS

Coracohumeral ligament. (Fig. 12–3.)   This is a broad band connecting the lateral border of the coracoid process with the anterior border of the greater tubercle of the humerus. It reinforces the upper anterior portion of the capsule.

Glenohumeral ligaments. (Fig. 12–2.)   These are three adjacent bands of fibers which blend with and strengthen the inner fibers of

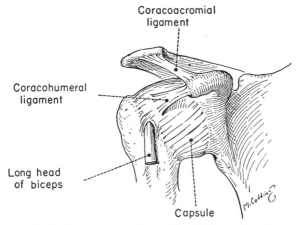

Figure 12–3. Anterior view of shoulder joint showing ligaments.

the front and lower parts of the capsule. They attach along the anterior edge of the glenoid fossa from the apex to the inferior rim. From here they pass in front of and beneath the shoulder joint, to attach to the anterior and inferior portions of the anatomic neck of the humerus.

Coracoacromial ligament. (Fig. 12–3.) Structurally, this ligament should be classed with those of the scapula, since both its attachments are on this bone. Functionally, however, it belongs with the ligaments of the shoulder joint. By connecting the acromion and coracoid processes, it forms a bridge over the top of the shoulder joint, and thus helps to protect this structure.

MUSCULAR REINFORCEMENTS (Fig. 12–4.)

1. Superior
   Supraspinatus
   Long head of biceps

The tendon of the long head of the biceps is unique in its relation to the joint in that it originates from within the joint capsule. It arises from the upper margin of the glenoid fossa as a continuation of the glenoid labrum, penetrates the capsule and passes through the intertubercular groove, which has been converted into a tunnel by the transverse humeral ligament. Its passage through the capsule, over the humeral head and between the two tubercles, is facilitated by a tubular sheath of synovial membrane.

2. Inferior
   Long head of triceps

3. Posterior
   Infraspinatus
   Teres minor

4. Anterior
   Subscapularis
   Fibrous prolongations of pectoralis major and teres major (these blend with the transverse humeral ligament)

The synovial membrane lines the capsule, folds back over the glenoid labrum, covers all but the upper portion of the anatomic neck of the humerus, and extends through the intertubercular groove in the form of a sheath for the tendon of the long head of the biceps. There are several bursae in the region of the shoulder joint. Among the larger are the one between the deltoid and the capsule, and the one on top of the acromion process.

Movements. The movements of the humerus are as follows:

FLEXION AND HYPERFLEXION. A forward upward movement in a plane at right angles to the plane of the scapula. If the movement exceeds 180 degrees, it is hyperflexion.

EXTENSION. Return movement from flexion.

HYPEREXTENSION. A backward movement in a plane at right angles to the plane of the scapula.

ABDUCTION. A sideward upward movement in a plane parallel with the plane of the scapula.*

---

*Some authorities interpret abduction as the sideward movement of the arm away from the body, thus including the action of the shoulder girdle. When reading the literature, one should note which interpretation is intended.

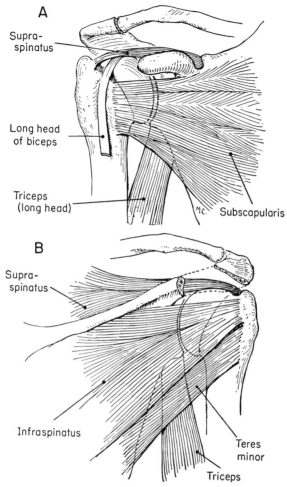

Figure 12–4. Muscular reinforcements of shoulder joint. *A,* Anterior view; *B,* posterior view.

ADDUCTION. Return movement from abduction.

OUTWARD ROTATION. A rotation of the humerus around its mechanical axis so that, when the arm is in its normal resting position, the anterior aspect turns laterally.

INWARD ROTATION. A rotation of the humerus around its mechanical axis so that when the arm is in its normal resting position, the anterior aspect turns medially.

HORIZONTAL FLEXION. A forward movement of the abducted humerus in a horizontal plane (i.e., from a plane parallel to the plane of the scapula to a plane at right angles to it).

HORIZONTAL EXTENSION. A backward movement of the flexed

humerus in a horizontal plane (i.e., from a plane at right angles to the plane of the scapula to a plane parallel to it).

CIRCUMDUCTION. A combination of flexion, abduction, extension, hyperextension and adduction, performed sequentially in either direction, so that the extended arm describes a cone, and the finger tips a circle.

Muscles. * The muscles of the shoulder joint may be classified according to their position in relation to the joint. This is not always clear cut, as may be seen from the illustrations.

Superior:
Middle deltoid
Supraspinatus
Inferior:
Latissimus dorsi
Teres major
Long head of triceps (primarily a muscle of the elbow joint)
Anterior:
Pectoralis major
Coracobrachialis
Anterior deltoid
Subscapularis
Biceps (primarily a muscle of the elbow joint)
Posterior:
Posterior deltoid
Infraspinatus
Teres minor

DELTOIDEUS (Figs. 12–6 and 12–7.)

Proximal attachments (O)
Anterior: Anterior border of outer third of clavicle.
Middle: Acromion process and outer end of clavicle.
Posterior: Lower margin of spine of scapula.

Distal attachment. (I) Lateral aspect of humerus, near midpoint.

Nerve supply. Axillary (circumflex) nerve.

Where to palpate
Anterior: In front of the head of the humerus and for a space of 2 or 3 inches below this.
Middle: Lateral surface of upper third of upper arm.
Posterior: Upper and lateral portion of posterior surface of scapula below scapular spine.

Action
Anterior: Flexion; horizontal flexion; inward rotation.
Middle: Abduction; horizontal extension.
Posterior: Extension; horizontal extension; outward rotation, especially when arm is below the horizontal.[13]

Comments. The deltoid muscle is complex in structure, con-

---

*Attention is called to the electromyographic investigations reported in the Supplementary Material at the end of this chapter.

sisting of several bundles of fibers. The extreme anterior and posterior bundles are of spindle or fusiform construction; the bundles composing the middle portion are multipenniform. This arrangement of the middle portion makes for great strength without resulting in too much bulk. The muscle is a powerful abductor of the humerus. In addition to raising the arm it is frequently called upon to hold the arm in an elevated position for long periods of time and thus make it possible for the hand to work at a height. The multipenniform arrangement of fibers also serves to compensate for the middle deltoid's poor angle of pull. This poor angle of pull, on the other hand, means that the muscle has a strong stabilizing component of force. This is fortunate, because in this position the shoulder joint depends more upon its muscles than upon its ligaments for holding the head of the humerus in the glenoid fossa.

The anterior portion of the deltoid aids in all forward movements of the arm and in inward rotation of the humerus. There is considerable disagreement in the literature concerning the movements effected by the posterior deltoid but there seems to be sufficient evidence to conclude that, in addition to the movements already mentioned, the lowest fibers, being situated below the axis of motion, assist in adducting the humerus from an overhead position. On the other hand, some of the upper fibers, that is, those closest to the middle deltoid, probably work with the latter in contributing to abduction. In fact, Shevlin, Lehmann and Lucci stated that in their experiments the posterior deltoid elevated the humerus in the frontal plane (i.e., abduction) at all the levels tested (45, 90 and 110 degrees of elevation). It is disappointing that they did not test above the 110 degree level, and also that they used only one electrode for the posterior deltoid, placed "in the middle of its bulk."[12]

SUPRASPINATUS (Figs. 12–4, 12–5 and 12–6.)

Proximal attachment. (O)   Medial two thirds of supraspinatus fossa above spine of scapula.

Distal attachment. (I)   Top of greater tuberosity of humerus.

Nerve supply.   Suprascapular nerve.

Where to palpate.   Above spine of scapula, provided scapula is supported, e.g., when armpit rests over back of chair.

Action.   Abduction; holds head of humerus against glenoid fossa during abduction.

Comments.   The supraspinatus has a particularly favorable angle of pull for initiating abduction. This compensates for the middle deltoid's poor angle. Steindler emphasizes the importance of the holding action of the supraspinatus and states that were it not for this, the deltoid would be unable to abduct the humerus.[13] Some authorities credit the muscle with two additional functions, namely lifting the capsule out of the way when the humerus is raised and contributing to outward rotation of the humerus.

By experimentally paralyzing the supraspinatus van Linge and Mulder found that the arm could still be raised through its full range, but not with its usual force and endurance. (See Basmajian, p. 166.[1])

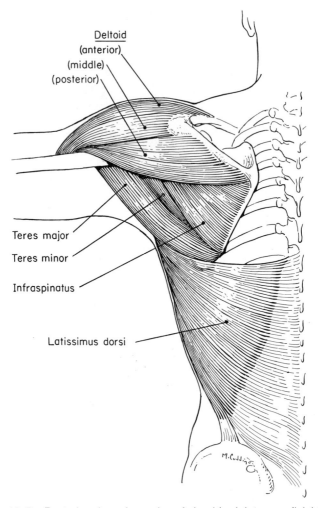

Deltoid
(anterior)
(middle)
(posterior)

Teres major

Teres minor

Infraspinatus

Latissimus dorsi

M. Cullings

Figure 12–5.   Posterior view of muscles of shoulder joint, superficial layer.

PECTORALIS MAJOR (Fig. 12–7.)

Proximal attachments. (O)   Medial two thirds of clavicle; anterior surface of sternum; cartilages of first six ribs; slip from aponeurosis of external oblique abdominal muscle.

Distal attachment. (I)   Lateral surface of humerus just below head by a flat tendon 2 to 3 inches wide.

Nerve supply.   Medial and lateral anterior thoracic nerves.

Where to palpate

> Clavicular: Just below the medial two thirds of the clavicle.
> Sternal: Lateral to the sternum, below clavicular portion.
> Both: Anterior border of axilla.

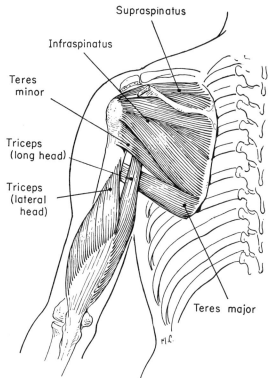

Figure 12–6. Posterior view of muscles of shoulder joint, deep layer.

Action

Upper or clavicular portion: Flexion; horizontal flexion; inward rotation, especially from a position of outward rotation; abduction when arm is well above the horizontal.

Lower or sternal portion: Adduction; horizontal flexion; inward rotation; extension.

Comments.   This large fan-shaped muscle of the chest converges to a flat tendon of insertion which twists on itself in such a way that the lowest fibers become the uppermost. The muscle is divided into three parts, the clavicular, the sternal and the abdominal, corresponding to its proximal attachments. Since the abdominal portion is relatively small and since it does not seem to have any unique function of its own, the common practice is to include it with the sternal portion. The clavicular portion lies close to the anterior deltoid muscle and works with it in the flexion, inward rotation and horizontal flexion of the humerus. Ordinarily the line of pull of the clavicular portion of the pectoralis major lies below the axis of the shoulder joint. When the arm is raised sideward well above the horizontal, however, as Steindler has explained, the line of pull of the upper clavicular fibers shifts to a position above the center of the shoulder

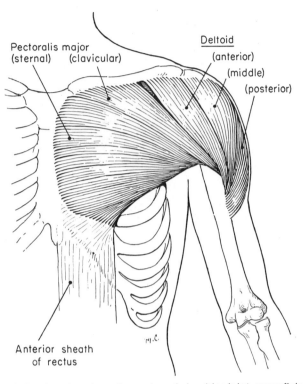

Figure 12–7.   Anterior view of muscles of shoulder joint, superficial layer.

joint and these fibers then cease to adduct and become abductors of the humerus.[13] The sternal portion acts only in downward and forward movements of the arm. The pectoralis major as a whole is particularly important in all pushing, throwing and punching activities. Scheving and Pauly found that it participates in inward rotation only when the movement is resisted. (See Basmajian, p. 163.[1])

CORACOBRACHIALIS (Fig. 12–8.)

Proximal attachment. (O)   Coracoid process of scapula.

Distal attachment. (I)   Inner surface of humerus opposite deltoid attachment.

Nerve supply.   Musculocutaneous nerve.

Where to palpate.   Anterior surface of upper arm, medial to short head of biceps. Forearm must be supported in flexed position and resistance given to lower end of humerus. Difficult to palpate.

Action.   Horizontal flexion; stabilization of shoulder joint; aids in flexion, adduction, inward rotation and in extension when the arm is raised overhead.

Comments.   Because the line of pull is so nearly parallel with the long axis of the humerus, the chief function of this muscle would seem to be stabilization of the shoulder joint.

SUBSCAPULARIS (Fig. 12–8.)

Proximal attachment. (O)   Entire anterior surface of scapula

Distal attachment. (I)   Lesser tuberosity of humerus.

Nerve supply.   Subscapular nerve.

Cannot be palpated.

Action.   Inward rotation; horizontal flexion; lower fibers aid in adduction when the arm is above the horizontal.

Comments.   Inward rotation is the chief action of the subscapularis. It performs this movement best when the arm is at the side or elevated backward. Another important function of this muscle is stabilization of the glenohumeral joint.

BICEPS BRACHII (Fig. 12–8.) (See also muscles of elbow.)

Proximal attachments. (O)   Long head from upper margin of glenoid fossa; short head from apex of coracoid process of scapula.

Distal attachment. (I)   Bicipital tuberosity of radius.

Nerve supply.   Musculocutaneous nerve.

Where to palpate.   Medial-anterior surface of upper arm, 3 or 4 inches above elbow.

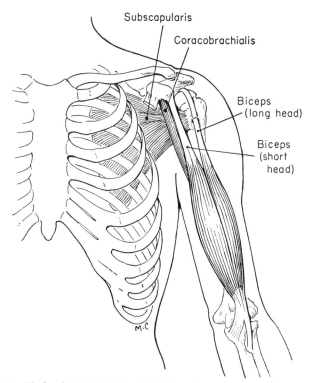

Figure 12–8.   Anterior view of muscles of shoulder joint, deep layer.

Action (at shoulder joint). Assists in flexion of the humerus, especially against resistance, in horizontal flexion, in adduction and in stabilization of the shoulder joint.

Comments. Inspection of Figure 12–8 shows that the short head of the biceps brachii and the coracobrachialis have almost identical lines of pull in relation to the shoulder joint. As one would expect, their actions at this joint are similar. One should keep the fact in mind, however, that the biceps is primarily a muscle of the elbow and radio-ulnar joints and its movements of the humerus are secondary. Further-more, the latter are influenced, if not actually determined, by the movements the forearm is undergoing and also by the position of both the humerus and the forearm with regard to rotation. These can significantly change the relation of the lines of pull of the two bicipital heads to the shoulder joint. Important points like this are not always taken into consideration in electromyographic investigations.

Wright, one of the most outstanding investigators of muscular action by means of palpation, has made some pertinent observations regarding the functions of the biceps muscle. She pointed out that, although the biceps is considered a flexor of the humerus, it is not active when shoulder flexion and forceful elbow extension occur simultaneously, such as when one pushes himself up from an armchair. She also noted that when the arm is raised forward with the elbow passively extended (apparently with the palm facing forward-upward) the biceps remains relaxed unless the forward elevation is strongly resisted, in which case it contracts, but not forcefully. She assumed that its function in this movement was simply protection of the elbow joint against strain of the anterior ligaments.[15]

The importance of considering all of the conditions when analyzing a movement cannot be overemphasized.

LATISSIMUS DORSI (Fig. 12–6.)

Proximal attachments. (O)   Spinous processes of lower six thoracic and all lumbar vertebrae; posterior surface of sacrum; crest of ilium; lower three ribs.

Distal attachment. (I)   Anterior surface of humerus below head, by a flat tendon, just anterior to and parallel with tendon of pectoralis major.

Nerve supply. Thoracodorsal (middle subscapular) nerve.

Where to palpate. Posterior border of axilla just below the teres major.

Action. Adduction; extension; hyperextension; horizontal extension; inward rotation.

Comments. This is a broad sheet of muscle which covers the lower and middle portions of the back. Coming mainly from the lower half of the thoracic portion of the spine, and the entire lumbar portion, the fibers gradually converge as they pass upward and laterally toward the axilla. Here the fibers twist on themselves in such a way that the lowest fibers become the uppermost. They end in the narrow flat tendon of the distal attachment. The muscle has a favorable angle of pull for depression of the arm, particularly when the latter is raised between 30 and 90 degrees.

TERES MAJOR (Figs. 12–5 and 12–6.)

Proximal attachment. (O) Posterior surface of inferior angle of scapula.

Distal attachment. (I) Anterior surface of humerus below head, just medial to tendon of latissimus dorsi.

Nerve supply. Lower subscapular nerve.

Where to palpate. Posterior border of axilla just above latissimus dorsi.

Action. Adduction; extension; hyperextension; inward rotation; horizontal extension.

Comments. In some respects the teres major may be thought of as the latissimus dorsi's "little helper." Judging by its relation to the shoulder joint it appears to be capable of effecting the same movements as the latter. Inman, Saunders and Abbott, in their electromyographic study, however, could detect no sign of contraction when these movements were being executed. They observed that the teres major contracted only in maintaining static positions and that it attained its maximum activity when the humerus was at approximately a 90 degree angle of elevation.[8]

INFRASPINATUS AND TERES MINOR (Figs. 12–4, 12–5 and 12–6.)

Proximal attachment. (O) Axillary border and posterior surface of scapula below scapular spine.

Distal attachment. (I) Posterior aspect of greater tuberosity of humerus.

Nerve supply. Suprascapular and axillary nerves.

Where to palpate. Posterior surface of scapula, medial and inferior to posterior deltoid muscle.

Action. Outward rotation; horizontal extension.

Comments. From the point of view of the kinesiologist there is no reason why these muscles should have separate names. They are as truly one muscle as are the two parts of the pectoralis major, or the three parts of the deltoid, in fact even more so because there is no difference in their function. Besides their powerful outward rotatory action, these muscles aid materially in holding the head of the humerus in the glenoid fossa. These two muscles, like all the muscles uniting the scapula with the humerus, act effectively to move the humerus only when the scapula is stabilized.

LONG HEAD OF TRICEPS BRACHII (Figs. 12–4 and 12–5.) (See also muscles of elbow.)

Proximal attachment. (O) Just below glenoid fossa of scapula.

Distal attachment. (I) Olecranon process of ulna.

Nerve supply. Musculospiral nerve.

Where to palpate. Posterior surface of arm close to shoulder joint.

Action (at shoulder joint). Stabilization of shoulder joint. Assists in adduction, extension and hyperextension.

THE SHOULDER GIRDLE (ACROMIOCLAVICULAR
AND STERNOCLAVICULAR ARTICULATIONS)

Structure of Acromioclavicular Articulation. (Fig. 12–9.) The articulation between the acromion process of the scapula and the outer end of the clavicle belongs to the diarthrodial classification. Within this group it is further classified as an irregular (arthrodial) joint. A small wedge-shaped disk may be found between the upper part of the joint surfaces, but this is frequently absent. The articular capsule is strengthened above by the acromioclavicular ligament, and behind by the aponeurosis of the trapezius and deltoid muscles. The clavicle is further stabilized by means of the coracoclavicular ligament, which, as the name suggests, binds the clavicle to the coracoid process.

LIGAMENTS

Acromioclavicular. This passes from the upper part of the outer end of the clavicle to the upper surface of the acromion process.

Coracoclavicular. This is actually two ligaments, the conoid and the trapezoid. The conoid ligament passes from the base of the coracoid process to the conoid tubercle on the under side of the clavicle. The trapezoid ligament extends from the top of the coracoid process to the trapezoid ridge on the under side of the clavicle.

Structure of Sternoclavicular Articulation. (Fig. 12–10.) The sternal end of the clavicle articulates with both the sternum and the cartilage of the first rib. It is classified as a double arthrodial joint because there are two joint cavities, one on either side of the articular disk. This round flat disk of white fibrocartilage is attached above to the upper and posterior border of the articular surface of the clavicle, and below to the cartilage of the first rib near its junction with the sternum. The articular capsule is thin above and below, but is thickened in front and behind by bands of fibers called the anterior and posterior sternoclavicular ligaments. The often overlooked impor-

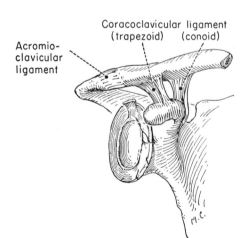

Acromio-
clavicular
ligament

Coracoclavicular ligament
(trapezoid)   (conoid)

Figure 12–9. Anterior view of acromioclavicular articulation.

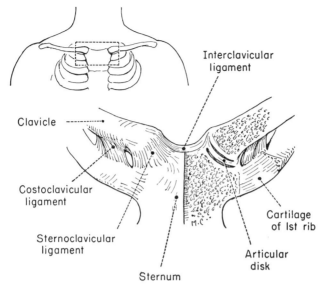

Figure 12–10. Anterior view of sternoclavicular articulation.

tance of this capsule was demonstrated by Bearn in a series of experiments involving the loading of the lateral end of the clavicle both before and after cutting various structures. He presented convincing evidence that it is the capsule, rather than the trapezius muscle, that provides the chief support for the clavicle.[2]

The movements of the clavicle at this joint are as follows: elevation and depression which occur approximately in the frontal plane about a sagittal-horizontal axis; horizontal forward-backward movements which occur in the horizontal plane about a vertical axis; and rotation forward and backward, very limited movements which occur approximately in the sagittal plane about the bone's own longitudinal axis. (In forward rotation the top of the clavicle revolves forward-downward.)

The sternoclavicular articulation is of great importance in the movements of the shoulder girdle and of the arm as a whole. It permits limited motion of the clavicle in all three planes and because of the bone's attachment to the scapula at its distal end, is partially responsible for the latter's movements.

LIGAMENTS

Anterior sternoclavicular. This is a band of fibers blending with the anterior fibers of the articular capsule.

Posterior sternoclavicular. The fibers forming this ligament blend with the posterior fibers of the articular capsule.

Interclavicular. This ligament consists of a flat band which passes across the upper margin of the sternum and attaches to the sternal end of each clavicle.

Costoclavicular. This is a short strong band of fibers which connects the upper border of the first costal cartilage with the costal tuberosity on the under side of the clavicle.

Movements. (Fig. 12–11.)   It is customary to define the movements of the shoulder girdle in terms of the movements of the scapulae. In doing this, there is some danger that the reader will visualize the movement as taking place solely in the joint between the scapula and the clavicle. It is well to emphasize the fact that *every movement of the scapula involves motion in both joints.*

The movements of the shoulder girdle, expressed in terms of the composite movements of the scapula, are as follows:

ELEVATION. (Fig. 12–11, *A*)   An upward movement of the scapula with the vertebral border remaining approximately parallel to the spinal column. The elevation of the scapula is the direct result of elevation of the outer end of the clavicle, a movement which takes place at the sternoclavicular joint. This occurs to a slight extent during elevation of the humerus and to a greater extent in lifting the shoulders in a hunching gesture. The farther the clavicles depart from the horizontal position, the closer the scapulae move toward each other. The latter movement might well be called passive adduction as it is caused by the movement of the clavicles rather than by the adductor muscles of the scapulae.

DEPRESSION.   The return from the position of elevation. There is no depression below the normal resting position.

ABDUCTION OR PROTRACTION. (Fig. 12–11, *B*.)   A lateral movement of the scapula away from the spinal column, with the vertebral border remaining approximately parallel to it. Pure abduction of the scapula is a hypothetical movement. Actually, because of two factors, (1) the rounded contour of the thorax and (2) the forward movement of the clavicle about a vertical axis at the sternoclavicular joint, a pure lateral movement of the scapula in the frontal plane is impossible. As the scapula abducts it turns slightly about its vertical axis in a movement known as a lateral tilt. This is characterized by a slight backward movement of the vertebral border and a corresponding forward movement of the axillary border. This causes the glenoid fossa to face slightly forward and the arms, if relaxed, to hang in a more forward position and in slight inward (medial) rotation.

ADDUCTION OR RETRACTION.   A medial movement of the scapula toward the spinal column combined with a reduction of lateral tilt.

UPWARD TILT. (Fig. 12–11, *D*.)   A turning of the scapula on its frontal-horizontal axis so that the posterior surface faces slightly upward and the inferior angle protrudes from the back. This is accompanied by a rotation of the clavicle about its mechanical axis so that the superior border turns slightly forward-downward and the inferior border backward-upward. It occurs only in conjunction with hyperextension of the humerus.

REDUCTION OF UPWARD TILT.   The return movement from upward tilt.

UPWARD ROTATION. (Fig. 12–11, *C*.)   A rotation of the scapula in

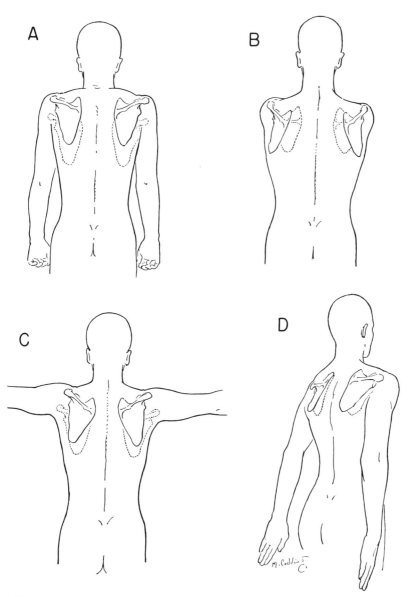

Figure 12–11. Movements of the shoulder girdle. *A,* Elevation; *B,* abduction (combined with lateral tilt and upward rotation); *C,* upward rotation; *D,* upward tilt.

the frontal plane so that the glenoid fossa faces somewhat upward. This movement occurs largely at the acromioclavicular joint but is accompanied by elevation of the outer end of the clavicle. Upward rotation is always associated with elevation of the humerus, either sideward or forward. It serves at least three useful purposes. (1) It puts the glenoid fossa in a favorable position for the upper extremity movement;[9] (2) by positioning the small glenoid fossa beneath the larger head of the humerus it contributes significantly to the stability of the shoulder joint,[7] and (3) by moving the origin of the deltoid medially at the same time that the latter muscle is elevating the humerus, the deltoid is prevented from shortening too much, thereby losing force too rapidly.[10]

DOWNWARD ROTATION.   The return from the position of upward rotation. There may be slight downward rotation beyond the normal resting position, so that the glenoid fossa faces slightly downward.

Muscles.*   The muscles of the shoulder girdle are classified as anterior or posterior muscles, according to their location on the trunk.

Anterior:	Posterior:
Subclavius	Levator scapulae
Pectoralis minor	Trapezius
Serratus anterior	Rhomboids

SUBCLAVIUS (Fig. 12–12.)

Proximal attachment. (O)   Upper surface of first rib at junction with cartilage.

Distal attachment. (I)   Under side of middle half of clavicle.

Nerve supply.   Branches from fifth and sixth cervical nerves. Cannot be palpated.

Action.   Depression of clavicle; stabilization of sternoclavicular joint.

Comments.   The fibers of the subclavius run almost parallel with the long axis of the clavicle. They have a slight downward and strong medialward pull. This would seem to indicate that, although the muscle is in a position to depress the outer end of the clavicle when necessary, its real function is to protect and stabilize the sterno-clavicular articulation. When the clavicle is fixed in elevation, the subclavius can aid slightly in lifting the first rib in forced inspiration.

PECTORALIS MINOR (Fig. 12–12.)

Proximal attachments. (O)   Anterior surface of third, fourth and fifth ribs near cartilages.

Distal attachment. (I)   Tip of coracoid process of scapula.

Nerve supply.   Medial anterior thoracic nerve.

Where to palpate.   Cannot be palpated when pectoralis major is contracting. May be palpated halfway between clavicle and nipple when arm is elevated backward as far as possible or against resistance. May also be palpated if subject sits with forearm resting on table

---

*Attention is called to the electromyographic investigations reported in the Supplementary Material at the end of this chapter.

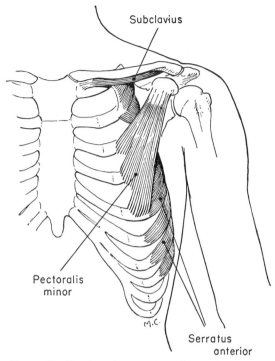

Figure 12–12. Anterior muscles of shoulder girdle.

at side of body and pushes both downward and laterally at the same time.

Action. Downward rotation; abduction and lateral tilt; upward tilt; depression.

Comments. Besides its action on the scapula, an important function of the pectoralis minor is its lifting effect on the ribs, both in forced inspiration and in maintaining good chest posture. When the scapulae are stabilized by the adductors, contraction of the pectoralis minor elevates the third, fourth and fifth ribs. Even without contracting, it exerts a slight upward and outward pull on these ribs if its tonus is good. Thus the pectoralis minor can contribute either to good posture or to poor, depending upon whether its more effective pull is on the ribs or on the scapula. The key to its function as a muscle of good posture is stabilization of the scapulae by the adductors – the rhomboids and the middle trapezius.

SERRATUS ANTERIOR (Fig. 12–12.)

Proximal attachments. (O) Outer surfaces of upper nine ribs at side of chest.

Distal attachment. (I) Anterior surface of vertebral border and inferior angle of scapula.

Nerve supply. Long thoracic nerve.

Where to palpate. Anterior-lateral surface of upper thorax, especially on a thin, muscular subject.

Action

Upper: Abduction and lateral tilt.

Lower: Upward rotation.

Both: A combination of the above plus a tendency to pull the vertebral border of the scapula inward toward the ribs.

Comments. The serratus anterior is made up of separate bands or bundles attached to the ribs, as the name suggests, in a saw-tooth arrangement. The first band, coming from the first two ribs, attaches to the uppermost portion of the vertebral border. The next two or three bands, coming from the second, third and occasionally fourth ribs, fan out to attach along almost the entire length of the vertebral border. These first four or five bands compose the upper serratus anterior, whose chief function is abduction of the scapula.

The lower portion consists of bands which come from the next four or five ribs and converge to attach to the anterior surface of the inferior angle of the scapula. Their function is to rotate the scapula upward.

LEVATOR SCAPULAE (Fig. 12–13.)   (See also muscles of neck.)

Proximal attachments. (O)   Transverse processes of first four cervical vertebrae.

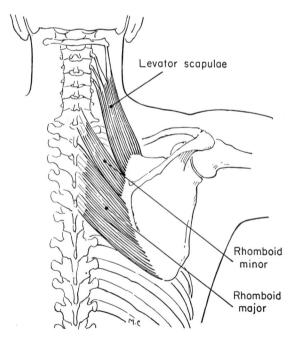

Figure 12–13. Posterior muscles of shoulder girdle, deep layer.

Distal attachment. (I) Vertebral border of scapula between medial angle and scapular spine.

Nerve supply. Dorsal scapular and branches from third and fourth cervical nerves.

Cannot be palpated.

Action (at scapula). Elevation; downward rotation; possibly slight adduction, especially when the body is in a horizontal position.

Comments. Bowen pointed out that, although one would expect the levator scapulae to elevate and adduct the scapula, actually it causes elevation and downward rotation when the trunk is in the erect position.[3] His explanation of this action is that the weight of the arm at the acromial end of the scapula pulls that end down at the same time that the levator is lifting the medial angle. Thus these two forces act as a force couple to rotate the scapula.

In more recent years Basmajian,[1] and Rasch and Burke,[11] who succeeded Bowen as authors of the textbook he originally wrote, appear to agree with him in attributing the levator scapulae's movement of downward rotation to the weight of the arm and to the scapula's consequent need of postural support. Another author sees this weight-supporting function as a cooperative action of the levator scapulae and the rhomboids lifting the medial border of the scapula, and of the upper trapezius lifting its lateral angle.[6] Still another claims that the levator, together with the rhomboid minor, tends to rotate the scapula downward in the early phase of contraction, preliminary to elevating it.[4]

If the levator scapulae rotates the scapula downward only when the weight of the arm prevents it from adducting the scapula, it would be assumed that the trunk must be in the erect position for gravity to have this effect. In other positions, as when a person is swimming, one would expect the levator to adduct, as well as to elevate, the scapula. It might be enlightening if an electromyographic study were to be made for the purpose of comparing the actions of the levator muscle when abduction of the humerus (and possibly other movements) is performed from two different starting positions—erect standing or sitting and prone lying.

TRAPEZIUS (Fig. 12–14.)

Proximal attachments. (O) Occipital bone; ligamentum nuchae; spinous processes of seventh cervical and all thoracic vertebrae.

Distal attachments (I)

Part I: Posterior border of lateral third of clavicle.

Part II: Top of acromion process.

Part III: Upper border of spine of scapula.

Part IV: Root of spine of scapula.

Nerve supply. Spinal accessory and branches from third and fourth cervical nerves.

Where to palpate. Kite-shaped area in upper back and neck (Fig. 12–14).

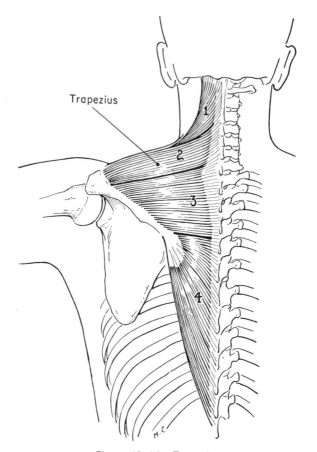

Figure 12–14. Trapezius.

Action
Part I: Elevation.
Part II: Elevation; upward rotation; assists in adduction.
Part III: Adduction.
Part IV: Upward rotation; depression; assists in adduction.

Comments. The trapezius is a fascinating muscle to study. As its location directly under the skin makes it easy to palpate, the student should investigate its actions for himself. While some anatomists treat the muscle in three parts, it is more accurate to consider separately the four parts listed above. Parts I and II comprise the upper trapezius, part III the middle and part IV the lower. The relation of the trapezius to the rhomboids and serratus is interesting. The rhomboids and part III of the trapezius both adduct the scapulae. In this action they are partners. Parts II and IV, however, rotate the scapulae upward; the rhomboids rotate them downward. In this respect, then, they are antagonists.

Trapezius II and IV are partners with the lower serratus with respect to upward rotation, but trapezius III and the upper serratus are antagonistic, the former adducting, and the latter abducting, the scapulae. Parts II and IV of the trapezius act on the scapula as a force couple to rotate the scapula upward, part II pulling up on the acromial end of the scapular spine, and part IV pulling down on the medial end or root. (See discussion of a force couple on page 100, and Figure 6–9 on page 99.)

Trapezius I and II have one important function which may be overlooked because there is little, if any, actual movement involved. This is support for the distal end of the clavicle and the acromion process of the scapula when a heavy weight is held by the hand with the arm down at the side. Anyone who has carried a heavy suitcase for a long distance has doubtless experienced tension and subsequent soreness in these parts of the muscle. When no weight is carried, however, the capsule of the sternoclavicular articulation provides all the support necessary for the fully depressed clavicle.[2]

These various combinations of function are an excellent illustration of the cooperative action of the muscles and of the astonishing versatility of the musculoskeletal mechanism.

RHOMBOIDEUS, MAJOR AND MINOR (Fig. 12–13.)

Proximal attachments. (O) Spinous processes of seventh cervical and first five thoracic vertebrae.

Distal attachment. (I) Vertebral border of scapula from spine to inferior angle.

Nerve supply. Dorsal scapular nerve.

Cannot be palpated.

Action. Downward rotation; adduction; elevation.

Comments. Functionally, the rhomboids may be regarded as one muscle. Their cooperative action with trapezius III, which has been discussed above, is an important factor in the maintenance of good shoulder posture. When the tonus of these two muscles is deficient, the unbalanced pull of the pectoralis minor and the serratus anterior results in habitually abducted and tilted scapulae. This in turn results in the failure of the pectoralis minor and serratus anterior to hold the chest in good posture. Thus one weak link in the chain of postural relationships leads to another.

MOVEMENTS OF THE ARM ON THE TRUNK

It has already been stated that the movements of the arm on the trunk do not take place at the shoulder joint alone, but that they involve movement of the shoulder girdle at both the acromioclavicular and sternoclavicular joints. In order to analyze correctly the movements of the upper extremity, it is necessary to understand the cooperative action of the shoulder joint and shoulder girdle. The fundamental movements of the arm, analyzed in terms of shoulder joint and shoulder girdle action, are stated below.

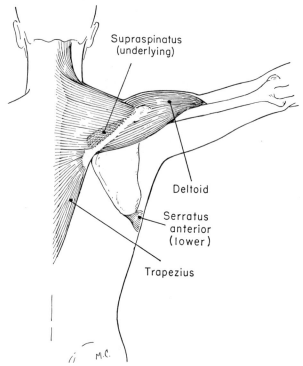

Figure 12–15.   Muscles which contract to produce sideward elevation of the arm.

SIDEWARD ELEVATION (Fig. 12–15.)
Shoulder joint.   Abduction of the humerus; outward rotation if the palms are turned to face each other in the overhead position.
Shoulder girdle.   Upward rotation, and slight elevation of the scapula, particularly after arm passes above the horizontal.
SIDEWARD DEPRESSION
Shoulder joint.   Adduction of the humerus; reduction of outward rotation.
Shoulder girdle.   Downward rotation of the scapula.
FORWARD ELEVATION   (To the horizontal.)
Shoulder joint.   Flexion of the humerus; slight outward rotation; abduction if scapula is laterally tilted (in which case glenoid fossa will be facing partly forward).
Shoulder girdle.   Slight upward rotation of the scapula; abduction and lateral tilt, unless inhibited.
FORWARD-UPWARD ELEVATION   (From the horizontal to the vertical and beyond.)
Shoulder joint.   Flexion and possibly hyperflexion of the humerus; slight outward rotation.
Shoulder girdle.   Upward rotation and some elevation of the scapula; reduction of abduction and lateral tilt.

FORWARD-DOWNWARD DEPRESSION (From the vertical to the starting position.)

Shoulder joint. Extension of the humerus; adduction; reduction of outward rotation.

Shoulder girdle. Downward rotation of the scapula; passes through position of abduction and lateral tilt, unless prevented by strong action of the scapular adductors.

BACKWARD ELEVATION (Fig. 12–16.)

Shoulder joint. Hyperextension of the humerus.

Shoulder girdle. Upward tilt of the scapula; elevation if movement is carried to extreme.

OUTWARD ROTATION (Fig. 12–17.)

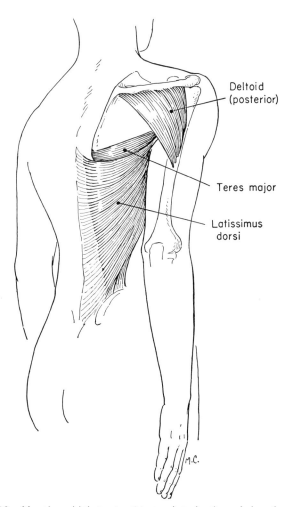

Deltoid (posterior)

Teres major

Latissimus dorsi

M.C.

Figure 12–16. Muscles which contract to produce backward elevation of the arm.

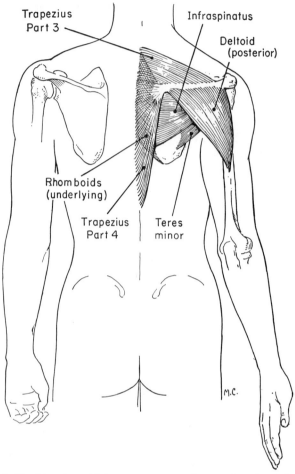

Figure 12–17. Muscles which contract to produce outward rotation of the arm and accompanying adduction of the scapula.

Shoulder joint. Outward rotation of the humerus; tendency toward hyperextension.

Shoulder girdle. Adduction of the scapula; reduction of any lateral tilt which may have been present.

INWARD ROTATION

Shoulder joint. Inward rotation of the scapula.

Shoulder girdle. Abduction and lateral tilt of the scapula; tendency toward elevation.

HORIZONTAL FORWARD SWING FROM POSITION OF SIDEWARD ELEVATION

Shoulder joint. Horizontal flexion of the humerus; slight inward rotation.

Shoulder girdle. Abduction and lateral tilt of the scapula; unless inhibited.

HORIZONTAL SIDEWARD-BACKWARD SWING FROM POSITION OF FORWARD ELEVATION

Shoulder joint. Horizontal extension of the humerus; slight outward rotation.

Shoulder girdle. Adduction and reduction of lateral tilt of the scapula.

SUPPLEMENTARY MATERIAL

Electromyographic Studies of the Muscles of the Shoulder Joint and Shoulder Girdle. In their extensive studies of the shoulder region, completed in 1944, Inman, Saunders and Abbott reported the actions of the muscles in sideward and forward elevation of the upper extremity. The highlights of their findings are briefly summarized below.[8]

ABDUCTORS AND FLEXORS OF THE HUMERUS

Deltoid: Greatest activity is between 90 and 180 degrees of elevation.

Supraspinatus: Acts with the deltoid throughout the entire range of motion.

Pectoralis Major: No activity was noted in sideward elevation. In forward elevation, the clavicular portion appeared to work synchronously with the anterior deltoid.

DEPRESSORS OF THE HUMERUS

Teres Major: No activity in movements of the upper extremity but only in the maintenance of static positions.

Subscapularis, Infraspinatus and Teres Minor: Continuous activity throughout both abduction and flexion.

SCAPULAR ROTATORS

Upper Trapezius, Levator Scapulae and Upper Serratus Anterior (acting as a unit): Passive support of the shoulder; active elevation of the shoulder girdle; constitute the upper component of a force couple in upward rotation of the scapula.

Lower Trapezius and Lower Four Digitations of Serratus Anterior: Constitute the lower component of a force couple in upward rotation of the scapula.

Middle Trapezius and Rhomboid Muscles: Act in abduction of the humerus to stabilize the scapula. Are only slightly active in flexion of the humerus; permit the scapula to rotate around the thorax. (This is the combination movement described in this text as abduction and lateral tilt. See page 192.)

Shevlin, Lehmann and Lucci made an electromyographic study in 1969 of the functions of the ten major muscles that cross the glenohumeral joint. Twelve persons, including both male and female, their ages ranging from 17 to 55 years, served as subjects. For the testing, the arm was raised in three different planes: forward (sagittal plane), sideward (lateral plane) and halfway between. These were designated respectively as 0, 90 and 45 degree planes. As the muscular contractions were isometric, no actual movements took place during the testing. In each of the three planes the arm was positioned at three levels of elevation, these being at 45, 90 and 110 degrees from the body.

In each of these nine positions four movements were attempted: elevation, depression, forward horizontal adduction, and backward horizontal abduction. The resistance given to these was of sufficient magnitude to prevent movement. This fact should be kept in mind when the results of the study are being considered.

The investigators made a statistical comparison between the amount of activity occurring during an attempted motion in one direction and an attempted motion in the opposite direction with the arm in the same position. They also compared the activity of a muscle contracting in the same direction with the arm in different positions. Their summary of these findings, which they believed offered new information, is as follows:

> The anterior deltoid was found to be significantly active in elevation of the humerus rather than in depression in all positions tested.
> The posterior deltoid was significantly active in elevation rather than depression in the frontal plane at all levels but only at the elevation of 110 degrees when the humerus was positioned at 45 degrees of horizontal abduction.
> The clavicular fibers of the pectoralis major in the frontal plane at the level of 110 degrees were significantly active in elevation.
> The supraspinatus and the middle deltoid functioned with statistically significant electrical activity in horizontal abduction rather than horizontal adduction.
> The subscapularis showed significantly more electrical activity in elevation than in depression of the humerus and in horizontal abduction than in horizontal adduction.[12]

In interpreting the results of this study it would be well for the reader to keep the following points in mind:

1. The illustrations in the article show that elevation of the arm in all three planes was performed with the palms down. This means that, in the 0 (sagittal) and 45 degree planes at least, the humerus was rotated inward and the forearm was pronated.

2. Since the contractions were isometric, no movement took place during the testing.

3. The highest elevation of the arm at which tests were made was 110 degrees. The average individual can raise the arm considerably higher than this, especially if he is permitted to rotate the arm outward. At the higher elevations some muscle fibers shift to the other side of the center of motion and, hence, reverse their action.

4. When a muscle is said to "participate" in a movement, this does not necessarily mean that it is acting as a mover for that movement. It may be stabilizing the joint or maintaining a position, e.g., rotation, when the part is being moved in the sagittal or in the frontal plane. This is especially likely to be the case when it seems to be implied that a muscle is taking part in antagonistic movements, such

as when it is stated that a certain muscle is "more active in flexion than in extension."

5. If these findings are to be compared with those of similar studies it is important to note the placement of the electrodes.

An Electromyographic Study of the Trapezius Muscle. In 1952 Wiedenbauer and Mortensen investigated the activity of the trapezius muscle in various movements of the scapula and arm.[14] Eleven men served as subjects, and the tests were made with the subjects seated. The trapezius showed definite activity during both elevation and retraction (adduction) of the scapula. In elevation, the upper portion showed the greatest activity, and in retraction, the middle and lower portions. During abduction of the humerus and the accompanying upward rotation of the scapula, the lower two-thirds of the trapezius was most active, and during flexion of the humerus, the lower third. The greatest activity of the trapezius as a whole was seen in abduction of the humerus.

Scapular Movements Accompanying Elevation of the Arm. In 1945 Wells investigated the movements of the scapula accompanying forward and sideward elevation of the arm, using a series of x-rays of one subject. Each x-ray was traced, and measurements were then made on the tracings. Abduction of the scapula was measured in terms of the horizontal distance between the midpoint of the vertebral border of the scapula and the near margin of the spinal column. (A line connecting the spinous processes would have been the logical reference line, but it could not be used, since many of the spinous processes did not show in the x-ray.) Rotation was measured, by means of a protractor, in terms of the angle formed between a continuation of the vertebral border and the margin of the spinal column (Fig. 12–18). The results were as follows:

Position of Arm	Scapular Abduction	Scapular Rotation
At rest	5.5 cm	−3° (downward rot.)
Sideward elev. about 45°	4.6 cm	0 (parallel)
Sideward elev. about 90°	5.6 cm	11° (upward rot.)
Sideward elev. about 135°	6.5 cm	36° (upward rot.)
Sideward elev. about 180°	7.3 cm	36° (upward rot.)
At rest	5.5 cm	−3° (downward rot.)
Forward elev. about 45°	7.2 cm	3.5° (upward rot.)
Forward elev. about 90°	10.1 cm	8° (upward rot.)
Forward elev. about 135°	9.3 cm	21° (upward rot.)
Forward elev. about 180°	8.2 cm	31.5° (upward rot.)

The reader should not make any generalizations from a study such as this which uses only one subject. In order to make a study from which generalizations can safely be made it would be necessary to standardize the methods of measurement and to use a large number of subjects selected at random. Even then, use of this type of measure-

Measurement of
upward rotation

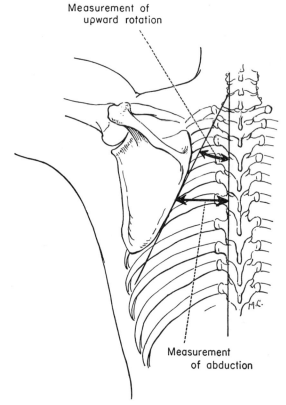

Measurement
of abduction

Figure 12–18. Measurements of the scapular movements accompanying sideward elevation of the arm. (The sketch is based on an x-ray.)

ment technique is a precarious practice because of the distortion present in x-rays.

In their more sophisticated investigation of the functions of the shoulder joint, Inman et al. noted that after 30 degrees of side elevation, and after 60 degrees of forward elevation of the arm, there appeared to be a constant two-to-one relationship between the movement of the humerus and that of the scapula. They observed that between 30 and 170 degrees of elevation, for every 15 degrees of total motion, abduction of the humerus (or flexion, in the case of forward elevation) was responsible for 10 degrees, and upward rotation of the scapula for 5 degrees. They stated that, in the early phase of elevation, the scapula seemed to be establishing a precise position of stability with reference to the humerus. The exact movement that occurs during this phase is apparently determined by the individual's habitual shoulder posture.[8]

In 1966 Freedman and Munro, using 61 male subjects with an age range of 17 to 24 years, made a roentgenographic study of sideward elevation of the arm. They investigated the relative amounts of scapular and glenohumeral movements with the arm at five stages of abduction, namely, 0, 45, 90 and 135 degrees and maximum abduction. They used the scapular plane as their point of reference in preference to the coronal (frontal) plane as Inman, Saunders and Abbott had done in their 1944 study. Their chief findings were as follows:

In the resting position the glenoid fossa faced slightly downward in over 80% of the subjects, the downward inclination amounting to slightly more than 5 degrees.

The total rotation of the scapula averaged 65 degrees and the total glenohumeral movement, 103 degrees.

For every two degrees of scapular rotation accompanying abduction of the humerus in the scapular plane, there was an average of three degrees of movement in the glenohumeral joint. During the final stage of abduction a relative increase of glenohumeral motion occurred.

Statistics indicated that there was a considerable amount of individual variation in the movements.[5]

DEMONSTRATIONS AND LABORATORY EXERCISES

Joint Structure and Function

1. Take a humerus and a scapula of the same side and "construct" a shoulder joint, using felt for the fibrocartilage and adhesive tape for the ligaments. Be accurate in the attachment of these structures. Two or three may work together on this project.

2. Using a form like that in Appendix B, record the essential information regarding the glenohumeral, acromioclavicular and sternoclavicular articulations. Study the movements of these joints both on the skeleton and on the living body.

3. In five different subjects measure the amount of abduction that occurs in the shoulder girdle (i.e., the separation of the scapulae) when the arms are raised to the forward-horizontal position. How much can this vary in one individual? In measuring the distance between the scapulae measure the horizontal distance between the midpoints of the vertebral borders.

4. Using a Lufkin rule or a protractor-goniometer, measure the amount of upward rotation of the scapula which occurs when the arm is raised sideward-upward to the overhead position. To make this measurement, center the instrument over the medial angle of the scapula, and adjust one of its arms in line with the normal resting position of the inferior angle and the other in line with the inferior angle after maximum upward rotation of the scapula has taken place.

Muscular Action. Record the results on the chart found in Appendix F.

Directions. Work in groups of three, one person serving as the subject, the second as an assistant, helping to support or steady the stationary part of the body and giving resistance to the moving part, and the third palpating the muscles and recording the results on the check list.

5. SIDEWARD ELEVATION OF THE ARM (shoulder joint: abduction and possibly outward rotation; shoulder girdle: upward rotation)

Subject: In erect position, raise arm sideward to shoulder level, keeping elbow straight.

Assistant: Resist movement by exerting pressure downward on subject's elbow. See to it that subject does not elevate shoulder.

Observer: Palpate the three portions of the deltoid and tell which portions contract. Palpate the four parts of the trapezius. Which parts contract? Does the pectoralis major contract during any part of the movement?

6. SIDEWARD DEPRESSION OF THE ARM (shoulder joint: adduction and possibly reduction of outward rotation; shoulder girdle: downward rotation)

Subject: In erect position with arm raised sideward to shoulder level, lower arm to side.

Assistant: Place hand under subject's elbow and resist movement (If no resistance is given, the muscle action will be the same as in elevation, except that the contraction will be eccentric instead of concentric.)

Observer: Palpate the latissimus dorsi, teres major, pectoralis major and posterior deltoid. Do they each contract, and, if so, during which part of the movement?

7. FORWARD ELEVATION OF THE ARM (shoulder joint: flexion and abduction; shoulder girdle: upward rotation and probably abduction)

Subject: In erect position, raise arm forward to shoulder level, keeping elbow straight.

Assistant: Resist movement by exerting pressure downward on the subject's elbow. See that subject does not elevate shoulder.

Observer: Palpate the anterior deltoid and the pectoralis major. Do both the sternal and clavicular portions of the latter muscle contract?

8. FORWARD DEPRESSION OF THE ARM (shoulder joint: adduction and extension; shoulder girdle: downward rotation and probably adduction)

Subject: In erect position with arm raised forward to shoulder level, lower it to the side.

Assistant: Resist movement at under side of elbow.

Observer: Palpate the latissimus dorsi and the pectoralis major. Do they contract with equal force throughout the movement?

9. BACKWARD ELEVATION OF THE ARM (shoulder joint: hyperextension; shoulder girdle: upward tilt)

Subject: Either in erect position or lying face down, raise arm backward, keeping elbow straight.

Assistant: Place hand over subject's elbow and resist movement.

Observer: Palpate the posterior deltoid, latissimus dorsi and teres major.

10. HORIZONTAL SIDEWARD-BACKWARD SWING OF THE ARM (from forward-horizontal position) (shoulder joint: horizontal extension and slight outward rotation; shoulder girdle: adduction and reduction of lateral tilt)

a. Subject: In erect position with arms raised forward to shoulder level, palms down, swing arms sideward in horizontal plane as far as possible.

Assistant: Stand facing subject between his arms and resist movement by grasping his elbows.

Observer: Palpate the posterior deltoid and latissimus dorsi. What other muscles can be palpated?

b. Subject: Lying face down on narrow plinth, or on table close to edge with arm hanging straight down, raise arm sideward as far above the horizontal as possible.

Assistant: Resistance may be given at elbow, but is not necessary, since gravity furnishes sufficient resistance.

Observer: Same as in *a*.

11. HORIZONTAL SIDEWARD-FORWARD SWING OF THE ARM (from side-horizontal position) (shoulder joint: horizontal flexion and slight inward rotation; shoulder girdle: abduction and lateral tilt)

a. Subject: In erect position with arm raised sideward to shoulder level, palm down, swing arm forward in horizontal plane.

Assistant: Stand behind subject's arm and resist movement by holding elbow.

Observer: Palpate pectoralis major and anterior deltoid.

b. Subject: Lie on back on table with arm extended sideward, palm up. Raise arm to vertical position, keeping elbow straight.

Assistant: Resistance may be given at elbow, but is not necessary, since gravity furnishes sufficient resistance.

Observer: Same as in *a*.

12. OUTWARD ROTATION OF ARM (shoulder joint: outward rotation; shoulder girdle: possibly adduction and reduction of lateral tilt)

Subject: Lie face down on table with upper arm at shoulder level, resting on table, and forearm hanging down off edge of table. Keeping forearm at right angles to upper arm, raise hand and forearm forward-upward to limit of motion, without allowing upper arm to leave table.

Assistant: Steady upper arm and resist movement of forearm by holding wrist.

Observer: Palpate infraspinatus and teres minor.

13. INWARD ROTATION OF ARM (shoulder joint: inward rotation; shoulder girdle: abduction and lateral tilt, and tendency toward elevation)

a. Subject: Same position as in 12. Raise forearm backward-upward.

Assistant: Steady upper arm and resist movement of forearm by holding wrist.

Observer: Palpate teres major and latissimus dorsi.

b. Subject: Lie on back on table with upper arm at shoulder level resting on table and forearm raised to vertical position. Lower forearm forward-downward to the limit of motion.

Assistant: Steady upper arm and resist forearm motion by holding wrist.

Observer: Palpate anterior deltoid and clavicular portion of pectoralis major.

14. ELEVATION OF SHOULDER

Subject: In erect position, lift shoulder toward ear, keeping arm muscles relaxed.

Assistant: Resist movement by pressing down on shoulder.

Observer: Palpate trapezius I and II.

15. DEPRESSION OF SHOULDER

a. Subject: In erect position with shoulder raised and elbow flexed. Push down with elbow, lowering shoulder to normal position.

Assistant: Resist movement by holding hand under elbow.

Observer: Palpate trapezius IV.

b. Subject: Take cross rest position between two chairs or parallel bars.

Observer: Palpate trapezius IV.

16. ADDUCTION OF SHOULDER GIRDLE (retraction)

Subject: In erect position with arms raised sideward, elbows flexed and fingers resting on shoulders, push elbows backward, keeping them at shoulder level.

Assistant: Stand facing subject and resist movement by pulling elbows forward.

Observer: Palpate middle and lower trapezius (parts III and IV). (This movement is somewhat similar to the one in 10, but here the emphasis is on the shoulder girdle rather than on the arm.)

17. ABDUCTION OF SHOULDER GIRDLE (protraction)

Subject: In erect position with arms raised sideward, elbows flexed and fingers resting on shoulders, pull elbows forward, attempting to touch them in front of chest.

Assistant: Stand behind subject and resist movement by pulling elbows back.

Observer: Palpate serratus anterior.

Action of the Muscles Other Than the Movers

18. STABILIZATION OF THE SCAPULA DURING FORCEFUL FORWARD DEPRESSION OF THE ARM

Subject: In erect position with arm raised forward above shoulder level, lower arm against strong resistance.

Assistant: Resist the arm movement by placing hand under the arm just above the subject's elbow.

Observer: Palpate trapezius IV. Explain.

19. STABILIZATION OF SCAPULA DURING OUTWARD ROTATION OF HUMERUS

Subject: Rotate the arm outward as it hangs at the side.

Observer: Palpate the scapular adductors. Explain.

20. ROTATION OF ARM IN POSITION OF SIDE ELEVATION

Subject: With one arm raised sideward to shoulder level, rotate it first outward, then inward.

Observer: Palpate middle deltoid. Explain its action.

21. VIGOROUS ARM-FLINGING SIDEWARD TO THE HORIZONTAL

Subject: Fling arm vigorously to the side horizontal position.

Observer: Palpate the adductors of the shoulder joint. Do they contract momentarily at the very end of the movement? Explain.

22. VIGOROUS ARM-FLINGING DOWNWARD

Subject: From an overhead position, fling arm vigorously forward-downward, stopping it at the body.

Observer: Palpate the flexors of the shoulder joint. Do they contract momentarily at the end of the movement? Explain.

23. REPEAT EXERCISE 9

Observer: Palpate pectoralis major. Explain.

REFERENCES

1. Basmajian, J. V.: Muscles Alive, 2nd ed. Baltimore, The Williams & Wilkins Company, 1967. Chapter 9. The Upper Limb.
2. Bearn, J. G.: Direct observations on the function of the capsule of the sternoclavicular joint in clavicular support. J. Anat., 101:159–170, 1967.
3. Bowen, W. P., and Stone, H. A.: Applied Anatomy and Kinesiology, 7th ed. Philadelphia, Lea & Febiger, 1953.
4. Brunnstrom, S.: Clinical Kinesiology, 2nd ed. Philadelphia, F. A. Davis Company, 1966.
5. Freedman, L., and Munro, R. R.: Abduction of the arm in the scapular plane; scapular and glenohumeral movements. J. Bone & Joint Surg., 48A:1503–1510, 1966.
6. Hollinshead, W. H.: Functional Anatomy of the Limbs and Back, 3rd ed. Philadelphia, W. B. Saunders Company, 1969.
7. Inman, V. T.: The shoulder as a functional unit. J. Bone & Joint Surg., 44A:977–978, 1962.
8. Inman, V. T., Saunders, J. B. deC. M., and Abbott, L. C.: Observations on the function of the shoulder joint. J. Bone & Joint Surg., 26:1–30, 1944.
9. Mollier, S.: On the Statics and Mechanics of the Human Shoulder Girdle under Normal and Pathological Conditions, trans. by F. E. Hastings and W. Skarstrom. Unpublished.
10. Ralston, H. J.: Mechanics of voluntary muscle. Am. J. Phys. Med., 32:166–184, 1953.
11. Rasch, P. J., and Burke, R. K.: Kinesiology and Applied Anatomy, 3rd. ed. Philadelphia, Lea & Febiger, 1967.
12. Shevlin, M. G., Lehmann, J. F., and Lucci, J. A.: Electromyographic study of the function of some muscles crossing the glenohumeral joint. Arch. Phys. Med. & Rehab., 50:264–270, 1969.
13. Steindler, A.: Kinesiology of the Human Body. Springfield, Ill., Charles C Thomas, Publisher, 1955.
14. Wiedenbauer, M. M., and Mortensen, O. A.: An electromyographic study of the trapezius muscle. Am. J. Phys. Med., 31:363–372, 1952.
15. Wright, W. G.: Muscle Function. New York, Hafner Publishing Company, 1962.

RECOMMENDED READINGS

Conway, A. M.: Movements at the sternoclavicular and acromioclavicular joints. Phys. Ther. Rev., 41:421–432, 1961.
Dempster, W. T.: Mechanisms of shoulder movement. Arch. Phys. Med. & Rehab., 46:49–70, 1965.
Inman, V. T.: The shoulder as a functional unit. Arch. Phys. Med. & Rehab., 44:67, 1963. (Abstr.)
Singleton, M. C.: Functional anatomy of the shoulder. J. Am. Phys. Ther. Assn., 46:1043–1051, 1966.

CHAPTER 13

The Upper Extremity: The Elbow Joint and Radioulnar Articulations

The elbow and the radioulnar joints work together to serve the hand in much the same way that the two joints of the shoulder girdle work together to serve the shoulder joint. Man's hand owes its usefulness to the variety of positions made possible by the joints of the elbow, the forearm and the shoulder. If, for instance, man were to lose the ability to rotate his forearm, the use of his hand would be so limited that he would have to change his whole mode of living. The shape of his tools, eating implements, door knobs and similar items, would have to be changed. Furthermore, his method of handling them would seem crude and clumsy compared with his present dexterity.

STRUCTURE OF THE ELBOW JOINT

The elbow joint consists of the articulation of the lower end of the humerus with the upper ends of the ulna and radius. Together they comprise a hinge joint whose only motions are flexion and extension. The rotatory movements of the forearm occur at the articulations between the radius and the ulna, not at the elbow joint. The semicircular structure at the upper end of the ulna is cupped around the back and under side of the spool-like process known as the trochlea, at the lower end of the humerus (Fig. 13–1). The inner surface of this semicircular structure is known as the semilunar notch. It terminates above and behind in the olecranon process, and below and in front in the coronoid process. Just lateral to the trochlea, on the lower end of the humerus, is the capitulum, the small spherical structure that articulates with the saucer-like surface of the radial head.

The two articulations of the elbow joint, as well as the proximal radioulnar articulation, are completely enveloped in an extensive capsule. The capsule is strengthened on all four sides by bands of fibers which are usually described respectively as the anterior, posterior, ulnar collateral and radial collateral ligaments (Figs. 13–2 and 13–3). Synovial membrane not only lines the capsule, but it also ex-

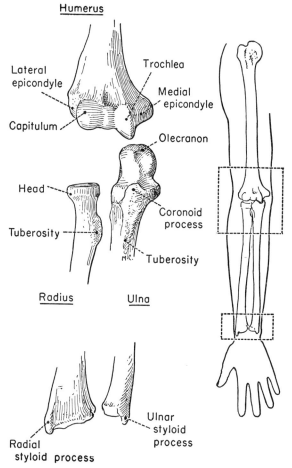

Figure 13–1. The bony structures of the elbow and radioulnar joints. (Anterior view.)

tends into the proximal radioulnar articulation, covers the olecranon, coronoid and radial fossae, and lines the annular ligament.

LIGAMENTS

Anterior. This is a broad, thin layer of fibers which blend with and thicken the anterior portion of the capsule.

Posterior. This is a thin, membranous layer of fibers which blend with and strengthen the posterior portion of the capsule.

Ulnar collateral. (Fig. 13–2.) This is a strong, thick triangular band, attached above by its apex to the medial epicondyle of the humerus, and below by its base to the medial margins of the coronoid and olecranon processes of the ulna, and the ridge between them.

Radial collateral. (Fig. 13–3.) This is a short fibrous band, attached above to the lower part of the lateral epicondyle of the hu-

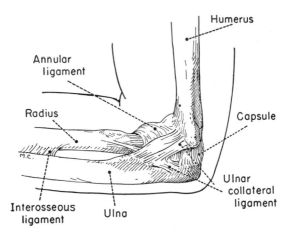

Figure 13–2.   Medial aspect of elbow joint showing ligaments.

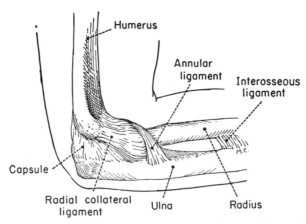

Figure 13–3.   Lateral aspect of elbow joint showing ligaments.

merus, and below to the lateral side of the annular ligament which encircles the head of the radius.

STRUCTURE OF THE RADIOULNAR JOINTS

Proximal Articulation. (Fig. 13–1.) The disk-shaped head of the radius fits against the radial notch of the ulna and is encircled by the annular ligament. The notch and the annular ligament together form a complete ring within which the radial head rotates. The articulation is classified as a pivot joint. It has no capsule of its own, but is enclosed within the capsule of the elbow joint.

ANNULAR LIGAMENT. (Figs. 13–2 and 13–3.) This is a strong band of fibers forming three quarters of the ring which encircles the radial head. It holds the radial head in close contact with the radial notch of the ulna. It is lined with a synovial membrane which is continuous with that of the elbow joint.

Distal Articulation. (Fig. 13–1.) At the distal end of the forearm the radius articulates, by means of a small notch, with the head of the ulna. A triangular shaped fibrocartilaginous disk lies between the head of the ulna and the carpal bones. It is attached by its apex to the styloid process of the ulna, and by its base to the medial margin of the lower end of the radius. It serves to reinforce the distal radioulnar joint and to separate this joint from the wrist. A loose articular capsule surrounds the joint.

LIGAMENTS

Volar radioulnar. This is situated on the volar (anterior) surface of the joint and is attached to the edge of the notch on the radius, the articular disk and the ulnar head.

Dorsal radioulnar. This lies behind the joint and is attached to the margin of the notch on the radius, the articular disk and the ulnar head.

Mid-Radioulnar Union. The shafts of the radius and ulna are united by means of the oblique cord and the interosseous membrane (Figs. 13–2 and 13–3).

Movements

ELBOW JOINT

Flexion. From the anatomic position (Fig. 1–1, B) this is a forward-upward movement of the forearm in the sagittal plane.

Extension. Return movement from flexion. A few individuals are able to hyperextend at the elbow joint. This ability is probably due to a short olecranon process, rather than to loose ligaments.

RADIOULNAR JOINTS

Pronation. This is a rotation of the forearm around its longitudinal axis, corresponding to inward rotation of the humerus. It usually accompanies the latter when the elbow is in extension.

Supination. This is a rotation of the forearm around its longitudinal axis, corresponding to outward rotation of the humerus. It usually accompanies the latter when the elbow is in extension. In the anatomic position of the arm (see page 8) the humerus is rotated outward and the forearm is supinated.

Pronation and supination of the forearm involve a rotation of the radial head within the ring formed by the ulnar notch and annular ligament at the proximal joint, and, at the distal joint, a rotation of the lower end of the radius around the outside of the ulnar head. Neither bone rotates about its own mechanical axis, as does the humerus, but each rotates about the mechanical axis of the forearm as a whole.

Muscles. The muscles of the elbow and radioulnar joints are classified below in two ways, first according to their action, and second according to their location.

MUSCLES LISTED ACCORDING TO ACTION

Elbow Joint

Flexors
    Biceps brachii
    Brachialis
    Brachioradialis
    Pronator teres
Extensors
    Triceps brachii
    Anconeus

Radioulnar Joints

Pronators
    Pronator teres
    Pronator quadratus

Supinators
    Supinator
    Biceps brachii

MUSCLES LISTED ACCORDING TO LOCATION

Anterior (elbow region)
    Biceps brachii
    Brachialis
    Brachioradialis
    Pronator teres

Anterior (wrist region)
    Pronator quadratus
Posterior
    Triceps brachii
    Anconeus
    Supinator

BICEPS BRACHII (Fig. 13–4.) (See also muscles of the shoulder joint.)
    Proximal attachments. (O)
        Long head: Upper margin of glenoid fossa.
        Short head: Apex of coracoid process of scapula.
    Distal attachment. (I)   Bicipital tuberosity of radius.
    Nerve supply. Musculocutaneous nerve.
    Where to palpate. Anterior surface of lower two thirds of upper arm.
    Action. Flexion at elbow joint; supination of forearm when elbow is flexed and when movement is resisted.[1]
    Comments. The biceps is a two-headed or twin spindle type of muscle. It is primarily a muscle of the elbow joint and of the proximal radioulnar articulation, but it also acts at the shoulder joint. Unless

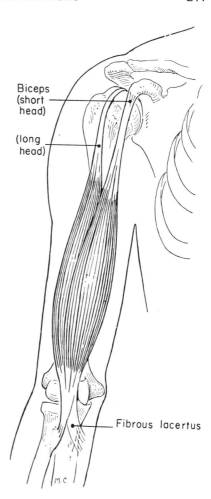

Figure 13–4. Biceps muscle of the arm.

prevented from doing so (by the action of neutralizers), the biceps simultaneously flexes and supinates the forearm (Fig. 13–5, A).

Some kinesiologists have been interested in the question as to whether the forcefulness of elbow flexion was related to the position of the forearm. Neither Beevor nor Wright could find any appreciable relation.[2, 12] Recent investigators have found that maximum strength was obtained when the forearm was either in the midposition or in supination.[4, 5, 8, 9] (See page 223.)

BRACHIALIS (Fig. 13–6.)

Proximal attachment. (O) Anterior surface of lower half of humerus.

Distal attachment. (I) Anterior surface of coronoid process of ulna.

Nerve supply. Musculocutaneous and branch from radial nerves.

Where to palpate. Just lateral to the biceps if the contraction

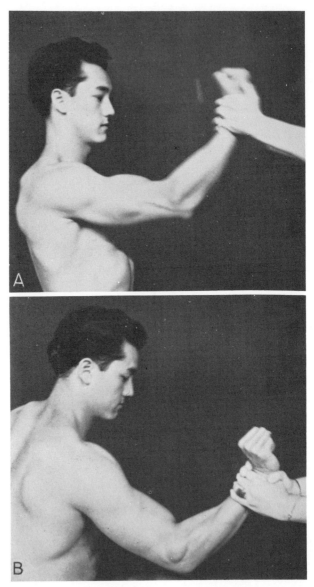

Figure 13-5. Flexion of the forearm. *A,* In a position of supination; *B,* in a position of pronation.

is sufficiently strong, and especially if the forearm is flexed in the pronated position.

Action.   Flexion at elbow joint.

Comments.   Basmajian reported that electromyographic investigations support the claim that the brachialis is an unexcelled flexor of the forearm under all conditions.[1] (See Fig. 13–6.)

BRACHIORADIALIS (Fig. 13–7.)

Proximal attachment. (O)   Upper two thirds of lateral supracondylar ridge of humerus.

Distal attachment. (I)   Lateral side of base of styloid process of radius.

Nerve supply.   Radial nerve.

Where to palpate.   On anterior-radial aspect of upper half of forearm.

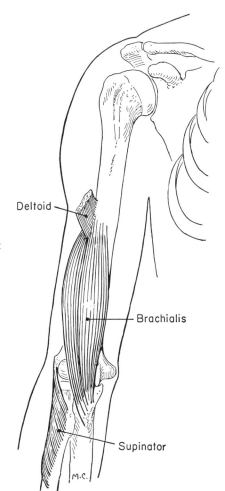

Figure 13–6.   Deep muscles on front of right arm.

Deltoid

Brachialis

Supinator

M.C.

Action. Flexion at elbow joint; may help to reduce pronation or supination of forearm during flexion.

Comments. The brachioradialis is primarily a flexor of the forearm. If the forearm is either pronated or supinated, however, it may help to "de-rotate" the forearm at the same time that it flexes it, but this has not been confirmed by electromyographic research. According to Basmajian and Latif, and DeSousa et al., the brachioradialis neither supinates nor pronates the fully extended forearm unless the movement is strongly resisted.[1, 3] It has also been noted that the brachioradialis is most active in quick movements (Travill and Basmajian).[1]

PRONATOR TERES (Fig. 13–7.)

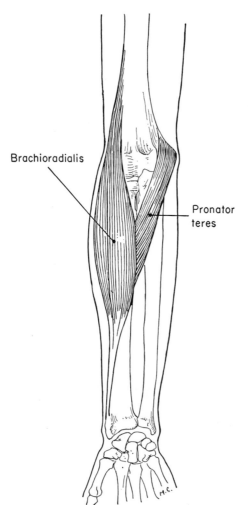

Brachioradialis

Pronator teres

Figure 13–7. Superficial muscles on front of right forearm.

Proximal attachments. (O) Medial epicondyle of humerus and medial side of coronoid process of ulna.

Distal attachment. (I) Lateral surface of radius near middle.

Nerve supply. Medial nerve.

Cannot be palpated.

Action. Pronation of forearm; assists in flexing forearm against resistance.[1]

Comments. Although the pronator teres is listed both with the pronators and with the flexors of the forearm, it is primarily a pronator.

PRONATOR QUADRATUS (Fig. 13–8.)

Medial attachment. (O) Anterior surface of lower fourth of ulna.

Lateral attachment. (I) Anterior surface of lower fourth of radius.

Nerve supply. Branch from median nerve.

Cannot be palpated.

Action. Pronation of forearm.

Comments. Experiments performed by Basmajian and Travill showed that the electrical activity of the pronator quadratus was definitely greater than that of the pronator teres, irrespective of the speed of the movement or the degree of elbow flexion.[1]

TRICEPS BRACHII (Figs. 13–9 and 13–10.)

Proximal attachments (O)

    Long head: Infraglenoid tuberosity.

    Lateral head: Posterior surface of upper half of humerus.

    Medial head: Posterior surface of lower two thirds of humerus.

Distal attachment. (I) Olecranon process of ulna.

Nerve supply. Radial nerve.

Where to palpate. Posterior surface of upper arm.

Action. Extension of forearm at elbow joint.

Comments. The triceps, virtually three muscles in one, covers the entire posterior surface of the upper arm. Only its long head crosses the shoulder joint. Its fibers are for the most part longitudinal,

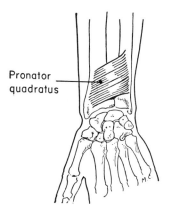

Figure 13–8. Anterior view of distal end of forearm showing pronator quadratus.

Pronator quadratus

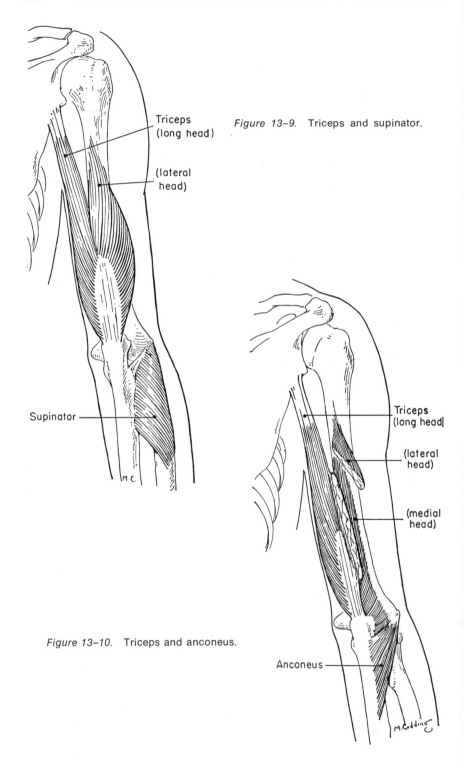

Figure 13–9. Triceps and supinator.

Figure 13–10. Triceps and anconeus.

running parallel with the long axis of the humerus. The medial and lateral portions run parallel to the long head at first, then turn toward it obliquely downward to unite with its broad flat tendon of attachment. The triceps is a forceful extensor of the forearm. Two factors contributing to its effectiveness are its large physiologic cross section (p. 91) and its favorable angle of pull (p. 92 ff.).

In a comparison of the three heads it was noted that the medial head appears to be the principal extensor of the forearm. It is usually accompanied by the lateral head, and by both the lateral and long heads against resistance.[1]

ANCONEUS (Fig. 13–10.)

Proximal attachment. (O)   Posterior surface of lateral epicondyle of humerus.

Distal attachment. (I)   Lateral side of olecranon process and posterior surface of upper part of ulna.

Nerve supply.   Branch from radial nerve.

Where to palpate.   Lateral margin of olecranon process of back of elbow.

Action.   Extension of forearm.

Comments.   In an electromyographic study of elbow joint muscles conducted in 1967, Pauly et al. found that the anconeus initiates extension of the forearm, helps to maintain the extended position, and appears to stabilize the elbow joint during other movements of the upper extremity. The investigators noted that it was particularly active during pronation of the forearm.[7]

SUPINATOR (Figs. 13–6 and 13–9.)

Proximal attachment. (O)   Lateral condyle of humerus; adjacent portion of ulna; radial collateral and annular ligaments.

Distal attachment. (I)   Lateral surface of upper third of radius.

Nerve supply.   Branch from deep radial nerve.

Cannot be palpated.

Action.   Supination of forearm under all conditions.

SUPPLEMENTARY MATERIAL

Relation of Forearm Position to the Strength of Elbow Flexion. Since the author's modest study[11] of this problem in which she adapted a grip dynamometer in a pull type holder to measure the strength of the elbow flexors of ten young women, there have been several reports of studies on larger numbers of subjects and using more appropriate equipment. With possibly one exception, these reverse her findings with respect to supination and the midposition of the forearm.

In 1952 Downer measured 30 female subjects, using a Beasley myodynemeter (an electronic instrument) in both a breaking point test and an isometric test. She found that the strongest contraction of the elbow flexors was obtained when the forearm was in the midposition and the least strong when the forearm was pronated.[4]

In 1955 Provins and Salter[8] measured eight male and four female subjects, and in 1956 Rasch[9] measured 24 male subjects. A strain gauge dynamometer was used in both investigations. In each study, as in Downer's, it was found that the greatest degree of elbow flexion strength was recorded when the forearm was in the midposition and the least when it was pronated.

The most recent study of the relation of forearm position to the strength of elbow flexion was made in 1969 by Larson. He stated two objectives: the first, "to determine if electromyograms obtained from surface electrodes overlying the areas of the biceps brachii, the brachialis, the brachioradialis, and the pronator teres muscles are affected by different forearm positions when performing several trials of maximal isometric elbow-flexor contractions," and the second, "to determine the effects of supination, pronation, and midposition on the force exerted by the elbow flexors during maximal isometric contractions." For subjects, he used thirty males with an age range of 17 to 31 years.

The subjects assumed the hook-lying position, the elbow was flexed to 65 degrees, the upper arm and elbow were fully supported on the table and the elbow was braced manually by an assistant. Instructions were given not to arch the back nor to raise the head or shoulders during maximal exertion. Maximal isometric elbow-flexor contractions were then performed three times in each of three forearm positions—supination, midposition and pronation. Cable-tensiometer scores were recorded and, at the same time, electromyographic recordings were obtained from the biceps-brachialis area, the brachioradialis area, and the pronator teres area. Larson assumed that the brachialis muscle was equally active in all three positions as it inserts into the ulna and would therefore not be affected by changes in the forearm position.

The results of this study led Larson to conclude that, within the scope of the study, (1) the biceps is most active electrically when the forearm is supinated, and least active when it is pronated, (2) the brachioradialis is most active electrically when the forearm is either in the midposition or in supination, and least active when the forearm is pronated, (3) the pronator teres, as a flexor, does not seem to be significantly affected by the position of the forearm, and (4) the isometric force exerted by the elbow flexors during maximal voluntary contractions is greatest when the forearm is supinated or in midposition, and least when the forearm is pronated.[5]

In their 1957 study of the biceps, brachialis and brachioradialis, Basmajian and Latif noted: (1) that the biceps flexed the supinated forearm and assisted in flexing the semiprone forearm when the movement was resisted; (2) that the brachialis flexed the forearm under all conditions, it being the "workhorse" of the elbow joint; and (3) that the brachioradialis was a rapid flexor of the forearm but that it also aided in slow flexion when the movement was resisted. They concluded that the three muscles act together with maximum electrical activity when the forearm is in the "semiprone" position; i.e., midposition, flexing against resistance.[1]

Relation of Different Forearm Positions to the Strength Exerted by the Elbow and Shoulder Muscles in Chinning. In 1963 McCraw, using 51 young men as subjects, investigated the effect of forearm positions (pronation, supination, mid-position, one forearm pronated and the other supinated) on the muscular strength used in chinning. An aircraft cable tensiometer was used to measure strength. He found that the variation in strength from position to position was no greater than that from trial to trial in the same position. He concluded from this that there appeared to be little justification for requiring a particular position of the forearms for pull-ups.[6]

His study is significant for at least two reasons, first his appreciation of the fact that the muscles used in extending the upper arms are as important in the performance of pull-ups as are the muscles that flex the elbows; and second, his recognition of the variations in day-to-day performance and his comparison of these with the variations due to the forearm position.

DEMONSTRATIONS AND LABORATORY EXERCISES

Joint Structure and Function

1. Using a form like the one in Appendix B, record the essential information regarding the two articulations of the elbow joint, likewise the two radioulnar articulations. Study the movements of these joints both on the skeleton and on the living body.

2. With a humerus, radius and ulna, "construct" an elbow joint, using felt for fibrocartilage and adhesive tape for ligaments. Attach these structures accurately. It is suggested that two or three students work together on this project.

3. Using a Lufkin rule or a protractor-goniometer, measure the range of motion in flexion, pronation and supination of the forearm on five different subjects.

Muscular Action. Record the results on the chart found in Appendix F.

4. FLEXION

Subject: Sit with entire arm resting on table. Flex forearm (*a*) with palm up (forearm supinated), (*b*) with thumb up (forearm in neutral position, and (*c*) with palm down (forearm pronated).

Assistant: Resist movement by holding wrist. Steady upper arm if necessary.

Observer: Palpate as many of the forearm flexors as possible. Do you notice any difference in the muscular action in *a, b* and *c*?

5. EXTENSION

a. Subject: Lie face down on table with arm raised to shoulder level, with upper arm resting on table, and with forearm hanging down. Extend forearm without moving upper arm.

Assistant: Steady upper arm and resist forearm at wrist.

Observer: Palpate the triceps and anconeus.

b. Subject: On hands and knees, bend and extend the elbows in a push-up exercise.

Observer: Palpate the triceps and anconeus.

6. SUPINATION

Subject: Assume hand-shaking position with assistant and turn forearm outward.

Assistant: Assume same position with subject and resist his movement.

Observer: Palpate and identify the muscles which contract.

7. PRONATION

Subject: Assume hand-shaking position with assistant and turn forearm inward.

Assistant: Assume same position with subject and resist movement.

Observer: Palpate and identify the muscles which contract. What is their function? Can you palpate the principal movers?

Action of Muscles Other Than Movers

8. SUPINATION WITHOUT FLEXION

Subject: Sit with arm supported, elbow in slightly flexed position and relaxed. Supinate forearm without increasing or decreasing flexion at elbow.

Observer: Palpate the triceps. Explain.

9. VIGOROUS FLEXION OF FOREARM

Subject: Flex forearm vigorously, then check movement suddenly before completing full range of motion.

Observer: Palpate the triceps. Does it contract during any part of the movement? Explain.

10. Perform a movement in which the supinator acts as a neutralizer.

REFERENCES

1. Basmajian, J. V.: Muscles Alive, 2nd ed. Baltimore, The Williams & Wilkins Company, 1967. Chapter 9, The Upper Limb.
2. Beevor, C.: The Croonian Lectures on Muscular Movements. Reprint. New York, The Macmillan Company, 1951.
3. DeSousa, O. M., DeMoraes, J. L., and Vieria, F. L. de M.: Electromyographic study of the brachioradialis muscle. Anat. Rec., *139*:125–131, 1961.
4. Downer, A. H.: Strength of the elbow flexor muscles. Phys. Ther. Rev., *33*:68–70, 1953.
5. Larson, R. F.: Forearm positioning on maximal elbow-flexor force. J. Am. Phys. Ther. Assn., *49*:748–756, 1969.
6. McCraw, L. W.: Effects of variations of forearm position in elbow flexion. Res. Quart. Am. Assn. Health, Phys. Ed. & Recrn., *35*:504–510, 1964.
7. Pauly, J. E., Rushing, J. L., and Scheving, L. E.: An electromyographic study of some muscles crossing the elbow joint. Anat. Rec. *159*:47–53, 1967.
8. Provins, K. A., and Salter, N.: Maximum torque exerted above the elbow joint. J. Appl. Physiol., *7*:393–398, 1955.
9. Rasch, P. J.: Effect of position of forearm on strength of elbow flexion. Res. Quart. Am. Assn. Health, Phys. Ed. & Recrn., *27*:333–337, 1956.
10. Steindler, A.: Kinesiology of the Human Body. Springfield, Ill., Charles C Thomas, Publisher, 1955.
11. Wells, K. F.: Kinesiology, 3rd ed. Philadelphia, W. B. Saunders Company, 1960, p. 165.
12. Wright, W. G.: Muscle Function. New York, Hafner Publishing Company, 1962.

CHAPTER 14

The Upper Extremity:
The Wrist and Hand

Philosophers and scientists alike have paid tribute to man's hand for the part it has played in human culture. Even the psalmist was indirectly honoring man's hand when he praised God's creations as "the work of thy fingers." With such an appreciation of the significance of the human hand as a background the student of kinesiology will find his study of the structure and movements of the hand to be more meaningful. No piece of modern machinery is more delicately constructed or more perfectly coordinated than the human hand. The extraordinary versatility of the hand is due largely to the thumb's ability to separate widely from the rest of the hand, to swing around in front of the palm, and to press with equal force against any one of the four fingers. Its action is like that of a crane which revolves on its base and then swings down and up to perform its task.

In a sense, the wrist is simply a mechanism for contributing to the usefulness of the hand, for it adds to the variety of positions in which the hand may be used. The same is true of the elbow joint and the radioulnar articulations, and even of the shoulder. In a sense, all the joints of the upper extremity may be looked upon as servants of the hand.

The hand and wrist owe their unusual mobility to their generous supply of joints (Fig. 14–1). The most proximal of these is the radiocarpal or wrist joint. Just beyond this are the two rows of carpal bones, each row consisting of four bones. The carpal joints include the articulations within each of these rows, as well as the articulations between the two rows. The carpometacarpal joints are located at the base of the hand. Closely associated with them are the intermetacarpal joints, those points of contact between the base of each metacarpal bone—except that of the thumb—and its neighbor. The fingers unite with the hand at the metacarpophalangeal joints. In the fingers themselves are the two sets of interphalangeal joints, the first between the proximal and middle rows of phalanges, and the second between the middle and distal rows. The thumb differs from the four fingers in having a more freely movable metacarpal bone and in consisting of two phalanges instead of three. The metacarpal bone of the thumb is so similar to a phalanx that it might well be described as a cross between a phalanx and a metacarpal.

Structure of the Wrist Joint.   The wrist joint is an ovoid (condyloid) joint formed by the union of the slightly concave, oval-shaped surface of the radius and articular disk with the slightly convex, oval-shaped surface of the proximal row of carpal bones (i.e., the navicular, lunate and triquetral bones, but not the pisiform). The distal radioulnar joint is in close proximity to the wrist joint and shares with it the articular disk which lies between the head of the ulna and the triquetral bone of the wrist. Yet it is not a part of the wrist joint, for each joint has its own articular capsule. The capsule of the wrist consists of four ligaments which merge to form a continuous cover for the joint (Fig. 14–1).

CAPSULAR LIGAMENTS

Volar radiocarpal. (Fig. 14–2.) A strong ligament, attached above to the anterior margin of the radius and articular disk, and below to both rows of carpal bones and to the volar intercarpal ligament.

Dorsal radiocarpal. (Fig. 14–3.) A thin, membranous ligament, attached above to the posterior margin of the radius and articular disk, and below to the proximal row of carpal bones.

Ulnar collateral ligament of the wrist. (Figs. 14–2 and 14–3.) A small fan-shaped ligament, attached above by its apex to the styloid process of the ulna and to the articular disk, and below by its base to the pisiform bone and the transverse carpal ligament (Fig. 14–14).

Radial collateral ligament of the wrist. (Figs. 14–2 and 14–3.) A

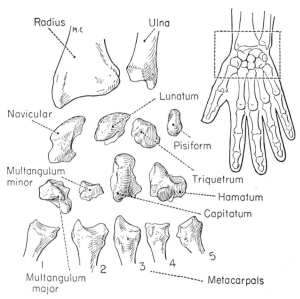

Figure 14–1.   Bones of the wrist. (Anterior view.)

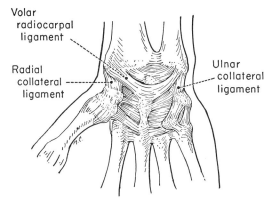

Figure 14–2.   Anterior view of right wrist joint showing ligaments.

small band of fibers, attached above to the styloid process of the radius, radiating downward to attach to the navicular, capitate and greater multangular bones.

Movements of the Wrist Joint

FLEXION.   From the anatomic position (Fig. 1–1, *B*) this is a forward-upward movement in the sagittal plane, whereby the palmar surface of the hand approaches the anterior surface of the forearm.

EXTENSION.   Return movement from flexion.

HYPEREXTENSION.   A movement in which the dorsal surface of the hand approaches the posterior surface of the forearm—the exact opposite of flexion.

RADIAL FLEXION (ABDUCTION).   From the anatomic position this is a sideward movement in the frontal plane, whereby the hand moves away from the body and the thumb side of the hand approaches the radial side of the forearm.

ULNAR FLEXION (ADDUCTION).   From the anatomic position this is a sideward movement in the frontal plane, whereby the hand

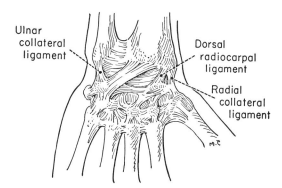

Figure 14–3.   Posterior view of right wrist joint showing ligaments.

moves toward the body and the little finger side of the hand approaches the ulnar side of the forearm.

CIRCUMDUCTION. A movement of the hand at the wrist whereby the finger tips describe a circle, and the hand as a whole describes a cone. It consists of flexion, radial flexion, hyperextension and ulnar flexion, taking place in sequence in either direction.

Structure and Movements of the Midcarpal and Intercarpal Joints. The articulation between the four carpal bones in the proximal row with the four in the distal row is known as the midcarpal articulation.* The joints between the bones within either row are known as the intercarpal joints of the proximal and distal rows, respectively.* All these joints are diarthrodial in structure, a joint cavity being present in each. Within this classification they belong to the non-axial group. This means that they permit only a slight gliding motion between the bones. Although this is the only type of motion that takes place in the individual joints composing the midcarpal articulation, these movements add up to a modified hinge type of movement for the midcarpal joint as a whole.

A further characteristic of the carpal region is that the bones are shaped and arranged in such a way that the anterior surface of the carpal region is slightly concave from side to side. This provides a protected passageway for the tendons, nerves and blood vessels supplying the hand. Among the many carpal ligaments, the radiate is the strongest. Its fibers radiate from the capitate to the navicular, lunate and triquetral bones on the anterior surface of the wrist.

Structure of the Carpometacarpal and Intermetacarpal Joints. (Fig. 14–4.) In many anatomy books the difference between the carpometacarpal joint of the thumb and that of the four fingers is emphasized. The former is described as a saddle joint, the latter as irregular (non-axial) joints. Morris, however, quotes Fick as describing the carpometacarpal joints of all the fingers as modified saddle joints, the joint of the little finger more nearly approaching a true saddle joint than any other except that of the thumb.[3] A careful inspection of these joints on the skeleton will probably lead the reader to agree with Fick. In regard to the carpometacarpal joint of the thumb, that is, the joint between the first metacarpal and greater multangular bones, there is no disagreement. It is clearly a saddle joint (Fig. 14–4). It is enclosed in an articular capsule which is stronger in back than in front. The capsule is thick but loose, and serves to restrict motion rather than to prevent it. There are no additional ligaments.

The carpometacarpal joints of the four fingers are not only encased in capsules, but are also protected by the dorsal, volar and interosseous carpometacarpal ligaments (Figs. 14–6 and 14–7). Closely associated with these joints are the intermetacarpal articulations, the joints between the bases of the metacarpal bones of the four fingers. These are irregular joints. They share the capsules of the carpometacarpal

---

*Anatomists differ in regard to these definitions. See both Gray's and Morris' Anatomy textbooks.[2, 3]

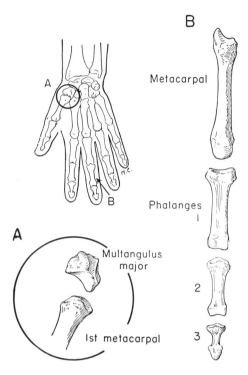

Figure 14-4. Bones of the hand showing selected joint surfaces. *A,* Carpometacarpal joint of thumb (a saddle joint). *B,* Metacarpal bone and phalanges of middle finger. (Anterior view.)

joints and are further reinforced by the dorsal, volar and interosseous basal ligaments, also by the transverse metacarpal ligament, a narrow fibrous band which connects the heads of the four outer metacarpal bones.

Movements of the Carpometacarpal and Intermetacarpal Joints: Carpometacarpal Joint of Thumb

ABDUCTION. (Fig. 14-5, *A.*) A forward movement of the thumb at right angles to the palm.

ADDUCTION. Return movement from abduction.

HYPERADDUCTION. (Fig. 14-5, *B.*) A backward movement of the thumb at right angles to the hand.

EXTENSION. (Fig. 14-5, *C.*) A lateral movement of the thumb away from the index finger.

FLEXION. (Fig. 14-5, *D.*) Return movement from extension.

HYPERFLEXION. (Fig. 14-5, *E.*) A medialward movement of the thumb from a position of slight abduction. The thumb slides across the front of the palm.

CIRCUMDUCTION. A movement in which the thumb as a whole describes a cone and the tip of the thumb describes a circle. It consists of all the movements described above, performed in sequence in either direction.

OPPOSITION. (Fig. 14-5, *F.*) This movement, which makes it possible to touch the tip of the thumb to the tip of any of the four fingers, is essentially a combination of abduction and hyperflexion and, according to some investigators, slight inward rotation. Others claim that what appears to be inward rotation of the metacarpal is actually a slight medial movement of the greater multangular bone with which the metacarpal articulates. The movements of the metacarpal are accompanied by flexion of the two phalanges, especially the distal. The apparent rotatory movement is explained in part by the oblique axis of motion about which abduction and adduction of the thumb take place, and in part by the movement of the greater multangular bone which accompanies flexion of the thumb. The total movement of the thumb in opposition might well be described as a movement of partial circumduction.

Movements of the Carpometacarpal and Intermetacarpal Joints of Fingers. The motion taking place in most of these joints is slight. It serves to supplement the movements of the wrist. The fifth carpo-

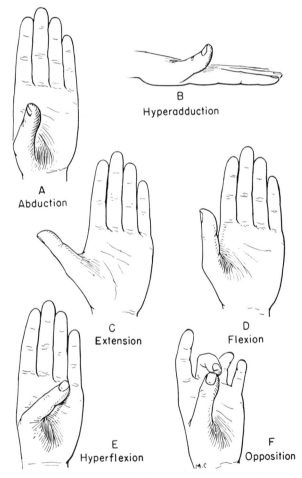

Figure 14–5.   Movements of the thumb at the carpometacarpal joint.

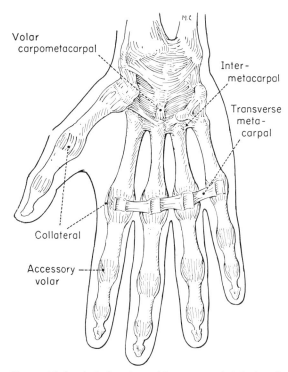

Figure 14–6.   Anterior view of ligaments of right hand.

metacarpal joint is slightly more mobile and permits a limited motion of the fifth metacarpal bone, somewhat resembling the motion of the thumb.

Structure of the Metacarpophalangeal Joints. (Figs. 14–4, 14–6 and 14–7.)   The joint at the base of each of the four fingers, uniting the proximal phalanx with the corresponding metacarpal bone, is an ovoid (condyloid) joint. The oval, convex head of the metacarpal fits into the shallow oval fossa at the base of the phalanx. The fossa is deepened slightly by the fibrocartilaginous volar accessory ligament. The joint is encased in a capsule and is protected on each side by strong collateral ligaments.

The metacarpophalangeal joint of the thumb has flatter joint surfaces than do the corresponding joints of the four fingers and has more of the characteristics of a hinge joint. In addition to the articular capsule, it is protected by a collateral ligament on each side and by a dorsal ligament.

Movements of the Metacarpophalangeal Joints of the Four Fingers

FLEXION.   The anterior surface of the finger approaches the palmar surface of the hand.

EXTENSION.   Return movement from flexion. Most individuals are able to achieve slight hyperextension in these joints.

ABDUCTION. For the fourth, fifth and index fingers this is a lateral movement away from the middle finger. This movement is limited and cannot be performed when the fingers are fully flexed.

ADDUCTION. Return movement from abduction.

Note: In place of abduction and adduction, the lateral movements of the middle finger are termed radial and ulnar flexion. These are comparable to radial and ulnar flexion at the wrist.

CIRCUMDUCTION. The combination of flexion, abduction, extension and adduction performed in sequence in either direction.

Movements of the Metacarpophalangeal Joints of the Thumb

FLEXION. The volar surface of the thumb approaches that of the thenar eminence (base of thumb).

EXTENSION. Return movement from flexion. Individuals vary greatly in their ability to hyperextend the thumb at this joint.

The Interphalangeal Joints. (Figs. 14–4, 14–6 and 14–7.)   As the name implies, these are the joints between the adjacent phalanges of the fingers or thumb. They are all hinge joints; hence their only movements are flexion and extension. These correspond to flexion and extension of the first phalanx at the metacarpophalangeal joints. Hyperextension is slight, if present at all. Each joint is enclosed within an articular capsule which is strengthened in front by an

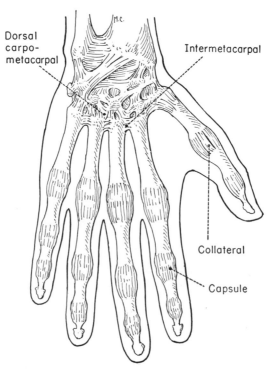

Figure 14–7.   Posterior view of ligaments of right hand.

accessory volar ligament and on each side by a strong collateral ligament.

Muscles of the Wrist, Fingers and Thumb. These muscles are treated in the same section because movement of the hand at the wrist joint is brought about almost as much by the forearm muscles of the fingers and thumb as by the wrist muscles proper. Certainly no analysis of wrist movements would be complete without mention of the finger and thumb muscles that assist the muscles of the wrist.

MUSCLES OF THE WRIST

Anterior	*Posterior*
Flexor carpi radialis	Extensor carpi radialis longus
Palmaris longus	Extensor carpi radialis brevis
Flexor carpi ulnaris	Extensor carpi ulnaris

MUSCLES OF THE FINGERS AND THUMB

Located on the Forearm	*Located in the Hand*
Fingers:	Fingers:
Flexor digitorum superficialis	Lumbricales manus
Flexor digitorum profundus	Interossei palmares
Extensor digitorum	Interossei dorsales manus
Extensor indicis	Abductor digiti minimi
Extensor digiti minimi	Flexor digiti minimi brevis
	Opponens digiti minimi
Thumb:	Thumb:
Flexor pollicis longus	Flexor pollicis brevis
Extensor pollicis longus	Abductor pollicis brevis
Extensor pollicis brevis	Opponens pollicis
Abductor pollicis longus	Adductor pollicis

FLEXOR CARPI RADIALIS (Fig. 14–8.)

Proximal attachment. (O) Medial epicondyle of humerus.

Distal attachment. (I) Anterior surface of base of second metacarpal.

Nerve supply. Median nerve.

Where to palpate. Anterior surface of wrist, just lateral to the tendon of palmaris longus.

Action. Flexion; assists in radial flexion of wrist.

PALMARIS LONGUS (Figs. 14–8 and 14–9.)

Proximal attachment. (O) Medial epicondyle of humerus.

Distal attachments. (I) Transverse carpal ligament and palmar aponeurosis.

Nerve supply. Median nerve.

Where to palpate. Anterior surface of wrist in exact center. It is the most prominent of the flexor tendons.

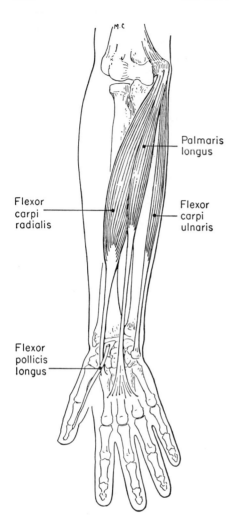

Palmaris
longus

Flexor
carpi
radialis

Flexor
carpi
ulnaris

Flexor
pollicis
longus

Figure 14–8. Superficial muscles on front of right forearm.

Action. Flexion of wrist.

FLEXOR CARPI ULNARIS (Fig. 14–8.)

Proximal attachments. (O) By two heads, from medial condyle of humerus and medial border of olecranon process of ulna.

Distal attachments. (I). Palmar surface of pisiform and hamate carpal bones, and base of fifth metacarpal.

Nerve supply. Ulnar nerve.

Where to palpate. Anterior surface of ulnar side of forearm. Tendon may be felt on medial side of anterior surface of wrist, just proximal to the pisiform bone.

Action. Flexion and ulnar flexion of wrist.

EXTENSOR CARPI RADIALIS LONGUS (Fig. 14–10, A.)

Proximal attachments. (O) Lateral epicondyle of humerus and supracondyloid ridge above it.

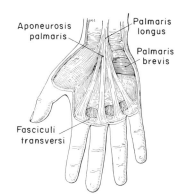

Figure 14–9. Palmar aponeurosis and palmaris muscles of right palm.

Distal attachment. (I)   Posterior surface of base of second metacarpal.

Nerve supply. Radial nerve.

Where to palpate.   Center of dorsal surface of forearm, about 2 inches below the elbow when forearm is in pronated position, as when palm rests on table. Also dorsal surface of wrist in line with index finger.

Action.   Extension and radial flexion of wrist; assists in flexion of forearm against resistance when forearm is pronated.

EXTENSOR CARPI RADIALIS BREVIS (Fig. 14–10, A.)

Proximal attachment. (O)   Lateral epicondyle of humerus.

Distal attachment. (I)   Posterior surface of base of third metacarpal.

Nerve supply.   Radial nerve.

Where to palpate.   Dorsal surface of forearm, slightly below the extensor carpi radialis longus. Difficult to distinguish from the latter.

Action.   Extension and radial flexion of wrist; assists in flexion of forearm against resistance when forearm is pronated.

EXTENSOR CARPI ULNARIS (Fig. 14–10, A.)

Proximal attachments. (O)   By two heads, from lateral epicondyle of humerus and middle third of posterior ridge of ulna.

Distal attachment. (I)   Posterior surface of base of fifth metacarpal.

Nerve supply.   Deep radial nerve.

Where to palpate.   Ulnar margin of posterior surface of forearm, halfway between elbow and wrist.

Action.   Extension and ulnar flexion of wrist; assists in flexion of forearm against resistance when forearm is pronated.

FLEXOR DIGITORUM SUPERFICIALIS (Fig. 14–11, A.)

Proximal attachments. (O)   Humero-ulnar head: Medial epicondyle of humerus, ulnar collateral ligament, medial margin of coronoid process.

Radial head: Oblique line on anterior surface of shaft of radius.

Distal attachments. (I)   By four tendons to the four fingers, each tendon splitting to attach to the sides of the base of the middle phalanx.

Nerve supply. Median nerve.

Where to palpate. Palm of hand.

Action. Flexion of middle phalanges of fingers; assists in flexion of first phalanges and of wrist.

FLEXOR DIGITORUM PROFUNDUS (Fig. 14–11, *B.*)

Proximal attachment. (O) Upper two thirds of anterior and medial surfaces of ulna.

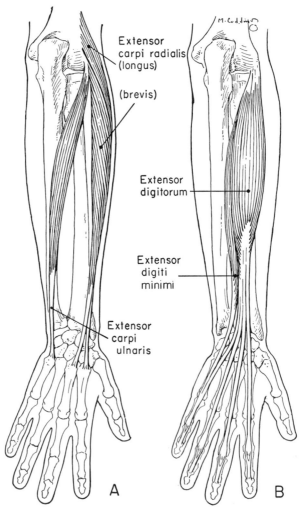

Figure 14–10. Muscles on back of right forearm. *A,* Extensor carpi radialis longus and brevis and extensor carpi ulnaris. *B,* Extensor digitorum and extensor digiti minimi.

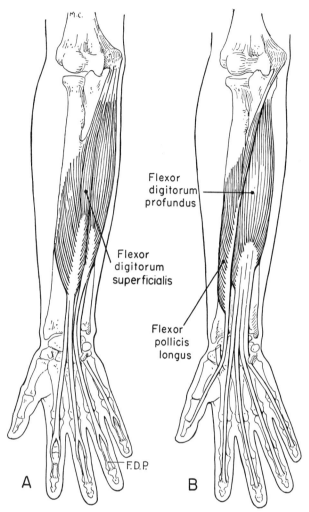

Figure 14–11. Deep muscles on front of right forearm. *A,* Flexor digitorum superficialis; *B,* flexor digitorum profundus and flexor pollicis longus.

Distal attachments. (I)   By four tendons to the four fingers, each
tendon passing through the corresponding tendon of the flexor
digitorum superficialis and attaching to the base of the distal phalanx.
   Nerve supply.   Interosseous branch of median nerve.
   Cannot be palpated.
   Action.   Flexion of distal phalanges of fingers; assists in flexion
of proximal middle phalanges and of wrist.
   FLEXOR POLLICIS LONGUS (Fig. 14–11, *B.*)
   Proximal attachment. (O)   Anterior surface of middle half of
radius.

Distal attachment. (I)   Anterior surface of base of distal phalanx of thumb.

Nerve supply. Volar interosseous branch of median nerve. Cannot be palpated.

Action.   Flexion of both phalanges of thumb; flexion of wrist; assists in adduction of thumb metacarpal.

EXTENSOR DIGITORUM (Fig. 14–10, *B.*)

Proximal attachment. (O)   Lateral epicondyle of humerus.

Distal attachments. (I)   By four tendons to the four fingers. Each tendon divides into three slips, the middle one attaching to the dorsal surface of the second phalanx and the other two uniting and attaching to the dorsal surface of the base of the distal phalanx.

Nerve supply.   Deep radial nerve.

Where to palpate.   Dorsal surface of hand and arm.

Action.   Extension of proximal phalanges of fingers; assists in extension of second and third phalanges and of wrist.

EXTENSOR INDICIS (Fig. 14–12.)

Proximal attachment. (O)   Dorsal surface of lower half of ulna.

Distal attachment. (I)   Unites with index finger tendon of extensor digitorum.

Nerve supply.   Deep radial nerve.

Cannot be palpated.

Action.   Extension of proximal phalanx of index finger; assists in extension of wrist.

EXTENSOR DIGITI MINIMI (Fig. 14–10, *B.*)

Proximal attachment. (O)   Proximal tendon of extensor digitorum.

Distal attachment. (I)   Unites with little finger tendon of extensor digitorum.

Nerve supply.   Deep radial nerve.

Cannot be palpated.

Action.   Extension of proximal phalanx of fifth finger; assists in extension of wrist.

EXTENSOR POLLICIS LONGUS (Fig. 14–12.)

Proximal attachment. (O)   Dorsal surface of middle third of ulna.

Distal attachment. (I)   Dorsal surface of base of distal phalanx of thumb.

Nerve supply.   Deep radial nerve.

Where to palpate.   If the hand is placed palm down on a table and the thumb raised as high as possible, the tendon may be clearly seen and palpated on the dorsal surface of the thumb and radial side of hand.

Action.   Extension of both phalanges of thumb; assists in adduction and, under some circumstances, extension of thumb metacarpal; assists in extension, and probably radial flexion, of wrist.

EXTENSOR POLLICIS BREVIS (Fig. 14–12.)

Proximal attachment (O)   Dorsal surface of radius below abductor pollicis longus.

Distal attachment. (I)   Dorsal surface of base of first phalanx.

Nerve supply.   Deep radial nerve.

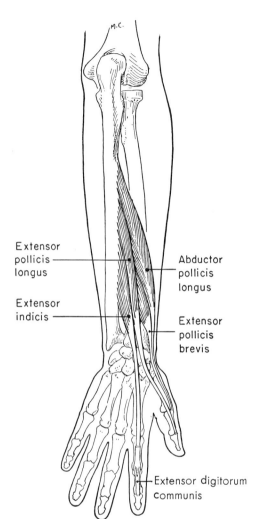

Figure 14–12.   Posterior muscles of the thumb and index finger.

Extensor pollicis longus

Extensor indicis

Abductor pollicis longus

Extensor pollicis brevis

Extensor digitorum communis

Where to palpate.   If the first phalanx is extended against resistance, the tendon stands out between the wrist and first metacarpophalangeal joint.

Action.   Extension of first phalanx of thumb; assists in extension and abduction of thumb metacarpal and in radial flexion of wrist.

Comments.   If the thumb is slightly hyperadducted and forcefully extended, both extensor tendons will stand out, leaving a deep hollow between them. This hollow has been called the anatomical snuff-box.

ABDUCTOR POLLICIS LONGUS (Fig. 14–12.)

Proximal attachment. (O)   Dorso-lateral surface of ulna below anconeus, dorsal surface of radius near center, and intervening interosseus membrane.

Distal attachment. (1)   Lateral surface of base of first metacarpal.
Nerve supply.   Deep radial nerve.

Where to palpate.   Just anterior to tendon of extensor pollicis brevis at base of metacarpal. The two tendons lie side by side.

Action.   Extension and abduction of thumb metacarpal; radial flexion of wrist; assists in flexion of wrist.

Comments on Flexion and Extension of Wrist and Fingers.   An interesting characteristic of the long finger muscles is the fact that they do not have sufficient length to permit the full range of motion in the joints of the fingers and wrist at the same time. For instance, it is impossible to achieve simultaneously complete flexion both of the fingers and of the hand because the antagonistic muscle, the extensor digitorum, will not stretch sufficiently to permit it. Likewise, it is impossible to achieve simultaneously complete extension of the fingers and hyperextension at the wrist because the two finger flexors, the digitorum superficialis and profundus, will not stretch sufficiently to permit it. Whether complete flexion is desired, or complete extension, in either case the antagonistic muscles act as a check rein. Thus, if complete flexion of the fingers is desired, the wrist can be flexed to only about half of its usual range, and if complete flexion at the wrist is desired, the fingers can be flexed only about half way.

Conversely, it is impossible to extend the fingers completely when the wrist is hyperextended to its limit of motion because of the pull on the finger flexors. This involuntary movement due to the tension of the opposing muscles is what is known as the tendon or pulley action of multijoint muscles (see p. 45). Because of this arrangement of the muscles the strongest finger flexion can be obtained when the wrist is held rigid in either a straight or slightly hyperextended position; the strongest finger extension, when the wrist is rigid in either a straight or slightly flexed position. The most powerful wrist action—either flexion or hyperextension—can take place only when the fingers are relaxed. In other words, strong finger action requires a rigid wrist; strong wrist action requires relaxed fingers. This aspect of wrist and finger action has been discussed exceptionally well by Wright.[4]

Muscles of the Fingers and Thumb Located in the Hand
ABDUCTOR DIGITI MINIMI MANUS (Fig. 14–13.)

Proximal attachments. (O)   Pisiform bone and tendon of flexor carpi ulnaris.

Distal attachments. (I)   Ulnar side of base of first phalanx of little finger and ulnar border of aponeurosis of extensor digiti minimi.

Nerve supply.   Ulnar nerve.

Where to palpate.   Ulnar border of hand.

Action.   Abduction of little finger; assists in flexion of first phalanx and extension of second and third phalanges.

FLEXOR DIGITI MINIMI BREVIS MANUS (Fig. 14–13.)

Proximal attachments. (O)   Hook of hamate bone and adjacent parts of transverse carpal ligament.

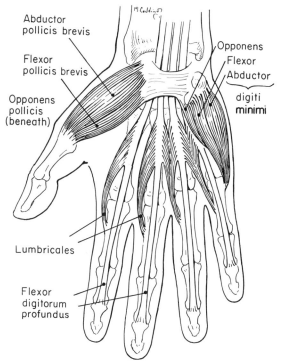

Figure 14-13. Muscles of right hand, anterior view.

Distal attachment. (I)   Ulnar side of base of first phalanx of little finger.

Nerve supply.   Palmar division of ulnar nerve.

Where to palpate.   On palm of hand just beside abductor digiti minimi. It is difficult to distinguish it from the latter muscle.

Action.   Flexion of proximal phalanx of little finger.

OPPONENS DIGITI MINIMI (Figs. 14–13 and 14–14.)

Proximal attachments. (O)   Hook of hamate bone and adjacent parts of transverse carpal ligament.

Distal attachment. (I)   Whole length of ulnar border of fifth metacarpal bone.

Nerve supply.   Deep palmar branch of ulnar nerve.

Cannot be palpated.

Action.   Combination of flexion and adduction of fifth meta-carpal bone, as in "cupping" the palm.

Comment.   This muscle is situated directly beneath the flexor brevis and abductor muscles for the same finger.

FLEXOR POLLICIS BREVIS (Fig. 14–13.)

Proximal attachments. (O)   Superficial head: Greater multangular bone and adjacent part of transverse carpal ligament. Deep head: Ulnar side of first metacarpal bone.

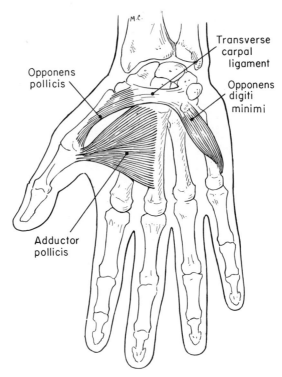

Figure 14–14.   Deep muscles of thumb and fifth metacarpal.

Distal attachments. (I) Superficial head: Radial side of base of first phalanx of thumb. Deep head: Ulnar side of base of first phalanx of thumb with adductor pollicis.

Nerve supply.   Median nerve.

Where to palpate.   The superficial head may be palpated along the ulnar margin of the anterior surface of the thenar eminence, but it is difficult to distinguish it from the abductor pollicis brevis.

Action.   Flexion of proximal phalanx of thumb; assists in abduction and hyperextension of thumb metacarpal.

Comment.   According to Basmajian, this muscle is dominant in maintaining a firm grip between the thumb and first two fingers, as when holding a cup by the handle.[1] The deep head is sometimes described as part of the palmar interossei. A sesamoid bone lies in the tendon of insertion of the superficial head.

ABDUCTOR POLLICIS BREVIS (Fig. 14–13.)

Proximal attachments. (O) Anterior surface of transverse carpal ligament, greater multangular bone and navicular bone.

Distal attachment. (I) Radial side of base of first phalanx of thumb.

Nerve supply.   Median nerve.

Where to palpate.   Anterior surface of thenar eminence.

Action. Abduction of thumb metacarpal; assists in flexion of proximal phalanx of thumb.

Comments. This is the most superficial muscle on the radial side of the thenar eminence.

OPPONENS POLLICIS (Figs. 14–13 and 14–14.)

Proximal attachments. (O) Anterior surface of greater multangular bone and transverse carpal ligament.

Distal attachment. (I) Whole radial border of anterior surface of first metacarpal.

Nerve supply. Median nerve.

Where to palpate. If the thumb is pressed hard against the middle finger, this muscle can be palpated along the lateral margin of the thenar eminence, close to the metacarpal bone.

Action. A combination of abduction, hyperflexion and possibly slight inward rotation of the thumb metacarpal, making it possible, when flexing the phalanges, to touch the tip of any of the four fingers.

ADDUCTOR POLLICIS (Fig. 14–14.)

Proximal attachments. (O) Carpal or oblique head: Deep carpal ligaments, capitate bone and bases of second and third metacarpal bones. Metacarpal or transverse head: Lower two thirds of anterior surface of third metacarpal bone.

Distal attachment. (I) Ulnar side of base of proximal phalanx of thumb.

Nerve supply. Deep palmar branch of ulnar nerve.

Where to palpate. On the inner anterior surface of the metacarpophalangeal joint of the thumb. It can easily be palpated when the thumb is pressed against one of the fingers.

Action. Adduction, flexion and hyperflexion of thumb metacarpal; flexion of proximal phalanx of thumb.

Comments. The two parts of this triangular shaped muscle are sometimes described as two separate muscles. A sesamoid bone is present in the tendon.

LUMBRICALES MANUS (Four in number) (Fig. 14–13.)

Proximal attachments. (O) Tendons of the flexor digitorum profundus in the middle of the palm.

Distal attachments. (I) Radial side of the tendons of the extensor digitorum.

Nerve supply. First and second lumbricales: Median nerve. Third and fourth lumbricales: Ulnar nerve.

Cannot be palpated.

Action. Flexion of proximal phalanges of fingers and extension of middle and distal phalanges.

Comments. The lumbrical muscles, so named because of their wormlike appearance, are situated deep in the palm of the hand.

INTEROSSEI PALMARES (Three in number) (Fig. 14–15.)

Proximal attachments (O)

> First: Ulnar side of second metacarpal bone.
> Second: Radial side of fourth metacarpal bone.
> Third: Radial side of fifth metacarpal bone.

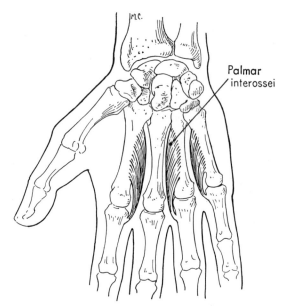

Figure 14–15.   Palmar interossei, right hand.

Distal attachments (I)

First: Ulnar side of base of first phalanx of index finger and expansion of extensor digitorum tendon.

Second: Radial side of base of first phalanx of fourth finger and expansion of extensor digitorum tendon.

Third: Radial side of base of first phalanx of fifth finger and expansion of extensor digitorum tendon.

Nerve supply.   Ulnar nerve.

Cannot be palpated.

Action.   Adduction and flexion of the second, fourth and fifth fingers at the metacarpophalangeal joints; extension of second and third phalanges of second, fourth and fifth fingers.

Comments.   These three small "between-the-bones" muscles are situated on the anterior surfaces of the second, fourth and fifth metacarpal bones on the side nearest the middle finger. A similar muscle, situated along the side of the first metacarpal bone, is sometimes described as one of the interossei palmares, sometimes as the deep head of the flexor pollicis brevis. (See description of the latter muscle.)

INTEROSSEI DORSALES MANUS (Four in number) (Fig. 14–16.)

Proximal attachments. (O)   By two heads from the adjacent sides of the metacarpal bones in each interspace.

Distal attachments. (I)   Base of proximal phalanx and aponeurosis of extensor muscles on each side of the middle finger, on the thumb side of the index finger and on the ulnar side of the fourth finger.

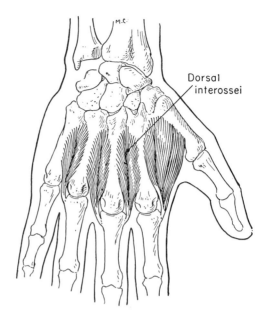

Figure 14–16. Dorsal interossei, right hand.

Nerve supply.   Palmar branch of ulnar nerve.
Cannot be palpated.
Action.   Abduction of index and fourth fingers; radial and ulnar
flexion of middle finger; flexion of proximal row of phalanges of
second, third and fourth fingers, and extension of middle and distal
rows.
Comments.   These are small bipenniform muscles. They occupy
the intervals between the metacarpal bones.

DEMONSTRATIONS AND LABORATORY EXERCISES

Joint Structure and Function
1. Using a form like the one in Appendix B, record the essential
information regarding the radiocarpal, the carpometacarpal, the metacarpophalangeal and the interphalangeal articulations. Study the
movements both on the skeleton and on the living body. Pay particular
attention to the carpometacarpal joint of the thumb.
2. With a Lufkin rule or protractor-goniometer measure the
amount of hyperextension possible at the wrist, (*a*) with the fingers
flexed; (*b*) with the fingers extended. Likewise measure the amount
of flexion possible at the wrist, (*a*) with the fingers flexed; (*b*) with the
fingers extended. Explain.
Muscular Action   (See check lists in Appendix F.) (If possible,
get someone who plays the piano to serve as subject.)
3. Flexion at Wrist
Subject: Sit with forearm resting on table with palm up. Flex hand
at wrist.

Assistant: Resist movement by holding palm.

Observer: Palpate, identify and explain the action of as many muscles as possible.

4. EXTENSION AND HYPEREXTENSION AT WRIST

Subject: Sit with forearm resting on table, palm down, hand hanging over edge of table. Extend hand at wrist.

Assistant: Resist movement by pressing on back of hand.

Observer: Palpate, identify and explain the action of as many muscles as possible.

5. RADIAL FLEXION AT WRIST

Subject: Sit with forearm resting on table, ulnar side (little finger side of hand) down. Keeping thumb against hand, raise hand from table without moving forearm.

Assistant: May give slight resistance to hand.

Observer: Palpate and identify the muscles responsible for radial flexion.

6. ULNAR FLEXION AT WRIST

Subject: Lie face down or bend forward in such a way that radial side of hand (thumb side) is on supporting surface, with forearm supported and wrist neither flexed nor hyperextended. Keeping little finger against hand, raise hand without moving forearm.

Assistant: May give slight resistance to hand.

Observer: Palpate and identify the muscles responsible for ulnar flexion.

7. FINGER FLEXION

Subject: Sit with forearm resting on table with palm up. Flex fingers without flexing at wrist.

Assistant: Resist movement by hooking own fingers over those of subject.

Observer: Palpate, identify and explain the action of as many muscles as possible.

8. FINGER EXTENSION

Subject: Sit with forearm resting on table with palm down, fingers curled over edge of table. Extend fingers.

Assistant: Resist movement by holding hand over subject's fingers.

Observer: Palpate, identify and explain the action of as many muscles as possible.

9. ABDUCTION OF THUMB

Subject: Place the hand on a table with the palm up and the thumb slightly separated from the index finger. Abduct the thumb at the carpometacarpal joint by raising it vertically upward.

Assistant: Give slight resistance to the thumb at the proximal phalanx.

Observer: Palpate the abductor pollicis brevis in the thenar eminence.

10. HYPERFLEXION OF THUMB IN POSITION OF SLIGHT ABDUCTION

Subject: Place the hand on a table with the palm up and the thumb slightly raised from the table. Hyperflex the thumb at the carpometacarpal joint.

Assistant: Give slight resistance to the proximal phalanx of the thumb.

Observer: Palpate the flexor pollicis brevis in the thenar eminence.

11. EXTENSION OF THUMB

Subject: Rest the fully extended hand on its ulnar border with the thumb uppermost. Extend the thumb as far as possible.

Observer: Identify the tendons of the abductor pollicis longus, the extensor pollicis longus and the extensor pollicis brevis.

12. OPPOSITION OF THUMB

Subject: Press the thumb hard against the tip of the middle finger.

Observer: Palpate and identify the opponens pollicis and adductor pollicis.

Action of Muscles Other Than Movers

13. Perform a movement in which the extensor carpi ulnaris and extensor carpi radialis longus and brevis act as neutralizers to prevent flexion at the wrist.

14. Perform a movement in which the extensor carpi ulnaris and flexor carpi ulnaris act as mutual neutralizers.

REFERENCES

1. Basmajian, J. V.: Muscles Alive, 2nd ed. Baltimore, The Williams & Wilkins Company, 1967, Chapter 10. Wrist, Hand and Fingers.
2. Goss, C. M.: Gray's Anatomy of the Human Body, 28th ed. Philadelphia, Lea & Febiger, 1966.
3. Schaeffer, J. P.: Morris' Human Anatomy, 11th ed. New York, McGraw-Hill, Inc., 1953.
4. Wright, W. G.: Muscle Function. New York, Hafner Publishing Company, 1962.

RECOMMENDED READINGS

(Particularly for Students of Physical and Occupational Therapy)

Eyler, D. L., and Markee, J. E.: The anatomy and function of the intrinsic musculature of the fingers. J. Bone & Joint Surg., *36A*:1–9, 1954.
Kendall, H. O., and Kendall, F. P.: Muscles: Testing and Function, 2nd ed. Baltimore, The Williams & Wilkins Company, 1970.
Long, C., Brown, M. E., and Weiss, G.: An electromyographic study of the extrinsic–intrinsic kinesiology of the hand: Preliminary report. Arch. Phys. Med. & Rehab., *41*:175–181, 1960.
Long, C.: Electromyographic kinesiology of the hand: Part II. Third dorsal interosseus and extensor digitorum of the long finger. Arch. Phys. Med. & Rehab., *42*:559–565, 1961.
Markee, J. E., and Eyler, D. L.: The Functional Anatomy of the Hand. Brochure to accompany film. Durham, N.C., Dept. of Anatomy, Duke University School of Medicine.

CHAPTER 15

The Lower Extremity: The Hip Joint and the Pelvic Girdle

The relationship between the hip joint and the pelvic girdle is somewhat similar to that between the shoulder joint and shoulder girdle. Just as the scapula tilts or rotates to put the glenoid fossa in a favorable position for the movements of the humerus, so the pelvic girdle tilts and rotates to put the acetabulum in a favorable position for the movements of the femur. There are these differences, however. Whereas the left and right sides of the shoulder girdle can move independently, the pelvic girdle can move only as a unit. Furthermore, whereas the movements of the shoulder girdle take place in its own joints (sternoclavicular and acromioclavicular), the pelvic girdle is dependent upon the lumbosacral joint and the hip joints for its movements. Hence an analysis of the movements of the pelvic girdle must always be in terms of spinal and hip action.

THE HIP JOINT

Structure. (Figs. 15–1, 15–2, 15–3, 15–4, 15–5.)   The hip joint is formed by the articulation of the spherical head of the femur with the deep cup-shaped acetabulum of the pelvis (Figs. 15–1 and 15–2). It is a typical ball-and-socket joint. The femoral head is completely covered with hyaline cartilage except for a small pit near the center, known as the fovea capitis, at which point the teres femoris is attached to the bone. The cartilage is thicker above and tapers to a thin edge at the circumference. Hyaline cartilage also lines the horseshoe-shaped surface of the acetabulum. It is thicker above than below. The center of the acetabulum is filled in with a mass of fatty tissue which is covered by synovial membrane. A flat rim of fibrocartilage, known as the glenoid labrum, is attached by its circumference to the margin of the acetabulum (Fig. 15–2). It covers the hyaline cartilage, and, since it is considerably thicker at the circumference than at the center, it serves to deepen the acetabulum. Also, since it is thicker above and behind, it serves to protect the acetabulum against the impact of the femoral head in forceful movements.

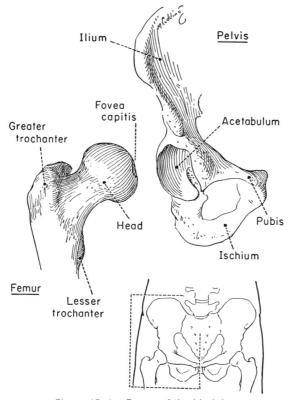

Figure 15–1.   Bones of the hip joint.

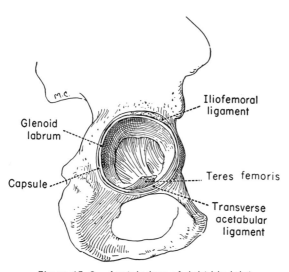

Figure 15–2.   Acetabulum of right hip joint.

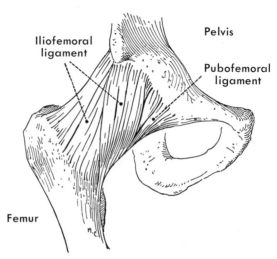

Figure 15-3. Anterior view of right hip joint.

The joint is enveloped in a loose, sleevelike capsule which is attached above to the margin of the acetabulum, and below to the distal margin of the anatomic neck of the femur. It is much thicker above and in front than it is below and behind. It consists of two sets of fibers, circular and longitudinal, and is reinforced by the iliofemoral, pubofemoral and ischiofemoral ligaments. It is lined with an extensive synovial membrane.

Ligaments

ILIOFEMORAL LIGAMENT. (Fig. 15-3.) This ligament, nicknamed the Y ligament because of its inverted Y shape, is an extraordinarily strong band of fibers located at the front of the capsule and intimately blended with it. Its shape is actually more that of a triangle or an inverted V than that of a Y. It is attached above to the anterior inferior spine of the ilium, and below by two divisions to the upper and the lower parts of the intertrochanteric line. It serves to check extension and both outward and inward rotation.

PUBOFEMORAL LIGAMENT. (Fig. 15-3.) This is a narrow band of fibers, attached above to the obturator crest and upper ramus of the pubis. Below, it blends with the fibers of the capsule. It prevents excessive abduction and helps to check extension and outward rotation.

ISCHIOFEMORAL LIGAMENT. (Fig. 15-4.) This is a strong triangular ligament on the back of the capsule. It is attached by its base to the ischium behind and below the margin of the acetabulum, and by its apex to the trochanteric fossa, the fibers blending with those of the capsule. It limits inward rotation and adduction in the flexed position.

TRANSVERSE ACETABULAR LIGAMENT. (Fig. 15-5.) This is a strong flat band of fibers, continuous with the glenoid labrum. It bridges the acetabular notch, thus completing the acetabular ring.

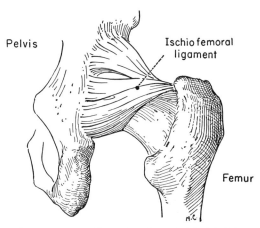

Figure 15-4.   Posterior view of right hip joint.

TERES FEMORIS. (Fig. 15-5.) This is a flat, narrow triangular band, sheathed in synovial membrane, lying within the hip joint. It is attached by its apex to the fovea capitis, the little pit near the center of the femoral head, and by its base to the margins of the acetabular notch and to the transverse acetabular ligament.

Position and Shape of Femur. The movements of the femur are similar to those of the humerus, but are not quite so free as the latter because of the deeper socket. In studying the movements of the femur the student should first be aware of the position of the femur in the fundamental standing position. If viewed from the front in this position, it is seen that the shaft of the femur is not vertical, but that it slants somewhat medialward. This serves to place the center of the knee joint more nearly under the center of motion of the hip joint.

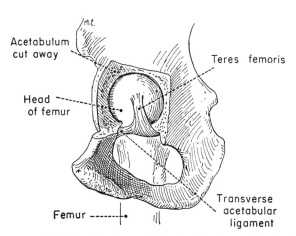

Figure 15-5.   Right hip joint from within, looking toward head of femur.

Hence the mechanical axis of the femur—a line connecting the center of the femoral head with the center of the knee joint—is almost vertical (Fig. 15–6). The degree of slant of the femoral shaft is related both to the size of the angle between the neck and shaft and to the width of the pelvis.

As seen from the side, the shaft of the femur bows forward. These characteristics of the femur—the obtuse neck-shaft angle and the forward bowing of the shaft—are, as Steindler has explained, provisions for resisting the strains and stresses sustained in walking, running and jumping, and for assuring the proper transmission of weight through the femur to the knee joint.

Movements of the Femur at the Hip Joint

FLEXION.   A forward movement of the femur in the sagittal plane. If the knee is straight, the movement is restricted by the tension of the hamstring muscles. In extreme flexion the pelvis tilts to supplement the movement at the hip joint.

EXTENSION.   Return movement from flexion.

HYPEREXTENSION.   A backward movement of the femur in the sagittal plane. This movement is extremely limited. Except in dancers and acrobats, it is possible only when the femur is rotated outward and is probably completely absent in many individuals. The restricting factor is the iliofemoral ligament at the front of the joint. The advantage of this restriction of movement is that it provides a stable joint for weight-bearing without the need for strong muscular contraction.

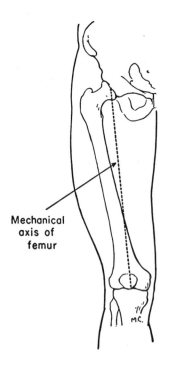

Mechanical
axis of
femur

Figure 15–6.   Mechanical axis of femur.

ABDUCTION. A sideward movement of the femur in the frontal plane so that the thigh moves away from the midline of the body. A greater range of movement is possible when the femur is rotated outward.

ADDUCTION. Return movement from abduction. Hyperadduction is possible only when the other leg is moved out of the way. In extreme hyperadduction the teres femoris becomes taut.

OUTWARD ROTATION. A rotation of the femur around its longitudinal axis so that the knee is turned outward.

INWARD ROTATION. A rotation of the femur around its longitudinal axis so that the knee is turned inward.

CIRCUMDUCTION. A combination of flexion, abduction, extension and adduction, performed sequentially in either direction.

Muscles. Several of the muscles which act at the hip joint act with equal or greater effectiveness at the knee joint. These are known as the two-joint muscles of the lower extremity. Only their action at the hip joint is recorded in this section.

Anterior:
  Iliopsoas
  Sartorius
  Pectineus
  Tensor fasciae latae
  Rectus femoris

Posterior:
  Gluteus maximus
  Biceps femoris ⎫
  Semitendinosus ⎬ "Hamstrings"
  Semimembranosus ⎭
  Six deep outward rotators

Lateral:
  Gluteus medius
  Gluteus minimus

Medial:
  Gracilis
  Adductor magnus
  Adductor longus
  Adductor brevis

ILIOPSOAS. (Fig. 15–7.) As the psoas major and iliacus muscles have a common distal attachment and act as one muscle at the hip joint, the usual practice of treating them as one muscle is followed here. The psoas is also included with the muscles of the spinal column.

Proximal attachments. (O) Psoas major: Sides of bodies and intervertebral cartilages of last thoracic and all lumbar vertebrae; front and lower borders of transverse processes of lumbar vertebrae. Iliacus: Anterior surface of ilium and base of sacrum.

Distal attachments. (I) Lesser trochanter of femur and for a short distance below along medial border of shaft.

Nerve supply. Femoral nerve.

Where to palpate. This muscle is almost impossible to palpate. The psoas major fibers may possibly be palpated on slender subjects who are able to keep the abdominal muscles relaxed during the testing. Two techniques are suggested.

1. The subject lies on his side, rolled toward the face, and flexes the thigh against resistance without contracting the abdominal muscles. The muscle may be palpated in the groin.

2. The subject lies on his back with the lower back arched as

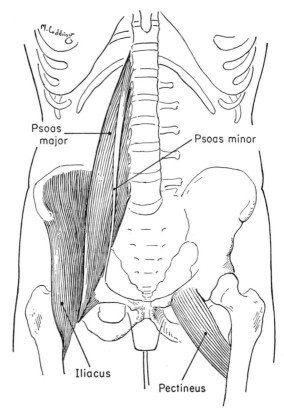

Figure 15–7. Anterior view of pelvic region showing psoas major and minor, iliacus and pectineus.

much as possible. From this position he flexes one thigh without contracting the abdominal muscles. An assistant should support the underside of the pelvis and try to prevent it from moving. The psoas may be palpated through the abdomen.

Action. Flexion of thigh on trunk; flexion of trunk (as a unit) on thighs when in supine lying position or in any position when movement is performed against resistance; probably helps to stabilize hip joint in standing position.

Comments. The iliopsoas is a strong hip flexor. There has been considerable disagreement concerning additional functions. There has been some evidence of both outward and inward rotation but it would be well to follow Basmajian's advice concerning this and abandon the controversy as there is insufficient evidence to support either side.

In regard to abduction or adduction, Steindler assumed that from its position the iliopsoas would *adduct* the femur but that such movement would be negligible. Basmajian quotes Close who stated at the conclusion of his EMG investigation that he found the iliopsoas to be definitely active in *abduction*, especially during extreme abduction. It may be of interest to the reader to look at Figure 15–6 which depicts the mechanical axis of the femur and to visualize the lines of pull of the iliopsoas. It will be noted that the only fibers that appear to be in a position to abduct are the outermost fibers of the iliacus which originate from the vicinity of the anterior superior iliac spine. It is the opinion of this author that conclusions regarding abduction or adduction should be postponed until additional investigations have been made.

SARTORIUS (Fig. 15–8.) (See also muscles of the knee.)

Proximal attachment. (O) Anterior superior iliac spine and upper half of notch below it.

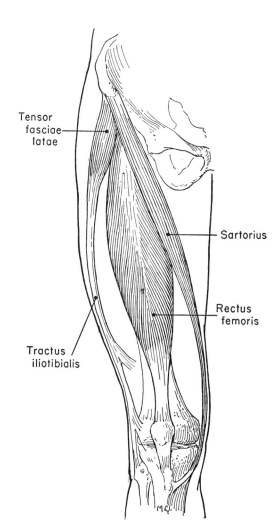

Tensor fasciae latae

Sartorius

Rectus femoris

Tractus iliotibialis

Figure 15–8. Muscles on front of right thigh.

Distal attachment. (I)   Anterior and medial surface of tibia just below condyle.

Nerve supply.   Femoral nerve.

Where to palpate.   At the anterior superior iliac spine. In a slender subject the entire muscle may be seen and palpated on the front of the thigh.

Action (at hip).   Flexion.

Comments.   This is a long, slender ribbon-like muscle, directed obliquely downward and inward across the front of the thigh. It is the most superficial of the anterior muscles of the thigh. Its name is derived from its supposed function of enabling one to sit with the legs folded in "tailor-fashion."

PECTINEUS (Fig. 15–7.)

Proximal attachment. (O)   Pectineal line between iliopectineal eminence and tubercle of pubis.

Distal attachment. (I)   Pectineal line of femur, between lesser trochanter and linea aspera.

Nerve supply.   Femoral nerve.

Where to palpate.   At the front of the pubis, just lateral to the adductor longus. Difficult to distinguish from the latter muscle.

Action.   Flexion; assists in adduction when hip is in flexed position. Whether it also contributes to outward rotation is debatable.

Comments.   This is a short, thick, quadrilateral muscle situated lateral and superior to the adductor longus and more or less parallel to it. It has a good angle of pull which, together with its internal structure, accounts for its ability to overcome considerable resistance.

TENSOR FASCIAE LATAE (Figs. 15–8 and 15–9.)

Proximal attachments. (O)   Anterior part of outer lip of iliac crest and outer surface of anterior superior iliac spine.

Distal attachment. (I)   Iliotibial tract of fascia lata on lateral-anterior aspect of thigh, about one third of the way down.

Nerve supply.   Superior gluteal nerve.

Where to palpate.   About 2 inches anterior to the greater trochanter.

Action.   Flexion; abduction; tenses the fascia lata. Whether or not it also contributes to inward rotation is debatable.

Comments.   This is a small muscle located close in front of, and slightly lateral to, the hip joint. Because its pull on the fascia lata is transmitted by means of the iliotibial tract down to the lateral condyle of the tibia, it helps to extend the leg at the knee. Together with the gluteus maximus, which also unites with the fascia lata, it helps to stabilize the knee joint in weight-bearing positions. When the lower extremities are fixed, both these muscles help to steady the pelvis and trunk on the thighs.

Not all kinesiologists agree that it contributes to inward rotation but Wheatley and Jahnke claimed that their electromyographic experiments showed it to be a medial (inward) rotator in all of the positions tested.[11]

RECTUS FEMORIS (Fig. 15–8.) (See also muscles of the knee.)

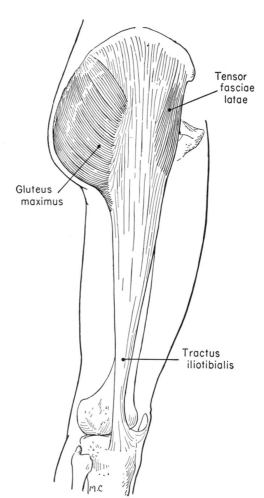

Figure 15–9. Lateral view of gluteus maximus, tensor fasciae latae and iliotibial tract.

Proximal attachments. (o) Anterior inferior iliac spine and groove above brim of acetabulum.

Distal attachment. (i) Base of patella. It may be said to attach indirectly, by means of the patellar ligament, to the tuberosity of the tibia.

Nerve supply. Femoral nerve.

Where to palpate. Anterior surface of thigh.

Action (at hip). Flexion.

Comments. This is a large bipenniform muscle, located superficially on the front of the thigh. It is the only one of the four muscles in the quadriceps femoris group that crosses the hip joint. It is therefore a two-joint muscle. For the pulley or tendon action of such muscles, see page 45.

GLUTEUS MAXIMUS (Figs. 15–9 and 15–10.)

Proximal attachments. (O)   Posterior gluteal line of ilium and adjacent portion of crest; posterior surface of lower part of sacrum and side of coccyx.

Distal attachments. (I)   Posterior surface of femur on ridge below greater trochanter; iliotibial tract of fascia lata.

Nerve supply.   Inferior gluteal nerves.

Where to palpate.   Posterior surface of buttock.

Action.   Extension; outward rotation in extended position; lower fibers assist in adduction and upper fibers in abduction.

Comments.   This large superficial muscle of the buttocks is a potentially powerful hip extensor. In order to understand all the movements it is capable of producing, it is helpful to study the position of the muscle with reference to the hip joint. A diagram such as that in Figure 15–11 makes clear the fact that about one third of the muscle

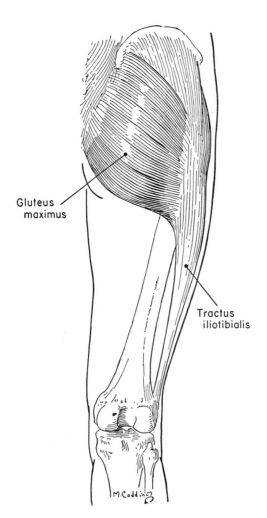

Gluteus
maximus

Tractus
iliotibialis

Figure 15–10.   Posterior view of gluteus maximus and iliotibial tract.

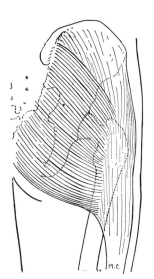

Figure 15–11. Diagram showing relation of gluteus maximus to hip joint.

lies above the center of motion, and two thirds of the muscle below it. Hence the gluteus maximus as a whole cannot be said either to abduct or to adduct the thigh. The uppermost fibers are in a position to abduct it; the lower portion of the muscle to adduct it.

In the light of findings from electromyographic investigations, earlier statements made in this text must now be modified. These findings are not in complete agreement, however. Basmajian agreed with Duchenne that ordinary walking is not affected by complete paralysis of this muscle.[2] Yet, the EMG study conducted by the Prosthetic Devices Research Project in Berkeley indicated that the muscle was active in the early part of the stance phase in both normal and fast walking on level ground.[1]

The latter study and one by Merrifield agree on its activity in stair climbing. It has also been found to be active in walking up an inclined plane, in extending the femur against resistance, in abducting the femur, especially against resistance and when rotated outward, and in adducting the femur against resistance when in an abducted position.[9] Surprisingly, Houtz and Fischer, the only investigators who have reported on its role in bicycling, stated that it was unimportant in this activity. (See Basmajian.[2]) In a later, more extensive study of gluteus maximus function, the same investigators had some additional surprising results. After testing their subjects in the performance of several exercises commonly prescribed for strengthening the gluteus maximus, they found that the movements which elicited the greatest electrical activity were as follows: hyperextension movements of the thigh performed against resistance from the erect standing position, muscle setting, and vigorous hyperextension of the trunk from an erect position. Furthermore, they found that lifting a 25 lb. weight from both a squat position and from a straight leg, trunk bend position, elicited relatively minor electrical activity.[6]

If a person stands erect with feet parallel, voluntary contraction of the gluteus maximus, achieved by "pinching the buttocks together," produces two interesting postural effects. The pull on the femur causes a slight outward rotation at the hip joint, but since friction between the soles of the feet and the floor prevents the feet from turning laterally, the rotatory force is transmitted from the femur to the talus, thence to the other tarsal bones, and results in supination of the foot and a lifting of the medial aspect of the longitudinal arch. At the same time the pull at the muscle's proximal attachment decreases the pelvic tilt, which in turn decreases the lumbar lordosis. This setting or tensing of the gluteus maximus is frequently advocated as a corrective exercise.

BICEPS FEMORIS, LONG HEAD (Fig. 15–12.) (See also muscles of the knee.)

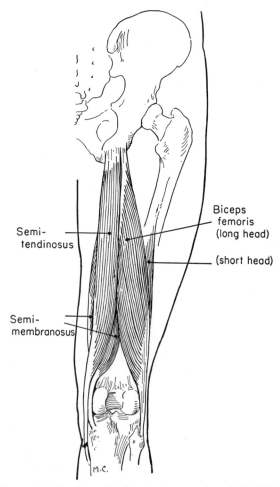

Figure 15–12. Superficial posterior muscles of right thigh.

Proximal attachment. (O) Lower and medial impression on tuberosity of ischium.

Distal attachments. (I) Lateral side of head of fibula and lateral condyle of tibia.

Nerve supply. Sciatic nerve.

Where to palpate. Lateral aspect of posterior surface of knee.

Action (at hip). Extension.

Comments. The biceps femoris forms the outer hamstring muscle. Only its long head crosses the hip joint. Its effectiveness as an extensor of the hip is in reverse proportion to the degree of flexion at the knee joint. If the knee is sharply flexed, the muscle has insufficient tension to act effectively at the hip joint. The tendon or pulley action of the two-joint muscles is discussed on page 45.

Basmajian reports that in addition to extension, some investigators include as functions of the long head of the biceps femoris lateral (outward) rotation of the extended hip, adduction against resistance of the abducted hip, and stabilization of the hip except in erect standing.[2]

SEMITENDINOSUS (Fig. 15–12.) (See also muscles of the knee.)

Proximal attachment. (O) Lower and medial impression on tuberosity of ischium with biceps femoris.

Distal attachment. (I) Upper part of medial surface of shaft of tibia.

Nerve supply. Sciatic nerve.

Where to palpate. Medial aspect of posterior surface of knee. The more lateral of the two small tendons which can be felt in this region.

Action (at hip). Extension.

Comments. See semimembranosus.

SEMIMEMBRANOSUS (Fig. 15–13.) (See also muscles of the knee.)

Proximal attachment. (O) Upper and lateral impression on tuberosity of ischium.

Distal attachment. (I) Horizontal groove on posterior surface of medial condyle of tibia.

Nerve supply. Sciatic nerve.

Cannot be palpated with certainty.

Action (at hip). Extension.

Comments. The semitendinosus and semimembranosus muscles form the inner component of the hamstring group. Their relation to the hip joint is similar to that of the long head of the biceps femoris.

Basmajian reports that some investigators found that all three hamstrings, in addition to extending the hip, help to stabilize it (except in the erect standing position); to adduct the femur from the abducted position when the movement is resisted; and to help rotate the extended femur, the long head of the biceps femoris rotating it laterally (outward) and the inner hamstrings rotating it medially (inward).[2]

THE SIX DEEP OUTWARD ROTATORS (Obturator externus and internus, gemellus superior and inferior, quadratus femoris, and piriformis) (Fig. 15–13.)

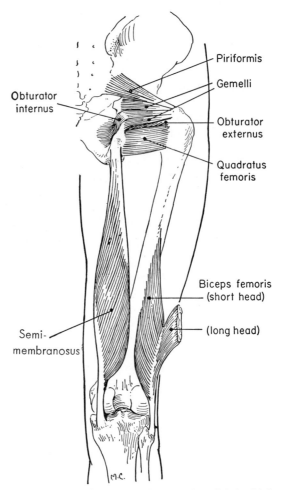

Figure 15–13. Deep posterior muscles of right thigh.

Proximal attachments. (o)   Outer and inner surfaces of sacrum and of pelvis in region of obturator foramen.

Distal attachment. (i)   Posterior and medial aspects of greater trochanter.

Nerve supply.   Third, fourth and fifth lumbar, and first and second sacral nerves.

Cannot be palpated.

Action.   Outward rotation.

Comments.   These muscles are situated behind the hip joint, the piriformis, the most superior, being slightly above it, and the obturator externus, the most inferior, being slightly below it. Some of the muscles in this group have a secondary function such as abduction or adduction, but neither of these functions compares in importance with that of outward rotation. All of these muscles appear to be favorably situated for helping to hold the head of the femur in the acetabulum.

GLUTEUS MEDIUS (Fig. 15–14, A.)

Proximal attachment. (O)   Posterior surface of ilium between crest, posterior gluteal line and anterior gluteal line.

Distal attachment. (I)   Oblique ridge on lateral surface of greater trochanter.

Nerve supply.   Superior gluteal.

Where to palpate.   About 2 or 3 inches above the greater trochanter.

Action.   Abduction; anterior fibers rotate inward.

Comments.   The gluteus medius is situated at the side of the hip between the iliac crest and the greater trochanter. The posterior portion lies beneath the gluteus maximus. The anterior portion is covered only by the fascia lata. The muscle is an important one in walking and in standing in good posture. When the weight is shifted onto one foot, tension of the gluteus medius and other abductors is an important factor in the stabilization of the hip. Lack of such stabilization results in an exaggerated sideward thrust of the supporting hip and drop of the pelvis on the opposite side. Paralysis of this muscle causes a typical limping gait known as the "gluteus medius gait." When the weight is borne on the affected side the trunk tilts strongly to that side and the opposite hip is thrust into prominence.

GLUTEUS MINIMUS (Fig. 15–14, B.)

Proximal attachment. (O)   Posterior surface of ilium between anterior and inferior gluteal lines.

Distal attachment. (I)   Anterior border of greater trochanter.

Nerve supply.   Superior gluteal nerve.

Cannot be palpated.

Action.   Inward rotation; abduction.

Comments.   This is a smaller muscle than the gluteus medius and is situated beneath it. Whereas the medius is primarily an

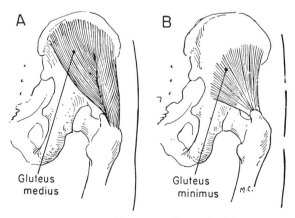

Figure 15–14.   Gluteus medius and minimus.

abductor and secondarily an inward rotator, the minimus is primarily an inward rotator and secondarily an abductor. The muscles work together as partners, each muscle acting as an assistant in the other's strongest action.

GRACILIS (Figs. 15–15, 16–8 and 16–9.) (See also muscles of the knee.)

Proximal attachment. (O)   Anterior aspect of lower half of symphysis pubis and upper half of pubic arch.

Distal attachment. (I)   Medial surface of tibia just below condyle.

Nerve supply.   Obturator.

Where to palpate.   Medial aspect of posterior surface of knee, immediately anterior to the semitendinosus tendon.

Action (at hip).   Adduction; assists in flexion.

Comments.   As the name indicates, this is a slender muscle. Being an adductor, it is sometimes called the adductor gracilis. Like the hamstrings, the sartorius and the rectus femoris, the gracilis is a muscle of the knee as well as of the hip joint. Wheatley and Jahnke found that it participates in hip flexion only when the knee is extended; also that it helps to rotate the femur medially (inward).[11]

ADDUCTOR MAGNUS (Fig. 15–15.)

Proximal attachments. (O)   Inferior rami of pubis and ischium and lateral border of inferior surface of ischial tuberosity.

Distal attachments. (I)   Linea aspera, medial supracondylar line, and adductor tubercle on medial condyle of femur.

Nerve supply.   Obturator and sciatic nerves.

Where to palpate.   Medial surface of middle half of thigh.

Action.   Adduction; extension; condyloid portion assists in inward rotation.

Comments.   As its name implies, this is the largest of the hip adductors. It is likewise the most powerful. It fans out from its relatively small origin on the lower arms of the pubis and ischium to its extensive attachment to the linea aspera along the whole length of the shaft of the femur. The upper portion, i.e., the portion attached to the lower ramus of the pubis, is sometimes described separately as the adductor minimus. Kinesiologists are not in agreement regarding its functions, other than that of hip adduction. Steindler observed that the upper part of the muscle acts as a flexor of the thigh, and the lower portion as an extensor.[10] Wright called the muscle a prime mover in the act of extension and claimed that it adducts only when the hip is in a position of extension.[12] They agreed on its inward rotatory action, but considered this very slight.

ADDUCTOR LONGUS (Fig. 15–15.)

Proximal attachment. (O)   Anterior surface of pubis.

Distal attachment. (I)   Medial lip of middle half of linea aspera.

Nerve supply.   Obturator nerve.

Where to palpate.   Just below its origin at the medial aspect of the groin.

Action.   Adduction; assists in flexion.

Comments.   Steindler has pointed out that while the adductor

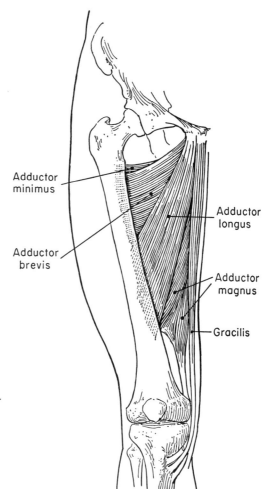

Adductor minimus

Adductor longus

Adductor brevis

Adductor magnus

Gracilis

Figure 15–15.   Adductor muscles of right thigh.

longus ordinarily helps to flex the thigh, when the flexion exceeds about 70 degrees this muscle becomes an extensor. This is due to the shift in the relationship between the muscle's line of pull and the joint's center of motion.

ADDUCTOR BREVIS (Fig. 15–15.)

Proximal attachments. (O)   Outer surface of body and inferior ramus of pubis.

Distal attachments. (I)   Line from lesser trochanter to linea aspera and upper fourth of linea aspera.

Nerve supply.   Obturator and accessory obturator nerves.

Cannot be palpated.

Action.   Adduction; assists in flexion.

Comments.   This lies just above the adductor longus. Like the latter, it acts as a flexor in the normal position, but later becomes an extensor after considerable hip flexion has been attained.

THE PELVIC GIRDLE

Structure. (Fig. 15–16.) Each hip bone (os innominatum) is made up of three bones—the ilium, ischium and pubis. These bones become fused into a single bone by about the time of puberty. The two hip bones together form the pelvic girdle. This bony girdle or basin, as it is sometimes called, is firmly attached to the sacrum at the sacroiliac articulation. The articulation is a difficult one to classify. It presents some of the characteristics of a diarthrodial joint, an articular cavity being present for part of the articulation. It is unlike other diarthrodial joints in one important respect, however. No movement can be voluntarily effected at the sacroiliac joint. Any movement which does occur is involuntary. Just how much motion can take place at the sacroiliac joint is a debatable matter. Some anatomists say that a slight "giving" may occur there as a shock absorption device; others claim that no motion occurs at the joint normally, except in women during pregnancy and parturition, when the ligaments relax in order to permit a slight spreading of the bones. (See report of study by Clayson et al., page 274.)

The sacrum is firmly bound to the two iliac bones by means of the anterior, posterior and interosseus sacroiliac ligaments (Figs. 15–17 and 15–18). It is further reinforced by the iliolumbar, sacrotuberous and sacrospinous ligaments and by the lower portion of the erector spinae muscle. Because of this firm attachment, the sacrum

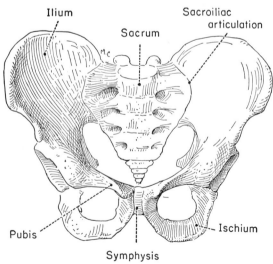

Figure 15–16.   Anterior view of pelvis.

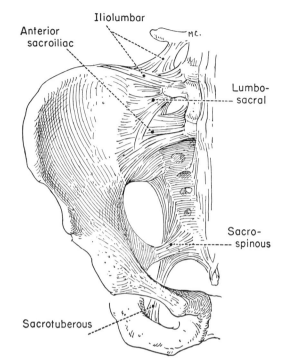

Figure 15–17. Anterior view of sacroiliac articulation showing ligaments.

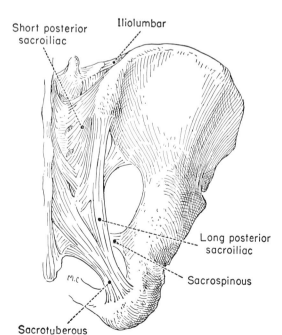

Figure 15–18. Posterior view of sacroiliac articulation showing ligaments.

might well be considered a part of the pelvic girdle. From the point of view of function it is more truly a part of the pelvis than of the spine.

The joints at which the movements of the pelvic girdle occur are the two hip joints and the joints of the lumbar spine, particularly the lumbosacral articulation.

Movements. The pelvic movements may be defined as follows:

1. Increased inclination (forward tilt) (Fig. 15–19, *C*). A rotation of the pelvis in the sagittal plane about a frontal-horizontal axis in such a manner that the symphysis pubis turns downward and the posterior surface of the sacrum turns upward.

2. Decreased inclination (backward tilt) (Fig. 15–19, *B*). A rotation of the pelvis in the sagittal plane about a frontal-horizontal axis in such a manner that the symphysis pubis moves forward-upward and the posterior surface of the sacrum turns somewhat downward.

3. Lateral tilt. A rotation of the pelvis in the frontal plane about a sagittal-horizontal axis in such a manner that one iliac crest is lowered and the other is raised. The tilt is named in terms of the side which moves downward. Thus in a lateral tilt of the pelvis to the left, the left iliac crest is lowered and the right is raised.

4. Rotation (lateral twist). A rotation of the pelvis in the horizontal plane about a vertical axis. The movement is named in terms of the direction toward which the front of the pelvis turns.

The Relationship of the Pelvis to the Trunk and Lower Extremities. Architecturally, the pelvis is strategically located. Linking the trunk with the lower extremities, it must cooperate with the motion of each, yet at the same time contribute to the stability of

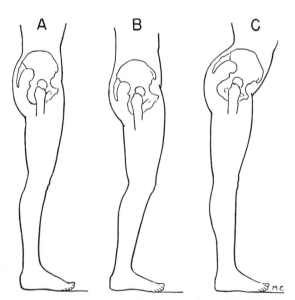

Figure 15–19. Anteroposterior inclinations of the pelvis. *A*, Mid-position; *B*, decreased inclination; *C*, increased inclination.

the total structure. When the body is in the erect standing position, the pelvis receives the weight of the head, trunk and upper extremities, divides it equally and transmits it to the two lower extremities. Whenever an individual stands on only one foot, the pelvis automatically adapts itself to this position and transmits the entire weight of the upper part of the body to one of the lower extremities. It requires a fine adjustment to do this in such a way that the balance of the total structure is preserved.

Since the pelvis depends upon the joints of the lower spine and those of the hips for its movements, it is not surprising that its motion is sometimes associated with the motion of the trunk or spine, and sometimes with that of the thighs. In such cases the movement of the pelvis may be said to be secondary to that of the spine, or of the thighs, as the case may be. In fact, most of its motion belongs in one or the other category. Occasionally, however, the movement seems to be initiated in the pelvis itself, with the spine and thighs cooperating with it. In such an event, the movement of the pelvis might be considered primary, and that of the spine and hips, secondary. One sees this type of movement when the individual "tucks his hips under" or makes other postural adjustments (see Fig. 15–19, B).

It is not always easy to judge the habitual tilt of the pelvis from the contours of the body. Prominent buttocks, heavy layers of fat or an unusually convex sacrum can easily mislead the observer. Figure 15–20 shows a sketch based on an x-ray which illustrates a type of build in which the contour of the lower back and pelvic region does not correspond to the bony structure. In this illustration the tilt, as

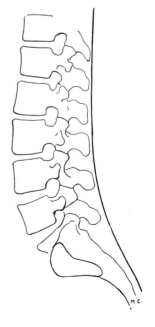

Figure 15–20. Lumbar and lumbosacral regions of the spine showing discrepancy in the lower lumbar curve as seen in the vertebral bodies and as seen in the contour of the back. (The sketch is based on an x-ray.)

judged by the position of the sacrum, is greater than it appears to be from the contour of the lower back. This observation is of importance to those who tend to place emphasis on the position of the pelvis in giving posture instruction.

The joint analysis of the primary movements of the pelvis, as performed when the person is in the fundamental standing position, is given below.

A movement of the pelvis which is *secondary to the movement of the lower extremity* is seen, for instance, in a high kick. (See Fig. 8–2.) In activities such as this the pelvis seems to move with the lower extremity for the purpose of increasing the latter's range of motion. Hence, when the thigh is flexed at the hip joint, the pelvic inclination is decreased; when the lower extremity is raised backward in apparent hyperextension, the pelvic inclination is increased; when one thigh is widely abducted, the pelvis tilts laterally; and when one leg is placed forward and the other backward as though taking a long stride, the pelvis rotates in the horizontal plane about a vertical axis.

Pelvic movements are *secondary to movements of the spine* when the latter are performed through the full range of motion. Thus complete flexion of the spine necessitates a decrease in the pelvic inclination; complete hyperextension necessitates an increased inclination; complete lateral flexion necessitates a lateral tilt; complete spinal rotation necessitates horizontal rotation of the pelvis.

It has already been stated that the movements of the pelvic girdle take place at the lumbar spine, the lumbosacral junction and the hip joints. The exact combination of movements of these joints depends upon whether the motion of the pelvis is primary, whether it is secondary to movements of the lower extremity or whether it is secondary to spinal movements.

Joint Analysis of Primary Movements of the Pelvis

Pelvis	Spinal Joints	Hip Joints
Increased tilt	Hyperextension	Slight flexion
Decreased tilt	Slight flexion	Complete extension
Lateral tilt to left	Slight lateral flexion right	R: Slight adduction / L: Slight abduction
Rotation to left (without turning the head or moving the feet)	Rotation right	R: Sl. outward rot. / L: Sl. inward rot.

Joint Analysis of Movements of the Pelvis Secondary to those of the Spine

Spine	Pelvis
Flexion	Decreased tilt
Hyperextension	Increased tilt
Lateral flexion to left	Lateral tilt to left
Rotation to left	Rotation to left

All the muscles which attach to the pelvic bones or to the sacrum serve either to initiate or to control pelvic movements. As one would expect, these are all muscles either of the hip joint or of the spine. (See Fig. 15–21.)

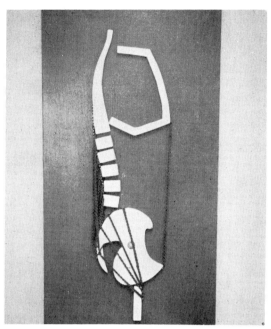

Figure 15–21. Visual aid demonstrating the motion of pelvic tilt and its effect on the lumbar spine. (From Holze, I.: Aid for teaching pelvic tilt. J. Am. Phys. Ther. Assn., *43*:114, 1963. Reproduced by permission of the author and of the editor of the Journal of the American Physical Therapy Association.)

SUPPLEMENTARY MATERIAL

Variations in Femoral and Tibial Torsion; Relation to Gait. Elftman investigated the torsion of both the femur and the tibia in 35 male cadavers. It was his opinion that extremes at either end of the scale might well account for peculiarities of gait. The possibility of femoral or tibial torsion should be taken into consideration when judging exaggerated toeing-in or toeing-out gaits. The results of Elftman's findings are recorded in Table 15–1.

An interesting study on the relation of femoral torsion to in-toeing and out-toeing was reported by Crane in 1959.[4] He noted that the out-toeing group was capable of 60 to 80 degrees of lateral rotation, but less than 20 degrees of medial rotation. The in-toeing group, on the other hand, was capable of only 10 to 20 degrees of lateral rotation and 60 to 80 degrees of medial rotation. X-rays showed abnormal

TABLE 15–1.　Measurements of Femoral and Tibial Torsion
(Elftman) (N = 35)

	Range	Mean	S.D.
Femoral torsion........................	0°–26°	11.86°	6.21 ± 0.74
Tibial torsion	12°–44°	27.40°	7.40 ± 0.89

femoral torsion in both of these groups. Although the cause could not be determined, Crane suggested that it might be traced either to fetal positions or, as was thought by Fitzhugh, to sleeping positions during infancy.

In comparing a group of "normal" children, aged 6 months to 9 years, with data on "normal" adults, he found that femoral torsion was three or four times greater during the first year of life than it was in adulthood and that the decrease in torsion occurred gradually.

A striking contrast was seen in a comparison of two young boys who had opposite patterns of sitting. Boy A, aged 7, habitually assumed a kneel-sitting position with the knees close and the feet widely separated and everted like a letter W. Boy B, aged 5, habitually assumed the familiar position known as "tailor sitting" or "Indian sitting." Their rotation and torsion measurements were as follows:

	Lat. Rot.	Med. Rot.	Femoral torsion (anteversion)
Boy A	5–10°	75°	R 50; L 53°
Boy B	80°	10°	Less than 10°

Movements of the Lower Spine and Pelvis. In 1962 Clayson and his co-workers reported their investigation of the mobility of the hip joints and lumbar vertebrae. Their subjects were 26 normal young women who had no history of disabilities of the back or hips. The movements studied were flexion and extension of the hip joint combined with flexion and extension of the lumbar spine. For their complete findings the reader is referred to their published report.[3]

A few of their measurements and observations were as follows:

Average maximum flexion and maximum extension of the hip joint, as measured by the pelvifemoral angle, were 60 ± 6.7° and 186 ± 6°, respectively.

The average pelvifemoral angle in the relaxed standing position was 175 ± 3.4°.

The greatest anteroposterior motion in the lumbar spine took place between the fifth lumbar vertebra and the sacrum.

In flexion, the lumbar curve became reversed in all but four subjects.

Anteroposterior motion at the sacroiliac joint ranged from 1° to 21°, the average being 8 ± 4.9°.

The combined anteroposterior motion taking place in the lumbar spine and hip joints together averaged 181° from maximum flexion to the relaxed standing position, and 41° from the latter to maximum extension, making a total average movement of 222°.

EMG Investigation of Iliopsoas Function.   Because of divergent opinions expressed by earlier investigators, LaBan, Raptou and Johnson undertook a study of the function of the iliopsoas muscle in 1965. They considered that their use of a flexible wire electrode had an advantage over the rigid ones used by previous investigators.

Using five subjects whose ages ranged from 20 to 29 years they tested the action of the iliopsoas in quiet standing, in walking at normal speed and in performing a number of movements from the long-lying and hook-lying supine positions. They detected no electrical activity of the iliopsoas during quiet standing. In the forward swing phase of walking they found considerable activity.

Their most interesting findings were from the comparison of sit-ups executed from the long-lying supine position with those done from the hook-lying (flexed knee and hip) supine position. They noted that the iliopsoas muscle showed considerable electrical activity throughout the entire range of movement when the sit-ups were performed from the hook-lying position, but in the straight leg lying position it showed little or no activity for the first 30 degrees of movement. After that it produced considerable activity. They assumed that the implication from this was that the abdominal muscles are responsible for the first 30 degrees of a sit-up performed from the long-lying position, with the rectus femoris being responsible for stabilizing the pelvis.[8]

DEMONSTRATIONS AND LABORATORY EXERCISES

Joint Structure and Function
1. Take a pelvic bone and a femur and "construct" a hip joint, using felt for the fibrocartilage and adhesive tape for the ligaments. Be as accurate as possible in the attachments of these structures. It is suggested that two or three students work together on this project.
2. Using a form like the one in Appendix B, record the essential information regarding the hip joint. Study the movements both on the skeleton and on the living body.
3. Using a Lufkin rule or a protractor type of goniometer, measure the range of motion in the following joint movements on five different subjects:
  a. Hip flexion, with straight knee.
  b. Hip flexion, with flexed knee.
  c. Total abduction of both thighs.
Muscular Action.   (See Appendix F for muscle check list.) Identify as many muscles as possible in the following experiments.
4. HIP FLEXION
  a. Subject: Sit on table with legs hanging over edge. Raise thigh.
  Assistant: Resist movement slightly by pressing down on knee.

Observer: Palpate pectineus, tensor fasciae latae, sartorius, rectus femoris and adductor longus. Does the gracilis contract?

b. Subject: Lie on one side, rolled toward face. Flex thigh of top leg, allowing knee to flex passively.

Assistant: Resist movement by pushing against knee.

Observer: Palpate iliopsoas.

5. HIP EXTENSION

a. Subject: Stand facing table with trunk bent forward until it rests on table. Grasp sides of table. Raise one leg, keeping the knee straight.

Assistant: Resist movement by pushing down on thigh close to knee. Second time, give resistance at heel.

Observer: Palpate gluteus maximus, adductor magnus and hamstrings.

b. Subject: Lie face down on table and raise one leg with knee straight.

Assistant: Resist movement by pushing down on knee.

Observer: Palpate same muscles as in *a.*

6. HIP ABDUCTION

Subject: Lie on one side and raise top leg.

Assistant: Resist movement by pushing down on knee.

Observer: Palpate gluteus maximus, gluteus medius and tensor fasciae latae.

7. HIP ADDUCTION

Subject: Lie on one side with top leg raised; then lower it.

Assistant: Resist movement by pressing up against knee.

Note: Unless resistance is applied, the action will be performed by means of the eccentric contraction of the abductors.

Observer: Palpate three adductors and name them.

8. OUTWARD ROTATION OF THIGH

Subject: Stand on one foot with the other knee bent at right angles so that the lower leg extends horizontally backward. Rotate the free thigh outward by swinging the foot medially.

Assistant: Steady subject's knee and resist movement of leg at ankle.

Observer: Palpate gluteus maximus.

9. INWARD ROTATION OF THIGH

Subject: Stand on one foot with other knee bent at right angles so that the lower leg extends horizontally backward. Rotate the free thigh inward by swinging the foot laterally.

Assistant: Steady subject's knee and resist movement of leg at ankle.

Observer: Palpate gluteus medius, tensor fasciae latae and lower adductor magnus.

10. DECREASE OF PELVIC INCLINATION

Subject: Lie on back with knees drawn up and feet resting on floor. Tilt pelvis in such a manner that lumbar spine becomes flatter.

Assistant: Kneeling at subject's head and facing his feet, place thumbs on his anterior superior iliac spines and fingers under his lower back. Resist movement by pushing iliac spines toward subject's feet.

Observer: Palpate rectus abdominis and gluteus maximus. Palpate the hamstrings. Do they contract?

11. INCREASE OF PELVIC INCLINATION

Subject: In erect standing position, stiffen knees and push buttocks as far to the rear as possible.

Observer: Palpate tensor fasciae latae, sartorius, pectineus and iliocostalis. Does the adductor longus or gracilis contract?

12. LATERAL TILT OF PELVIS

Subject: Stand on stool on one foot, with other leg hanging free. Pull free hip up as far as possible.

Assistant: Give slight resistance by holding ankle down.

Observer: Palpate oblique abdominals, iliocostalis, adductor magnus, adductor longus and gracilis on side of free leg.

REFERENCES

1. Advisory Committee on Artificial Limbs; National Research Council: The Pattern of Muscular Activity in the Lower Extremity During Walking. Berkeley, Cal., Prosthetic Devices Research Project, Institute of Engineering Research, University of California. Series II, 1953.
2. Basmajian, J. V.: Muscles Alive, 2nd ed. Baltimore, The Williams & Wilkins Company, 1967.
3. Clayson, S. J., Newman, I. M., Debevec, D. F., Anger, R. W., Skowland, H. V., and Kottke, F. J.: Evaluation of mobility of hip and lumbar vertebrae of normal young women. Arch. Phys. Med. & Rehab., *43*:1–8, 1962.
4. Crane, L.: Femoral torsion and its relation to toeing-in and toeing-out. J. Bone & Joint Surg., *41A*:421–428, 1959.
5. Elftman, H.: Torsion of the lower extremity. Am. J. Phys. Anthrop., *3* (new series): 255–265, 1945.
6. Fischer, F. J., and Houtz, S. J.: Evaluation of the function of the gluteus maximus muscle. Am. J. Phys. Med., *47*:182–191, 1968.
7. Holze, I.: Aid for teaching pelvic tilt. J. Am. Phys. Ther. Assn., *43*:114, 1963.
8. LaBan, M. M., Raptou, A. D., and Johnson, E. W.: Electromyographic study of function of iliopsoas muscle. Arch. Phys. Med. & Rehab., *46*:676–679, 1965.
9. Merrifield, H. H.: An electromyographic study of the gluteus maximus, the vastus lateralis and the tensor fasciae latae. Diss. Abstr., *21*:1833, 1961.
10. Steindler, A.: Kinesiology of the Human Body. Springfield, Ill., Charles C Thomas, Publisher, 1955.
11. Wheatley, M. D., and Jahnke, W. D.: Electromyographic study of the superficial thigh and hip muscles in normal individuals. Arch. Phys. Ther., *31*:508–522, 1951.
12. Wright, W. G.: Muscle Function. New York, Hafner Publishing Company, 1962.

RECOMMENDED READINGS

Inman, V. T.: Functional aspects of the abductor muscles of the hip. J. Bone & Joint Surg., *29A*:607–619, 1947.
Mendler, H. M.: Relationship of Hip Abductor Muscles to Posture. J. Am. Phys. Ther. Assn., *44*:98–102, 1964.
Williams, M., and Lissner, H. R.: Biomechanics of Human Motion. Philadelphia, W. B. Saunders Company, 1962, pp. 44, 45.

CHAPTER 16

The Lower Extremity:
The Knee Joint

The knee joint is a masterpiece of anatomic engineering. Placed midway in each supporting column of the body, it is subject to severe stresses and strains in its combined functions of weight-bearing and locomotion. As Steindler has pointed out, it meets the requirements made of it with remarkable efficiency.[8] To take care of the weight-bearing stresses it has massive condyles; to facilitate locomotion it has a wide range of motion; to resist the lateral stresses due to the tremendous lever effect of the long femur and tibia, it is reinforced at the sides by strong ligaments; to combat the downward pull of gravity and to meet the demands of such violent locomotor activities as running and jumping, it is provided with powerful musculature. It would be difficult, indeed, to find a mechanism better adapted for meeting the combined requirements of stability and mobility than the knee joint.

In this connection, however, mention should be made of two forms of malalignment at the knee joint, one of which is common. These are the conditions popularly known as "knock-knees" and "bowlegs." In "knock-knees" (genu valgum) the knees are nearer the midline of the body than is normal. In the standing position the knees are closer together than the feet, so that when the feet are placed side by side, the knees are either pressed together or "staggered" with one slightly behind the other. Mechanically, the condition means that the weight-bearing line of the lower extremity passes lateral to the center of the knee joint. This puts the medial ligament (tibial collateral) under increased tension and subjects the lateral meniscus to increased pressure and friction. Such a joint is an unstable one. Not only is it more prone to injury than a well-aligned joint, but in all weight-bearing positions postural strains are constantly present. The condition of "bowlegs" (genu varum) is just the reverse of "knock-knees," with the additional complication that the long bones themselves are curved laterally.

Structure. Although the knee is classified as a hinge joint, its bony structure resembles two ovoid or condyloid joints lying side by side. The lateral flexion which is permitted in a single ovoid joint is not possible in the knee joint because of the presence of the second

278

condyle. The two rocker-like condyles of the femur rest on the two slightly concave areas on the top of the tibia's broad head (Fig. 16–1). These articular surfaces of the tibia are separated by a roughened area, called the intercondyloid eminence, which terminates both anteriorly and posteriorly in a slight hollow, but rises at the center to form two small tubercles not unlike miniature twin mountain peaks (Fig. 16–2). The medial articular surface is oval; the lateral is smaller and more nearly round. Each is overlaid by a somewhat crescent-shaped fibrocartilage, known as a semilunar cartilage or meniscus.

The lower end of the femur terminates in the two rocker-like condyles already mentioned. The lateral condyle is broader and more prominent than the medial. The medial condyle projects downward farther than the lateral. This, however, is evident only when a disarticulated femur is held vertically. In its normal position in the body the femur slants inward from above downward. This slant is known as the obliquity of the femoral shaft. Observation of the mounted skeleton will show that the downward projection of the medial condyle compensates for the obliquity of the femoral shaft.

Another interesting feature of the condyles is that they are not quite parallel. While the lateral condyle lies in the sagittal plane, the medial condyle slants slightly medially from front to back. This is an important factor in the movements of the knee.

Anteriorly, the two condyles are continuous with the smooth, slightly concave surface of the patellar facet for the articulation of the patella. The patella, or knee cap, is a large sesamoid bone located slightly above and in front of the knee joint. It is held in place by the quadriceps tendon above, by the patellar ligament below, and by the intervening fibers which form a pocket for the patella (Fig. 16–3).

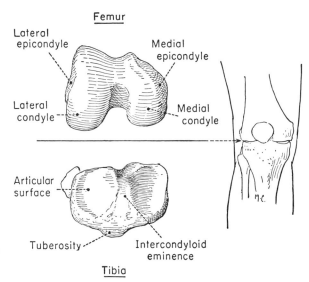

Figure 16–1. Articulating surfaces of knee joint.

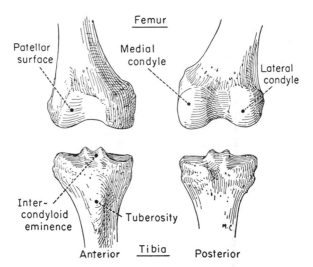

Figure 16–2.   Anterior and posterior views of bones of knee joint.

The articular cavity is enclosed within a loose membranous capsule which lies under the patella and folds around each condyle, but which excludes the intercondyloid tubercles and the cruciate ligaments. It is supplemented by expansions from the fascia lata, iliotibial tract and various tendons. The oblique popliteal ligament covers the posterior surface of the joint completely, shielding the cruciate ligaments and other structures not enclosed within the capsule (Fig. 16–4).

The synovial membrane of the knee joint is the most extensive of any in the body. It folds in and around the joint in a manner far too complicated to attempt to describe here. There are numerous bursae in the vicinity of the knee joint, among the largest and most important being the prepatellar, infrapatellar and suprapatellar bursae.

The Semilunar Cartilages. (Fig. 16–5.) These cartilages, or menisci as they are called, are somewhat circular rims of fibrocartilage, situated on the articular surfaces of the head of the tibia. They are relatively thick at their peripheral borders, but taper to a thin edge at their inner circumferences. Thus they deepen the articular facets of the tibia and, at the same time, serve in a shock absorbing capacity. The inner edges are free, but the peripheral borders are attached loosely to the rim of the head of the tibia by fibers from the inner surface of the capsule.

The lateral semilunar cartilage forms an incomplete circle, conforming closely to the nearly round articular facet. Its anterior and posterior horns, which almost meet at the center of the joint, are attached to the intercondyloid eminence.

The medial cartilage is shaped like a large letter C, broader toward the rear than in front. Its anterior horn tapers off to a thin strand which is attached to the anterior intercondyloid fossa. It is not so freely movable as the lateral cartilage, one reason for this being its secure anchorage to the tibial collateral ligament at the medial side of the knee. Largely because of this point of attachment, the medial cartilage is more frequently injured than the lateral. One of the most common injuries is caused by either a sudden twist or a lateral blow when the knee is bearing weight in a flexed position. In either case the tibial collateral ligament is wrenched, and instead of pulling loose from the medial cartilage, it pulls the medial cartilage loose from the head of the tibia. Once the cartilage is loose, it tends to slip around and get jammed in the joint, making it impossible to extend the knee completely. The usual remedy for this type of injury is removal of the meniscus. Surprisingly enough, the joint loses little of its usefulness when this is done.

Ligaments of the Knee

PATELLAR LIGAMENT. (Fig. 16–3.) This is a strong flat ligament

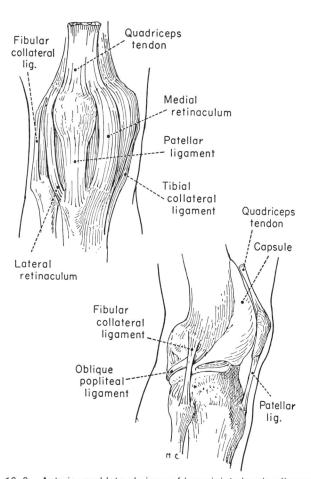

Figure 16–3. Anterior and lateral views of knee joint showing ligaments.

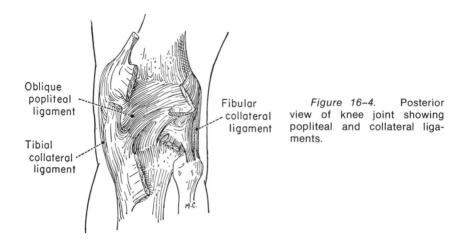

Oblique
popliteal
ligament

Tibial
collateral
ligament

Fibular
collateral
ligament

Figure 16–4. Posterior view of knee joint showing popliteal and collateral ligaments.

connecting the lower margin of the patella with the tuberosity of the tibia. The superficial fibers, passing over the front of the patella, are continuations of the central fibers of the quadriceps femoris tendon.

COLLATERAL TIBIAL LIGAMENT. (Figs. 16–3, *A*, 16–4 and 16–6.) This is a broad, flat, membranous band on the medial side of the joint. It is attached above to the medial epicondyle of the femur below the adductor tubercle, and below to the medial condyle of the tibia. It is firmly attached to the medial meniscus. This fact should be noted because of its significance in knee injuries. It serves to check extension and to prevent motion laterally.

COLLATERAL FIBULAR LIGAMENT. (Figs. 16–3, 16–4 and 16–6.) This is a strong, rounded cord, attached above to the back of the lateral epicondyle of the femur, and below to the lateral surface of the head of the fibula. It serves to check extension and to prevent motion medially.

OBLIQUE POPLITEAL LIGAMENT. (Figs. 16–3, *B*, and 16–4.)   This is a broad, flat ligament, covering the back of the knee joint. It is attached above to the upper margin of the intercondyloid fossa and posterior surface of the femur, and below to the posterior margin of the

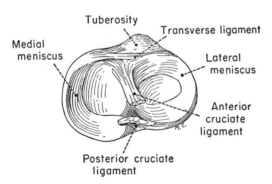

Tuberosity

Transverse ligament

Medial
meniscus

Lateral
meniscus

Anterior
cruciate
ligament

Posterior cruciate
ligament

Figure 16–5. The menisci (semilunar cartilages) of the knee joint.

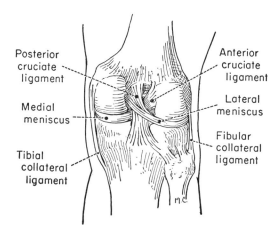

Posterior
cruciate
ligament

Anterior
cruciate
ligament

Figure 16-6. Posterior view of knee joint showing cruciate ligaments.

Medial
meniscus

Lateral
meniscus

Fibular
collateral
ligament

Tibial
collateral
ligament

m.c.

head of the tibia. Medially, it blends with the tendon of the semi-membranosus muscle, and laterally with the lateral head of the gastrocnemius.

THE CRUCIATE LIGAMENTS. (Fig. 16-6.) These are two strong, cordlike ligaments situated within the knee joint, although not enclosed within the joint capsule. They are called cruciate from the fact that they cross each other and are further designated anterior and posterior, according to their attachments to the tibia. They serve to check certain movements at the knee joint. They limit extension and prevent rotation in the extended position. They also check the forward and backward sliding of the femur on the tibia, thus safeguarding the anteroposterior stability of the knee.

ANTERIOR CRUCIATE LIGAMENT. (Fig. 16-6.) This passes upward and backward from the anterior intercondyloid fossa of the tibia to the back part of the medial surface of the lateral condyle of the femur.

POSTERIOR CRUCIATE LIGAMENT. (Fig. 16-6.) This is a shorter and stronger ligament than the anterior. It passes upward and forward from the posterior intercondyloid fossa of the tibia to the lateral and front part of the medial condyle of the femur.

TRANSVERSE LIGAMENT. (Fig. 16-5.) This is a short, slender cordlike ligament, connecting the anterior convex margin of the lateral meniscus to the anterior end of the medial meniscus.

THE ILIOTIBIAL TRACT. (Figs. 15-9 and 15-10.) The iliotibial tract is said to act like a tense ligament which connects the iliac crest with the lateral femoral condyle and the lateral tubercle of the tibia. At the knee joint the tract serves as a stabilizing ligament between the lateral condyle of the femur and the tibia. The attachment to the femoral condyle is then a fixed point and the distal end moves forward in knee extension and backward in knee flexion.[4]

Movements. The movements which occur at the knee joint are primarily flexion and extension. A slight amount of rotation can take place when the knee is in the flexed position.

FLEXION AND EXTENSION.   The movements of flexion and exten-sion at the knee are not so simple as are those of a true hinge joint. This can be demonstrated in the classroom by holding a disarticulated femur and tibia together in a position of extension, then, holding the tibia stationary, flexing the femur on the tibia as though the individual were assuming a squat or sitting position. If no other adjustment is made, the femoral condyles will roll back completely off the top of the tibia. What prevents this in real life is the fact that as the condyles roll backward they simultaneously glide forward, and thus remain in contact with the menisci throughout each phase of the movement. Conversely, when the femur extends on the tibia, the forward roll of the femoral condyles is accompanied by a backward glide.

Because the femoral condyles are not quite parallel, and differ in size, a slight degree of rotation occurs during the initial phase of flexion and the final phase of extension. This can be readily seen on the living subject if he stands with the knees slightly flexed and then extends them completely. The patellae are seen to turn slightly medialward, indicating slight inward rotation of the thighs. Because of the inequality of the two condyles, the medial condyle continues to roll forward after the lateral condyle has ceased its movement. The inward rotation of the femur which accompanies the completion of extension is commonly known as "locking" the knees. In persons who tend to hyperextend their knees habitually the rotation is more pronounced.

When the leg is flexed or extended in a non-weight-bearing posi-tion, the tibia rotates on the femur, instead of vice versa. The final phase of extension is accompanied by slight outward rotation of the tibia. At the beginning of flexion the tibia rotates inward until the mid-position is attained.[7]

The rotation which occurs in the final stage of extension and the initial phase of flexion is an inherent part of these movements and should not be confused with the voluntary rotation that can be performed when the leg is not bearing weight and the knee is in a flexed position.

INWARD AND OUTWARD ROTATION IN THE FLEXED POSITION. When the leg has been flexed at the knee to a right angle and beyond, it is possible to rotate the leg on the thigh through a total range of about 50 degrees. This can occur, however, only when the leg is not bearing the body weight. It is impossible, for instance, to rotate either the leg or the thigh in this manner when the body is in a stooping position. A good way to demonstrate rotation of the tibia is to sit on a chair with the heel resting lightly on the floor. In this position, with the knee and thigh held motionless, the foot should be turned first in and then out. The action will be that of inward and outward rotation of the tibia. The movement taking place within the foot itself should be discounted.

Muscles.   The muscles acting on the knee joint are classified as anterior or posterior according to the relation of their distal tendons to the transverse axis of the joint.

Anterior:
  Rectus femoris
  Vastus intermedius
  Vastus lateralis
  Vastus medialis

Posterior:
  Biceps femoris
  Semimembranosus ⎫
  Semitendinosus ⎬ "Hamstrings"
  Sartorius   ⎭
  Gracilis
  Popliteus
  Gastrocnemius

RECTUS FEMORIS (Fig. 16–7.) (See also muscles of the hip.)
Proximal attachments. (O) Anterior inferior iliac spine and groove above brim of acetabulum.
Distal attachment. (I) Base of patella, as part of the quadriceps

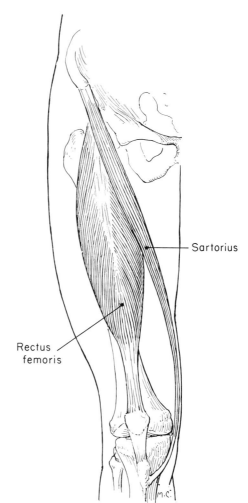

Figure 16-7. Front of thigh showing rectus femoris and sartorius muscles.

Sartorius

Rectus femoris

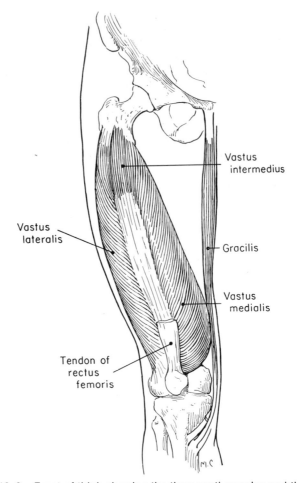

Figure 16–8. Front of thigh showing the three vasti muscles and the gracilis.

femoris tendon. It may be said to attach indirectly to the tuberosity of the tibia by means of the patellar ligament.

Nerve supply. Femoral nerve.

Where to palpate. Anterior surface of thigh.

Action (at knee). Extension.

THE THREE VASTI (VASTUS LATERALIS, VASTUS INTERMEDIUS, VASTUS MEDIALIS) (Fig. 16–8.)

Proximal attachment (O):

Vastus Lateralis: Upper part of intertrochanteric line; anterior and lower borders of greater trochanter; lateral lip of gluteal tuberosity and upper half of linea aspera.

Vastus Intermedius: Anterior and lateral surfaces of upper two thirds of shaft of femur.

Vastus Medialis: Lower half of intertrochanteric line; medial lip of linea aspera; and upper part of medial supracondylar line.

Distal attachment. (I) The tendons of three vasti muscles unite with that of rectus femoris to form the quadriceps femoris tendon. This attaches to the base of the patella, and indirectly, by means of the patellar ligament, to the tuberosity of the tibia.

Nerve supply. Femoral nerve.

Where to palpate. Vastus lateralis may be palpated on the anterolateral aspect of the thigh, lateral to the rectus femoris, and vastus medialis on the anteromedial aspect of the lower third of the thigh, medial to the rectus femoris. Vastus intermedius cannot be palpated.

Action. Extension.

Comments on the quadriceps femoris. The rectus femoris, situated on the front of the thigh, is the most superficial of the quadriceps group and is the only one of the four which also acts at the hip joint. According to Wright, the rectus femoris also serves as an anterior ligament of the hip.[10]

The vastus lateralis and vastus medialis are superficially located except for the anterior portions, which are covered by the rectus femoris. The vastus intermedius lies beneath the rectus and is completely covered by it. The three vasti muscles, with their fibers converging toward the patella, serve to steady the knee joint in all weight-bearing positions and to maintain a balanced tension on the patella. Being one-joint muscles, the vasti are powerful knee extensors, regardless of the position of the hip joint.

Static contraction of the quadriceps, when the knee is fully extended, serves to pull up or "set" the patella. These muscles are not active in ordinary standing.[1]

Pocock concluded from his investigation of the quadriceps muscles that they function as a unit and do not have any particular timing pattern as had been previously suggested.[6]

Hollinshead made the interesting observation that, because of the close relationship between hip, knee and ankle action when the weight is on the feet, the gluteus maximus, gastrocnemius and soleus could be said to help extend the knees.[3]

BICEPS FEMORIS (Fig. 16–9.) (See also muscles of the hip.)

Proximal attachments. (O) Long head: Lower and medial impression on tuberosity of ischium.

Short Head: Lateral lip of linea aspera.

Distal attachments. (I) Lateral side of head of fibula and lateral condyle of tibia.

Nerve supply. Sciatic nerve.

Where to palpate. Lateral aspect of posterior surface of knee.

Action (at knee). Flexion of leg at knee; outward rotation of tibia when knee is in non-weight-bearing flexed position.

Comments. This is the outer hamstring muscle.

SEMIMEMBRANOSUS (Fig. 16–9.) (See also muscles of the hip.)

Proximal attachment. (O) Upper and lateral impression on tuberosity of ischium.

Distal attachment. (I) Horizontal groove on posterior surface of medial condyle of tibia.

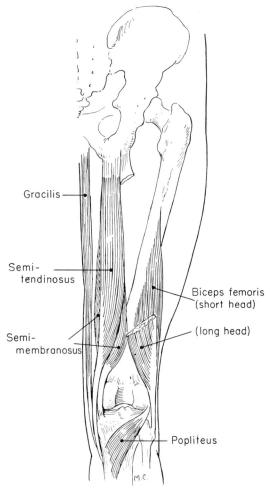

Figure 16–9.   Posterior muscles of thigh and knee.

Nerve supply.   Sciatic nerve.

Where to palpate.   The tendon lies beneath the tendons of gracilis and semitendinosus at the knee, and is difficult to identify.

Action (at knee).   Flexion of leg at knee; inward rotation of tibia when knee is in non-weight-bearing flexed position.

Comments.   This is one of the two inner hamstring muscles.

SEMITENDINOSUS (Fig. 16–9.) (See also muscles of the hip.)

Proximal attachment. (o)   Lower and medial impression on tuberosity of ischium, together with biceps femoris.

Distal attachment. (i)   Upper part of medial surface of shaft of tibia.

Nerve supply.   Sciatic nerve.

Where to palpate.   Medial aspect of posterior surface of knee.

It is the most posterior of the two small tendons which can be felt in this region.

Action (at knee). Flexion of leg at knee; inward rotation of tibia when knee is in non-weight-bearing flexed position.

Comments. This is one of the two inner hamstring muscles.

Comments on the hamstrings. The hamstrings, so named from their large, cordlike tendons behind the knee joint, consist of the biceps femoris, semimembranosus and semitendinosus muscles. Although the biceps femoris constitutes the lateral hamstring, its long head lies approximately along the midline of the posterior aspect of the thigh, as far down as the popliteal space. At about this level the two heads unite to form their common tendon of attachment. The long head is fusiform in construction; the short head, penniform.

The semimembranosus and semitendinosus constitute the medial hamstrings. The former lies deeper than the latter and attaches higher on the tibia. The semitendinosus is attached to the medial surface of the tibia below the head, just below the attachment of the gracilis and behind that of the sartorius. Few writers mention any difference in the actions of these two muscles, but Bowen stated that the semimembranosus has more powerful action at the hip than does the semitendinosus.[2]

Although the hamstrings act at both the knees and the hips, their primary function is knee flexion. Wright called attention to the usefulness of the hamstrings in preventing hyperextension at the knee, and in unlocking the knee (i.e., reducing hyperextension) when one is returning from a position in which the line of gravity falls in front of the knee joints (e.g., inclining the trunk forward without bending the knees).[10] Nearly everyone is familiar with the limiting effect of the hamstrings. The difficulty experienced by most people in touching the toes with the fingers without bending the knees, and in sitting erect on the floor with the legs extended straight forward, is due to the fact that the hamstrings are frequently not long enough to permit such extreme stretching at the hips and knees simultaneously.

SARTORIUS (Fig. 16–7.) (See also muscles of the hip.)

Proximal attachment. (O) Anterior superior iliac spine and upper half of notch below it.

Distal attachment. (I) Anterior and medial surface of tibia just below condyle.

Nerve supply. Femoral nerve.

Where to palpate. At the anterior superior iliac spine. The entire muscle may be seen and palpated on the front of the thigh in a slender subject.

Action (at knee). Flexion of leg at knee; assists in inward rotation of tibia when knee is flexed.

Comments. This superficial, ribbon-like muscle runs obliquely downward and medialward across the front of the thigh. On its way to its distal attachment it curves around behind the bulge of the medial condyles in such a way that its line of pull is posterior to the axis of the knee joint. Thus, in spite of the fact that at least two thirds of the muscle — including its proximal and distal attachments — lies on the anterior aspect of the lower extremity, its action at the knee joint is not extension, but flexion.

GRACILIS (Figs. 16–8 and 16–9.) (See also muscles of the hip.)

Proximal attachment. (O)   Anterior aspect of lower half of symphysis pubis and upper half of pubic arch.

Distal attachment. (I)   Medial surface of tibia just below condyle.

Nerve supply.   Obturator nerve.

Where to palpate.   Medial aspect of posterior surface of knee, anterior to the semitendinosus tendon, but close to it.

Action (at knee).   Flexion of leg at knee; assists in inward rotation of tibia when knee is in flexed position.

Comments.   This is a long slender muscle situated on the medial side of the thigh.

POPLITEUS (Fig. 16–9.)

Proximal attachment. (O)   Lateral surface of lateral condyle of femur.

Distal attachment. (I)   Posterior surface of tibia, above popliteal line.

Nerve supply.   Tibial nerve.

Cannot be palpated.

Action.   Inward rotation of tibia; assists in flexion of leg at knee.

Comments.   The popliteus may be thought of as the "pronator teres" of the leg because of the similarity in structure and function. It "unlocks" the knee joint at the beginning of flexion and it serves to protect and stabilize the knee joint when a squatting position is assumed and maintained.[1]

GASTROCNEMIUS (Fig. 17–11.) (See also muscles of the ankle.)

Proximal attachments. (O)   Posterior surface of each femoral condyle and adjacent parts, by two separate heads.

Distal attachment. (I)   Posterior surface of calcaneus by means of calcaneal tendon (tendon of Achilles).

Nerve supply.   Tibial nerve.

Where to palpate.   Calf of leg and back of ankle.

Action (at knee).   Assists in flexion of leg at knee.

Comments.   Although this is primarily a muscle of the ankle joint, it is mentioned here because of its relation to the knee joint. As Wright pointed out, more important than its ability to help flex the leg at the knee joint is its function as a posterior ligament to protect the joint in movements of violent extension, such as running and jumping.[10]

SUPPLEMENTARY MATERIAL

Vulnerability of the Knee Joint.   Several writers have called attention to the strains and stresses to which the knee is subject and have emphasized the need for physical therapists and physical educators to be aware of the relation of these forces to knee function.

Williams and Lissner have pointed out the demands made on the quadriceps muscles when the knee is flexed in the weight bearing position, as when climbing stairs, seating oneself and rising from a chair, and deep knee bending. They have described methods for analyzing both tension and compression forces acting on the structures of the knee and have suggested the application of these to exercise procedures.[9]

Some denounce the use of deep squat exercises as taught in weight training and other conditioning programs and suggest that they be eliminated. Such exercises, they believe, tend to weaken the ligaments and increase the vulnerability of the joint.[5]

Although such criticism would appear to be valid when applied to the *misuse* or *overuse* of deep knee bending movements, the author is not convinced that all such exercises should be condemned. After all, the squatting, rather than the sitting, position has been used by many generations of children and primitive people, apparently with no harmful effects. Judging by past and present habits it appears to be a "natural" position for human beings.

DEMONSTRATIONS AND LABORATORY EXERCISES

Joint Structure and Function
1. Take a femur and a tibia and "construct" a knee joint, using felt for the fibrocartilage and adhesive tape for the ligaments. Be accurate in attaching these structures. It is suggested that two or three students work together on this project.

2. Using a form like that in Appendix B, record the essential information regarding the knee joint. Study the movements both on the skeleton and on the living body.

Muscular Action   (See Appendix F for muscle check list.)
3. FLEXION AT KNEE
Subject: Lie face down and flex leg at knee by raising foot.
Assistant: Steady subject's thigh and resist movement by pushing down on ankle.
Observer: Palpate biceps femoris, semitendinosus, gracilis, sartorius and gastrocnemius.
4. EXTENSION AT KNEE
a. Subject: Rise from a squat position.
Observer: Palpate quadriceps femoris.
b. Subject: Sit on table with legs hanging over edge. Extend leg.
Assistant: Steady subject's thigh and resist movement by holding ankle down.
Observer: Palpate quadriceps femoris.
5. OUTWARD ROTATION OF LEG WITH KNEE IN FLEXED POSITION
Subject: Sit on table with legs hanging over edge. Turn foot laterally as far as possible without moving thigh.
Assistant: Steady subject's thigh and give slight resistance by holding foot.

Observer: Palpate biceps femoris.

6. INWARD ROTATION OF LEG WITH KNEE IN FLEXED POSITION
Subject: Sit on table with legs hanging over edge. Turn foot medially as far as possible without moving thigh.

Assistant: Steady subject's thigh and give slight resistance by holding foot.

Observer: Palpate semitendinosus, gracilis and sartorius.

REFERENCES

1. Basmajian, J. V.: Muscles Alive, 2nd ed. Baltimore, The Williams & Wilkins Company, 1967.
2. Bowen, W. P., and Stone, H. A.: Applied Anatomy and Kinesiology, 7th ed. Philadelphia, Lea & Febiger, 1953.
3. Hollinshead, W. H.: Functional Anatomy of the Limbs and Back, 3rd ed., Philadelphia, W. B. Saunders Company, 1969.
4. Kaplan, E. B.: The iliotibial tract. J. Bone & Joint Surg., *40A*:817–832, 1958.
5. Klein, K. K.: The knee and the ligaments. J. Bone & Joint Surg., *44A*:1191–1192, 1962.
6. Pocock, G. S.: Electromyographic study of the quadriceps during resistive exercise. J. Am. Phys. Ther. Assn., *43*:427–434, 1963.
7. Schaeffer, J. P.: Morris' Human Anatomy, 11th ed. New York, McGraw-Hill, Inc., 1953.
8. Steindler, A.: Kinesiology of the Human Body. Springfield, Ill., Charles C Thomas, Publisher, 1955.
9. Williams, M., and Lissner, H. R.: Biomechanical analysis of knee function. J. Am. Phys. Ther. Assn., *43*:93–99, 1963.
10. Wright, W. G.: Muscle Function. New York, Hafner Publishing Company, 1962.

RECOMMENDED READING

Markee, J. E., et al.: Two joint muscles of the thigh. J. Bone & Joint Surg., *37A*:125–142, 1955.

CHAPTER 17

The Lower Extremity: The Ankle and Foot

The foot has two functions of tremendous importance — support and propulsion. In studying the structure of the foot, these functions should be kept constantly in mind, for only by seeing the foot in terms of the combined static and dynamic demands made upon it can one fully appreciate its intricate mechanism.

The foot is united with the leg at the ankle joint. Within the foot itself are the seven tarsal bones. Two of the joints in this region are of sufficient importance to the kinesiologist to merit special description. These are the subtalar and the midtarsal joints, the latter including the talonavicular and calcaneocuboid articulations. The movements within the foot occur mainly at these two joints.

The structure of the ankle, the tarsal joints and the toes will be described separately, but the muscles of these three regions will be discussed together, since many of them act on more than one joint.

Structure of the Ankle. (Figs. 17–1, 17–2 and 17–3.) The ankle is a hinge joint. It is formed by the articulation of the talus (astragalus) with the malleoli of the tibia and the fibula. The latter bones, bound together by the transverse tibiofibular ligament, the anterior and posterior ligaments of the lateral malleolus (tibiofibulare anterius and posterius), and the interossei, constitute a mortise into which the upper, rounded portion of the talus fits. The joint is surrounded by a thin, membranous capsule which is thicker on the medial side of the joint. In the back it is a thin mesh of membranous tissue. It is not continuous like most capsules. It is reinforced by several strong ligaments.

Ligaments

MEDIAL (MEDIALE). (Fig. 17–2.) This is a triangular ligament, attached by its apex to the medial malleolus and radiating downward to a broad attachment. It consists of four bands. The tibiotalaris posterior, or posterior talotibial ligament, slants backward to its attachment on the talus. The tibiocalcanea, or calcaneotibial ligament, passes downward to the sustentaculum tali on the medial side of the calcaneus. The tibionavicularis, or tibionavicular ligament, passes downward and slightly forward to the navicular bone and the calcaneonavicular ligament. The tibiotalaris anterior, or anterior talotibial ligament, comes from the anterior margin of the malleolus

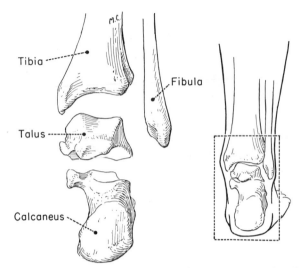

Figure 17–1. Bones of ankle and subtalar joints, posterior view.

and is attached below to the front of the talus close to the joint. The medial ligament as a whole is a strong mass of fibers protecting the medial side of the ankle joint.

LATERAL. (Fig. 17–3.)   These are three ligaments on the lateral side of the joint, the calcaneofibular and the anterior and posterior talofibular. All are attached above to the lateral malleolus. The anterior talofibular ligament is a short flat band which crosses in front of the talofibular articulation to attach to the front of the talus. The calcaneofibular is a strong, cordlike ligament, coming from the tip of the lateral malleolus and passing downward and slightly backward to its attachment on the lateral surface of the calcaneus. The posterior talofibular ligament is a strong thick band which runs almost horizon-

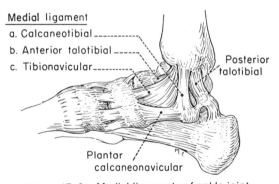

Figure 17–2. Medial ligaments of ankle joint.

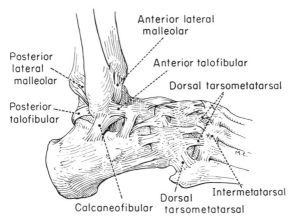

Figure 17–3.   Lateral ligaments of ankle joint.

tally from the posterior margin of the lateral malleolus to a tubercle on the back of the talus.

Movements.   The movements of the ankle joint occur about an axis which is usually described as frontal-horizontal, but which is actually slightly oblique, as evidenced by the fact that the lateral malleolus is slightly posterior to the medial. This is of minor significance, but it explains the tendency of the foot to turn out when it is fully elevated, and to turn in when fully depressed.

DORSAL FLEXION (FLEXION).   A forward-upward movement of the foot in the sagittal plane, so that the dorsal surface of the foot approaches the anterior surface of the leg.

PLANTAR FLEXION (EXTENSION).   A forward-downward movement of the foot in the sagittal plane, so that the dorsal surface of the foot moves away from the anterior surface of the leg.

Structure of the Foot. (Figs. 17–4 and 17–5.)   The foot is made up of seven tarsal bones, five metatarsals and fourteen phalanges. The most posterior of the tarsals is the calcaneus, or heel bone. The knobby, irregular-shaped talus sits above and partly medial to it. It is supported medially by the shelflike projection of the calcaneus, called the sustentaculum tali. The navicular (scaphoid) is anterior to the talus, and the cuboid projects further forward than does the navicular. On the medial side of its anterior portion and in front of the navicular, the three cuneiform bones lie side by side. The first metatarsal articulates with the first cuneiform, the second metatarsal with the second cuneiform, the third metatarsal with the third cuneiform, and the fourth and fifth metatarsals with the cuboid. The phalanges are somewhat similar to those of the thumb and fingers, there being two in the great toe and three in each of the four lesser toes.

The foot as a whole is usually described as an elastic arched structure, the keystone of the arch being the talus. This bone has several marks of distinction. Aside from being the connecting link between the foot and the leg, it is distinguished by having no muscles attached to it and by receiving and transmitting the weight of the entire body (with the exception of the foot itself), a function which requires great strength and firm support.

The foot has two arches, a longitudinal and a transverse. The longitudinal arch passes from the heel to the heads of the five metatarsals. It is sometimes described as being made up of an inner and an outer component. The outer component includes the calcaneus, cuboid and fourth and fifth metatarsals (Fig. 17–5, A). The inner component consists of the calcaneus, talus, navicular, three cuneiforms and the three medial metatarsals (Fig. 17–5, B). The outer component has a nearly flat contour and lacks mobility, hence is better adapted to the function of support, whereas the inner component, with its greater flexibility and its curving arch, is adapted to the function of shock absorption, so important in all forms of locomotion. Contrary to popular opinion, the height of the longitudinal arch is not indicative of the strength of the arch. Thus a low arch is not necessarily a weak one, *provided it is not associated with a pronated (i.e., abducted and everted) foot.*

The transverse arch is the side-to-side concavity on the under

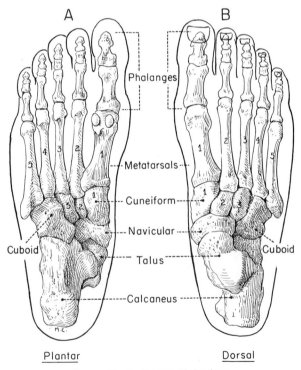

Figure 17–4. Bones of the foot.

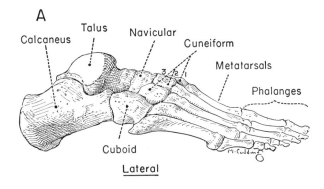

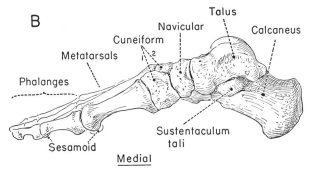

Figure 17–5. Bones of the foot.

side of the foot formed by the anterior tarsal bones and the metatarsals. The anterior boundary of this arch, under the metatarsal heads, is known as the metatarsal arch. There is considerable controversy as to whether or not this should be called an arch, since, under the pressure of the body weight in standing and in walking, it flattens completely. The metatarsal arch exists, therefore, only in non-weight-bearing positions.

The toes, especially the large and powerful "big toe," are largely responsible for propulsion. They provide the "push off" at the end of the step. Their use in locomotion is directly proportional to the vigor and speed of the walk or run.

The strength and elasticity of the foot are due in large measure to the ligaments which bind the bones together and to the muscles which work to preserve the balance of the foot. Thus the ligaments and the muscles share the responsibility for maintaining the integrity of the arches.

The two tarsal joints to be considered here are the subtalar and the midtarsal.

SUBTALAR JOINT. The subtalar joint consists of the articulation of the inferior surface of the talus bone with the superior and anterior surfaces of the calcaneus and the superior surface of the calcaneo-navicular ligament. Ordinarily the point of contact between a bone and a ligament is not considered part of the articulation, but in this case it is, because of the presence of a cartilaginous articular facet which is lined with synovial membrane. The articulations are reinforced by the anterior, posterior, lateral and medial talocalcaneal ligaments and the talocalcaneal interosseus ligament (Fig. 17–6). They permit slight forward, backward and lateral gliding, also very slight inversion and eversion.

Plantar calcaneonavicular ligament (the spring ligament). (Fig. 17–6.) This ligament forms an inherent part of the subtalar joint. By connecting the sustentaculum tali of the calcaneus with the under side of the navicular, it forms a sling to give support to the talus. For the latter purpose it is covered with a fibrocartilaginous articular facet which has a smooth surface and is lined with synovial mem-

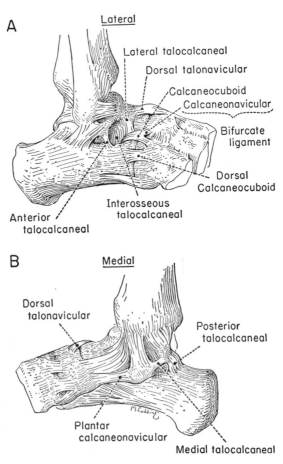

A   Lateral

Lateral talocalcaneal
Dorsal talonavicular
Calcaneocuboid
Calcaneonavicular
Bifurcate ligament
Dorsal Calcaneocuboid
Interosseous talocalcaneal
Anterior talocalcaneal

B   Medial

Dorsal talonavicular
Posterior talocalcaneal
Plantar calcaneonavicular
Medial talocalcaneal

Figure 17–6.   Ligaments of tarsal joints.

brane. It is called the spring ligament because it contains yellow elastic fibers and has considerable elasticity. The importance of this can be readily seen when one remembers that the talus receives the weight of the entire body and is in turn supported largely by the spring ligament. The shock absorbing function of this arrangement is obvious. It is also fairly obvious that excessive prolonged pressure of this ligament (through improper use of the feet) will cause it to stretch permanently and will result in a lowered arch.

MIDTARSAL JOINT (TRANSVERSE TARSAL; CHOPART'S). This consists of two articulations, the lateral one being the calcaneocuboid joint, and the medial one, the talonavicular. On looking down at these joints from above, the continuous line of articulation—the talonavicular and calcaneocuboid—is seen to form a somewhat flattened letter S (Figs. 17–4, B and 17–7). The talonavicular joint may be described as a shallow ball-and-socket joint. It permits movements about three axes. The calcaneocuboid joint is non-axial and permits only slight gliding motions. These would seem to be supplementary or secondary to the freer motions of the talonavicular joint. The movements of the midtarsal articulation, particularly on the talonavicular joint, are as follows:

Very slight dorsal and plantar flexion. These movements supplement dorsal and plantar flexion at the ankle joint.

Slight abduction and adduction of the front part of the foot on the rear part.

Very slight inversion and eversion of the front part of the foot on the rear.

Ligaments of the midtarsal joint. (Figs. 17–6 and 17–8.) The midtarsal joint is reinforced above by three dorsal ligaments—the dorsal talonavicular, the calcaneocuboidal part of the bifurcate ligament and the dorsal calcaneocuboid—and below by the long and short plantar ligaments. The short plantar ligament, also called the plantar calcaneocuboid, is a short, wide, thick ligament of great strength. It

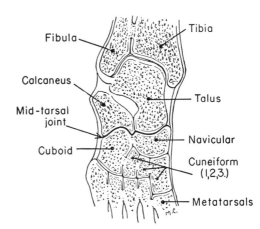

Figure 17–7. Oblique section of tarsal bones showing midtarsal joint.

Fibula

Tibia

Calcaneus

Talus

Mid-tarsal joint

Cuboid

Navicular

Cuneiform (1,2,3.)

Metatarsals

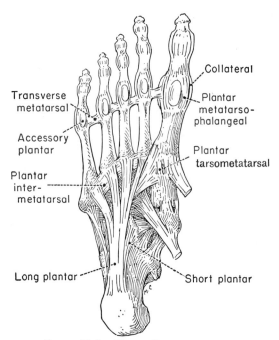

Figure 17–8.   Plantar ligaments of foot.

extends from the tubercle at the anterior end of the plantar surface of the calcaneus to the plantar surface of the cuboid behind the oblique ridge. The long plantar ligament is a longer, more superficial, but equally strong and dense band. It extends from the plantar surface of the calcaneus in front of the tuberosity to the oblique ridge on the plantar surface of the cuboid, with prolongations to the bases of the second, third, fourth and medial half of the fifth metatarsal bones.

THE TARSOMETATARSAL JOINTS. (Figs. 17–6 and 17–8.)   These are all non-axial joints, with the possible exception of the first, which presents a slightly saddle-shaped appearance. They are reinforced by the dorsal and plantar tarsometatarsal and the interosseous ligaments. The movements are of a gliding nature, resembling a restricted form of flexion, extension, abduction and adduction.

THE INTERMETATARSAL ARTICULATIONS. (Figs. 17–3 and 17–8.) These include two sets of side-by-side articulations, those between the bases and those between the heads of the metatarsal bones. They are all non-axial joints, permitting only slight gliding movements. The bases of the metatarsals are united by the dorsal and plantar intermetatarsal and the interosseous ligaments. The heads of the metatarsals are connected by the transverse metatarsal ligament. The articulations between the heads of the metatarsal bones are an important part of the metatarsal arch. The total result of the movements occurring there is a spreading or flattening of the arch when the weight is on it and a return to its plantar concavity when the weight is taken off it.

THE METATARSOPHALANGEAL JOINTS. (Fig. 17–8.) These may best be described as a modified form of ovoid joints. They are reinforced by the dorsal and plantar metatarsophalangeal, and the collateral ligaments. The movements are flexion, extension and limited abduction and adduction. The joint of the great toe differs somewhat from the corresponding joint in each of the four lesser toes. It is considerably larger than the others and it has two sesamoid bones under it in place of the plantar ligament.

THE INTERPHALANGEAL JOINTS. These are all hinge joints, permitting only flexion and extension. The ligaments reinforcing them are the dorsal and plantar interphalangeal and the collateral.

SUMMARY OF MOVEMENTS OF THE FOOT

Ankle Joint. Dorsal and plantar flexion (dorsal surface of foot moves toward and away from anterior surface of leg)

Tarsal Joints (especially subtalar and midtarsal)

Dorsal and plantar flexion (correspond to ankle joint movements)

Inversion and eversion (medial, lateral border of foot is raised)

Abduction and adduction (front part of foot bends laterally and medially)

Note: The terms "pronation" and "supination" of the feet represent composite movements, pronation being the combination of abduction and eversion; supination, the combination of adduction and inversion. Because of the structure of the joints, these movements always occur together in this manner.

Toes. Flexion and extension (toes curl under; toes straighten out)

Muscles. The muscles of the ankle and foot, classified according to their location, are as follows:

Muscles on anterior aspect of leg:
  Tibialis anterior
  Extensor digitorum longus
  Extensor hallucis longus
  Peroneus tertius
Muscles on posterior aspect of leg:
  Gastrocnemius
  Soleus
  Tibialis posterior
  Flexor digitorum longus
  Flexor hallucis longus
Muscles on lateral aspect of leg:
  Peroneus longus
  Peroneus brevis

Intrinsic muscles of the foot:
  Extensor digitorum brevis
  Flexor digitorum brevis
  Quadratus plantae
  Lumbricales
  Abductor hallucis
  Flexor hallucis brevis
  Adductor hallucis
  Abductor digiti minimi
  Flexor digiti minimi brevis
  Dorsal interossei
  Plantar interossei

TIBIALIS ANTERIOR (Fig. 17–9, A.)

Proximal attachments. (O) Lateral condyle and upper two thirds of lateral surface of tibia.

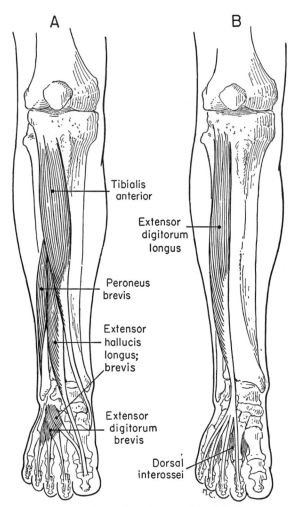

Figure 17–9.   Anterior muscles of the leg.

Distal attachments. (1)   Plantar surface of base of first meta-tarsal and medial surface of first cuneiform.

Nerve supply.   Deep peroneal nerve.

Where to palpate.   Anterior surface of leg, just lateral to tibia.

Action

      Ankle: Dorsal flexion.

      Foot: Dorsal flexion; supination (adduction and inversion).

Comments.   About two thirds of the way down the leg the tibialis anterior becomes tendinous. The tendon crosses over to the medial side of the leg and passes in front of the malleolus on its way to the first cuneiform.

In her electromyographic study of the action of the leg muscles in movements of the free foot (the subject standing on the other foot), O'Connell found that dorsiflexion was initiated by the tibialis anterior.[5]

EXTENSOR DIGITORUM LONGUS (Fig. 17–9, B.)

Proximal attachments. (O) Lateral condyle of tibia and upper three fourths of anterior surface of fibula.

Distal attachments. (I) Dorsal surface of second and third phalanges of four lesser toes.

Nerve supply. Deep peroneal nerve.

Where to palpate. Anterior surface of ankle and dorsal surface of foot, lateral to tendon of extensor hallucis longus.

Action

Ankle: Dorsal flexion.

Foot: Dorsal flexion; assists in eversion and abduction.

Toes: Extension of four lesser toes.

Comments. This is a penniform muscle and is situated lateral to the tibialis anterior in the upper part of the leg and lateral to the extensor hallucis longus in the lower part. Just in front of the ankle joint the tendon divides into four tendons, one for each of the four lesser toes.

EXTENSOR HALLUCIS LONGUS (Fig. 17–9, A.)

Proximal attachment. (O) Middle half of anterior surface of fibula.

Distal attachment. (I) Dorsal surface of base of distal phalanx of hallux (great toe).

Nerve supply. Deep peroneal nerve.

Where to palpate. Dorsal surface of foot and great toe.

Action

Ankle: Helps in dorsal flexion.

Foot: Dorsal flexion.

Toes: Extension and hyperextension of great toe.

Comments. Like the preceding muscle, this is penniform in structure. Its upper portion lies beneath the tibialis anterior and extensor digitorum longus, but about halfway down the leg the tendon emerges between these two muscles, thus becoming superficial. After it has reached the ankle the tendon slants medially across the dorsal surface of the foot to the top of the great toe.

PERONEUS TERTIUS (Fig. 17–10.)

Proximal attachment. (O) Anterior surface of lower third of fibula.

Distal attachment. (I) Dorsal surface of base of fifth metatarsal.

Nerve supply. Deep peroneal nerve.

Where to palpate. Dorsal surface of foot close to base of fifth metatarsal.

Action

Ankle: Dorsal flexion.

Foot: Dorsal flexion; pronation (eversion and abduction).

Comments. This little muscle lies lateral to the extensor digitorum longus and is sometimes described as the fifth tendon of the latter muscle.

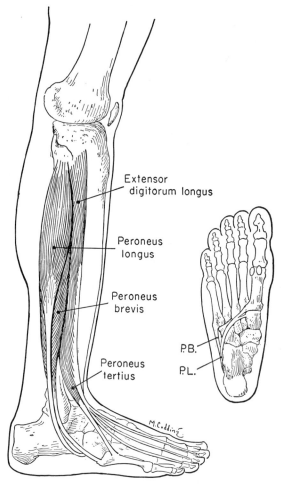

Extensor
digitorum longus

Peroneus
longus

Peroneus
brevis

Peroneus
tertius

P.B.

P.L.

M.Codding

Figure 17–10.   Lateral muscles of the leg. (*P.B.* = Peroneus brevis; *P.L.* = peroneus longus.)

PERONEUS LONGUS (Fig. 17–10.)

Proximal attachments. (O)   Lateral condyle of tibia; lateral surface of head and upper two thirds of fibula.

Distal attachments. (I)   Lateral margin of plantar surface of first cuneiform and base of first metatarsal.

Nerve supply.   Superficial peroneal nerve.

Where to palpate

Muscle belly: Lateral surface of upper half of leg.

Tendon: Lateral surface of lower half of leg and just above and behind lateral malleolus.

Action

Ankle: Plantar flexion.

Foot: Plantar flexion; pronation (eversion and abduction).

Comments. This muscle is situated superficially on the lateral aspect of the leg. Its distal tendon passes behind the lateral malleolus and proceeds forward and downward to the margin of the foot where it passes behind the tuberosity of the fifth metatarsal. At this point it turns under the foot, passes through the peroneal groove of the cuboid, and slants forward across the plantar surface of the foot to its attachment at the base of the first metatarsal and first cuneiform, not far from the attachment of the tibialis anterior.

PERONEUS BREVIS (Figs. 17–9, A and 17–10.)

Proximal attachment. (O) Lateral surface of lower two thirds of fibula.

Distal attachment. (I) Tuberosity on lateral side of base of fifth metatarsal.

Nerve supply. Superficial peroneal nerve.

Where to palpate. Lateral margin of foot just posterior to base of fifth metatarsal.

Action

    Ankle: Assists in plantar flexion.

    Foot: Plantar flexion; pronation (eversion and abduction).

Comments. This is a penniform muscle, lying beneath the peroneus longus on the lower half of the lateral aspect of the leg. Its tendon passes behind the lateral malleolus immediately anterior to the tendon of longus and continues forward just above the longus tendon to its attachment on the tuberosity of the fifth metatarsal, below the attachment of peroneus tertius.

GASTROCNEMIUS (Fig. 17–11.) (See also muscles of the knee.)

Proximal attachments. (O) Posterior surface of each femoral condyle and adjacent parts, by two separate heads.

Distal attachment. (I) Posterior surface of calcaneus by means of calcaneal tendon (tendon of Achilles).

Nerve supply. Tibial nerve.

Where to palpate. Calf of leg and back of ankle.

Action. Plantar flexion of foot at ankle.

Comments. The gastrocnemius is the large superficial muscle on the back of the leg and can be seen as two bulges in the upper part of the calf when it is well developed. Its two heads, together with the soleus, constitute the triceps surae. The lateral and medial portions of the muscle remain distinct from each other as far down as the middle of the back of the leg. Then they fuse to form the broad tendon of Achilles.

This muscle is a powerful plantar flexor of the ankle joint whose most familiar function is to enable one to rise on the toes. Many anatomists have thought that it acted only when the movement was resisted, but Sheffield, Gersten and Mastellone found that it was active in unresisted movements of plantar flexion with the subjects in a supine position.[6] It has a large angle of pull, approximately 90 degrees when the foot is in its fundamental position. Its internal structure and its leverage combine to make it an exceedingly powerful muscle. Herman and Bragin, in a 1967 study, concluded that its

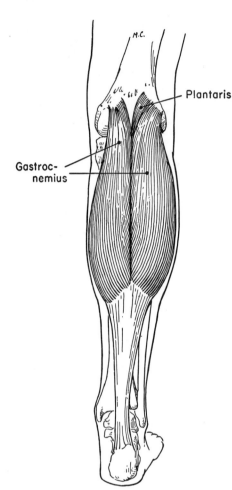

Figure 17–11.   Gastrocnemius.

most important role was plantar flexion in large contractions and in the rapid development of tension.[2]

SOLEUS (Fig. 17–12.)

Proximal attachments. (O)   Posterior surface of head of fibula and upper two thirds of shaft; popliteal line and medial border of middle third of tibia.

Distal attachment. (I)   Posterior surface of calcaneus by means of calcaneal tendon (tendon of Achilles).

Nerve supply.   Tibial nerve.

Where to palpate.   Slightly lateral to and below the lateral bulge of the gastrocnemius.

Action.   Plantar flexion of foot at ankle.

Comments.   The soleus lies beneath the gastrocnemius, except along the lateral aspect of the lower half of the calf, where a portion of it lies lateral to the upper part of the calcaneal tendon. Its fibers are inserted into the calcaneal tendon in a bipenniform manner. In an electromyographic study of the leg muscles when the subjects balanced on one foot, Sheffield, Gersten and Mastellone found that the soleus was consistently more active than the gastrocnemius.[6] Herman and Bragin stated that it was most active in minimal contractions and when the foot was "at dorsiflexion." The latter would seem to imply that it was especially active in the reduction of dorsiflexion.[2]

TIBIALIS POSTERIOR (Fig. 17–13.)

Proximal attachments. (O) Posterior surface of upper two thirds of tibia beginning at popliteal line; medial surface of upper two thirds of fibula.

Distal attachments. (I) Tuberosity of navicular bone with branches to sustentaculum tali of calcaneus, to the three cuneiforms, to cuboid and to the bases of the three middle metatarsal bones.

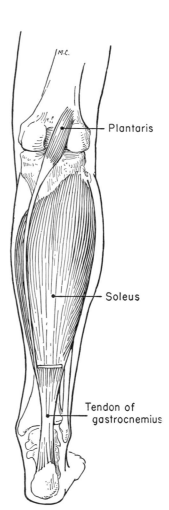

Figure 17–12. Posterior muscles of the leg, middle layer.

Plantaris

Soleus

Tendon of
gastrocnemius

Nerve supply. Tibial nerve.
Cannot be palpated.
Action

 Ankle: Assists in plantar flexion.

 Foot: Supination (inversion and adduction); plantar flexion.

Comments. This is the deepest of the muscles on the back of the leg. The main part of the muscle covers the intermuscular septum between the tibia and fibula. In the lower fourth of the leg its tendon slants across to the medial side of the ankle, passes behind the medial malleolus and above the sustentaculum tali, then turns under the foot around the medial margin of the navicular bone to insert into its under side. The muscle is penniform in structure. Because of its direction of pull and its numerous attachments on the plantar surface of the tarsal bones, an important function of this muscle is maintenance of the longitudinal arch.

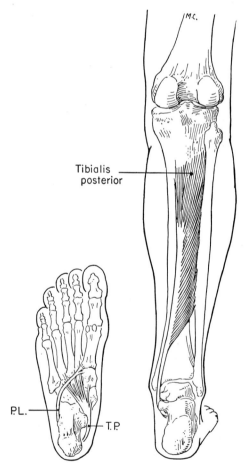

Figure 17–13. Tibialis posterior. (*P.L.* = Peroneus longus; *T.P.* = tibialis posterior.)

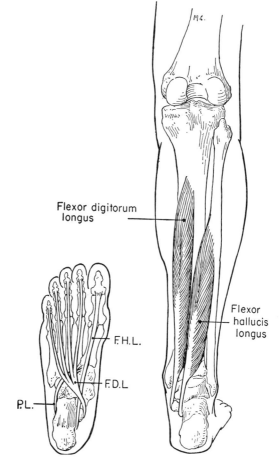

Figure 17–14. Flexor digitorum longus and flexor hallucis longus. (*F.H.L.* = Flex. hal. long.; *F.D.L.* = flex. dig. long.; *P.L.* = per. long.)

FLEXOR DIGITORUM LONGUS (Fig. 17–14.)

Proximal attachment. (O) Posterior surface of middle three fifths of tibia.

Distal attachments. (I) Plantar surface of base of distal phalanx of each of the four lesser toes.

Nerve supply. Tibial nerve.

Cannot be palpated.

Action

Ankle: Assists in plantar flexion.

Foot: Plantar flexion; assists in supination (inversion and adduction).

Toes: Flexion of four lesser toes.

Comments. This muscle is situated on the medial side of the back of the leg, behind the tibia. It is penniform in structure. Its distal tendon passes behind the medial malleolus between the tendons of tibialis posterior and flexor hallucis longus. Beneath the tarsal bones it divides into four tendons which go to the distal phalanx of each of the four lesser toes. Sheffield, Gersten and Mastellone found it to be a strong supinator in the non-weight-bearing position.[6] Its supinatory action in weight-bearing is yet to be investigated electromyographically.

FLEXOR HALLUCIS LONGUS (Fig. 17–14.)

Proximal attachment. (O)   Posterior surface of lower two thirds of fibula.

Distal attachment. (I)   Plantar surface of base of distal phalanx of hallux (great toe).

Nerve supply.   Tibial nerve.

Where to palpate.   Medial border of calcaneal tendon close to the calcaneus.

Action

Ankle: Assists in plantar flexion.

Foot: Plantar flexion; assists in supination (inversion and adduction).

Toes: Flexion of great toe.

Comments.   The flexor hallucis longus is situated on the lateral side of the back of the leg behind the fibula and the lateral portion of the tibia. The fibers unite with the distal tendon in a penniform manner. The tendon crosses behind the ankle to the medial side, passes behind and beneath the sustentaculum tali, the little shelflike projection on the medial side of the calcaneus, and runs forward under the medial margin of the foot to the distal phalanx of the great toe. It is the most posterior of the three tendons that pass behind the medial malleolus. One of its important functions is to provide the "push off" in walking, running and jumping.

PLANTAR FASCIA. (Fig. 17–15.)   On the plantar surface of the foot the muscles are covered by fascia. This is divided into medial, central and lateral portions. The central portion, known as the plantar aponeurosis, is particularly strong and fibrous. It extends under the whole length of the foot, connecting the tuberosity of the calcaneus with the bases of the proximal phalanges of the five toes. This is an exceedingly strong band which serves as an effective binding rod for the longitudinal arch.

INTRINSIC MUSCLES OF THE FOOT. (Figs. 17–16, 17–17 and 17–18.)   These muscles will be treated as a group, rather than individually. All their attachments are within the foot itself. They are innervated by the deep peroneal, medial plantar and lateral plantar nerves. As is to be expected, these muscles are much more highly developed in primitive people than in people who wear shoes habitually.

In a recent study on phasic activity of the intrinsic muscles of the foot, Mann and Inman concluded that these muscles act as a functional unit, also that they have a significant role in stabilization of the foot during propulsion.[4] Since habitually pronated feet are known to be unstable, it is not surprising that these investigators found the intrinsic muscles to be more active in such feet than they are in

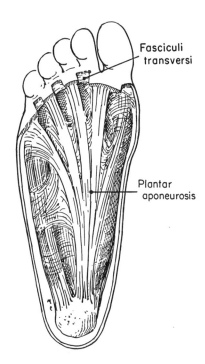

Fasciculi
transversi

Plantar
aponeurosis

Figure 17–15.   Plantar fascia of the foot.

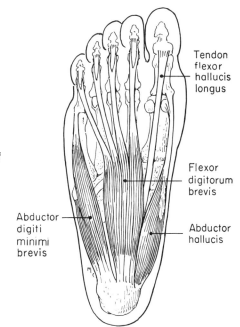

Tendon
flexor
hallucis
longus

Flexor
digitorum
brevis

Abductor
hallucis

Figure 17–16.   Plantar muscles of
the foot, superficial layer.

Abductor
digiti
minimi
brevis

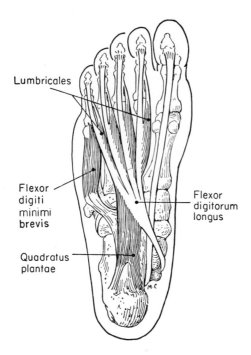

Lumbricales

Flexor
digiti
minimi
brevis

Flexor
digitorum
longus

Quadratus
plantae

Figure 17–17.   Plantar muscles
of the foot, middle layer.

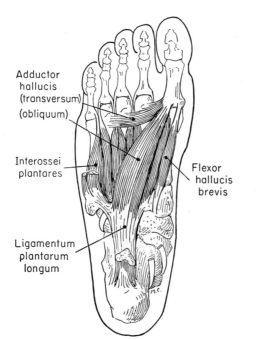

Adductor
hallucis
(transversum)
(obliquum)

Interossei
plantares

Flexor
hallucis
brevis

Ligamentum
plantarum
longum

Figure 17–18.   Plantar muscles
of the foot, deep layer.

"normal" feet. In relaxed standing, however, no activity of these muscles was detected in either pronated or normal feet.

Basmajian, Smith and other investigators similarly concluded from their EMG investigations that the intrinsic muscles of the foot are not active in the normal *static* support of the longitudinal arches.[1] Definite activity was noted, however, in rising on the toes and in voluntarily attempting to increase the height of the arches.

A more recent investigation of the mechanics of arch support is reported below.

SUPPLEMENTARY MATERIAL

Action of the Muscles in the Support of the Arches. In 1963 Basmajian and Stecko reviewed the question of the mechanics of arch support and investigated three theories regarding the maintenance of the arches. These are that they are maintained by muscular contraction alone, by bones and ligaments alone or by the combination of muscular contraction and passive structures.

Using 20 young men as subjects, they investigated six muscles electromyographically. These were the tibialis anterior, tibialis posterior, peroneus longus, flexor hallucis longus, abductor hallucis and flexor digitorum brevis. They found that the men could support loads of 100–200 lbs. standing on one foot without any evidence of muscular action, and that with loads of 400 lbs. some muscles became active, but many still remained inactive. They concluded from these findings that the arches' first line of defense is ligamentous and that the muscles constitute a dynamic reserve which is called into action reflexively when the load is excessive.[1]

Flexibility and Stability of Feet. In a study of the flexibility and stability and other characteristics of the feet of 100 young women, Lawrence noted that there was no significant relationship between flexibility and stability, also that the size and weight of the body had very little effect upon the measurements of foot size, flexibility, stability or degree of out-toeing. Lawrence also observed that long, narrow feet tended to be more flexible, but less stable, than feet of other proportions.[3]

Action of the Muscles in Movements of the Free Foot. Basmajian and O'Connell, in independent studies, reached similar conclusions regarding the action of muscles in movements of the non-weight-bearing foot. Briefly, these are as follows:

1. Dorsiflexion is initiated by tibialis anterior and assisted by extensor digitorum longus and extensor hallucis longus.

2. Plantar flexion is initiated either by peroneus longus or soleus.

3. Tibialis anterior is definitely active in inversion of the foot only when the latter movement is accompanied by dorsiflexion.[1, 5]

Action of the Foot and Ankle Muscles in Standing. Although their studies were not entirely comparable, some investigators found that the gastrocnemius was active in relaxed standing and others found that the soleus was active, but the gastrocnemius was not unless the body swayed forward. Several investigators agreed that the tibialis anterior and peroneus longus were not active in relaxed standing but noted that the tibialis anterior became active when the body swayed backward.[1]

For additional findings the reader is referred to *Muscles Alive* by Basmajian or to the original reports listed in the back of that book.

DEMONSTRATIONS AND LABORATORY EXERCISES

Joint Structure and Function
1. Using forms like the one in Appendix B, record the essential information regarding the ankle joint, the subtalar joint and the mid-tarsal joints. Study the movements of these joints both on the skeleton and on the living body.

2. Using a Lufkin rule or a protractor-goniometer, measure the range of motion at the ankle joint with the knee straight and with the knee flexed. Measure ten subjects.

Muscular Action (See Appendix F for muscle check list.)

3. PLANTAR FLEXION

Subject: (*a*) Stand and rise on the toes. (*b*) Hold one foot off the floor and extend it vigorously.

Observer: Compare the muscular action of the leg in (*a*) and (*b*).

4. DORSIFLEXION

Subject: Sit on a table with the legs straight and with the feet over the edge. Dorsiflex one foot as far as possible.

Assistant: Resist the movement by holding the foot.

Observer: Identify the tibialis anterior, peroneus tertius, extensor digitorum longus and extensor hallucis longus.

5. PRONATION (EVERSION AND ABDUCTION)

Subject: In same position as in 4, turn one foot laterally without extending it.

Assistant: Steady the leg at the ankle and resist the movement by holding the foot.

Observer: Identify the muscles that contract.

6. SUPINATION (INVERSION AND ADDUCTION)

Subject: In same position as in 4 and 5, turn one foot medially as far as possible.

Assistant: Steady the leg at the ankle and resist the movement by holding the foot.

Observer: Identify the muscles that contract.

REFERENCES

1. Basmajian, J. V.: Muscles Alive, 2nd ed., Baltimore, The Williams & Wilkins Company, 1967.
2. Herman, R., and Bragin, S. J.: Function of the gastrocnemius and soleus muscles. J. Am. Phys. Ther. Assn., 47:105–113, 1967.

3. Lawrence, S.: A Study of the Flexibility and the Stability of the Feet of College Women. Unpublished master's thesis, Smith College, 1955.
4. Mann, R., and Inman, V. T.: Phasic activity of intrinsic muscles of the foot. J. Bone & Joint Surg., 46A:469–481, 1964.
5. O'Connell, A. L.: Electromyographic study of certain leg muscles during movements of the free foot and during standing. Am. J. Phys. Med., 37:289–301, 1958.
6. Sheffield, F. F., Gersten, J. W., and Mastellone, A. F.: Electromyographic study of the muscles of the foot in normal walking. Am. J. Phys. Med., 35:223–236, 1956.

RECOMMENDED READINGS

Bettmann, E. H.: The human foot. Arch. Phys. Ther. 25:13–26, 1944.
Jones, R. L.: The human foot: An experimental study of its mechanics and the role of its muscles and ligaments in the support of the arch. Am. J. Anat., 68:1–39, 1941.
Kelly, E. D.: A comparative study of structure and function of normal, pronated and painful feet among children. Res. Quart. Am. Assn. Health, Phys. Ed. & Recrn., 18:291–312, 1947.

CHAPTER 18

The Spinal Column

If one were faced with the problem of devising a single mechanism that would *simultaneously* (1) give stability to a collapsible cylinder; (2) permit movement in all directions, yet always return to the fundamental starting position; (3) support three structures of considerable weight—a globe, a yoke and a cage; (4) provide attachment for numerous flexible bands and elastic cords; (5) transmit a gradually increasing weight to a rigid basin-like foundation; (6) act as a shock absorber for cushioning jolts and jars; and (7) encase and protect a cord of extreme delicacy, he would be staggered by the immensity of the task. Yet the spinal column fulfills all these requirements with amazing efficiency. It is at the same time an organ of stability and mobility, of support and protection, of resistance and adaptation. It is an instrument of great precision, yet of robust structure. Its architecture and the manner in which it performs its many functions are worthy of careful study. From the kinesiologic point of view, we are interested in the spine chiefly as a mechanism for maintaining erect posture and for permitting movements of the head, neck and trunk.

In order to understand these functions of the spine, it is necessary to have a clear picture, first of the spinal column as a whole, and second of the distinguishing characteristics of the different regions. The spinal column, consisting of seven cervical, twelve thoracic and five lumbar vertebrae, the sacrum and the coccyx, presents four curves as seen from the side. The cervical and lumbar curves are convex forward, the thoracic and sacrococcygeal curves convex to the rear (Fig. 18–1). The thoracic and sacrococcygeal curves are called primary curves because they exist before birth. The cervical and lumbar curves develop during infancy and early childhood, hence are called secondary curves. From the first cervical to the fifth lumbar vertebrae, the vertebral bodies become increasingly larger, an important factor in the weight-bearing function of the spine.

There are two sets of interspinal articulations, those between the vertebral bodies and those between the vertebral arches. The latter are in pairs, there being one on either side of each vertebra. The articulations of the first two vertebrae are atypical and will be described

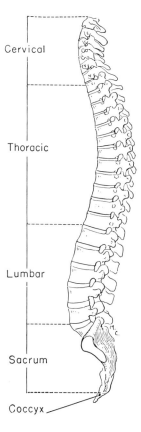

Cervical

Thoracic

Figure 18–1. Lateral view of the spinal column showing anteroposterior curves.

Lumbar

Sacrum

Coccyx

separately. The articulation of the sacrum with the ilia is discussed on page 268 in the section on the pelvic girdle.

There is such a close relationship between the structure of the spinal column and the movements that take place in its different regions that the student will find it well worth the effort to acquire a thorough grasp of the structure before proceeding to the movements. If possible, he should refer frequently both to a skeleton and to a strung set of vertebrae while studying spinal structure.

Articulations of the Vertebral Bodies. (Fig. 18–2.) These joints are classified as synchondroses, or cartilaginous joints. The bodies of the vertebrae are united by means of fibrocartilages, otherwise known as intervertebral disks. These correspond to the surfaces of the adjacent vertebral bodies, except in the cervical region, where they are smaller from side to side. They adhere to the hyaline cartilage both above and below, there being no articular cavity in this type of joint. In thickness they are fairly uniform in the thoracic region, but in the cervical and lumbar regions they are thicker in front than in back. Altogether they constitute one fourth of the length of the spinal column. Each disk consists of two parts, an outer fibrous rim and an

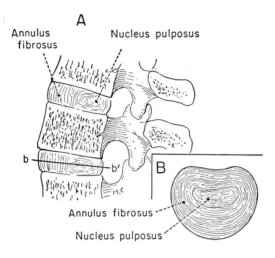

Figure 18–2. A, Sagittal section of lumbar vertebrae and intervertebral fibrocartilages. *B,* Transverse section of intervertebral fibrocartilage.

inner pulpy nucleus, known as the nucleus pulposus. This is a ball of firmly compressed elastic material, not unlike the center of a golf ball. It constitutes a pivot of motion and permits compression in any direction, as well as torsion. The intervertebral disks are also important as shock absorbers.

Ligaments of the Vertebral Bodies.

ANTERIOR LONGITUDINAL LIGAMENT. (Fig. 18–3.) This ligament extends from the inner surface of the occipital bone down the front of the spinal column to the sacrum. It starts as a narrow band and widens as it descends. It is thinnest in the cervical region and thickest in the thoracic.

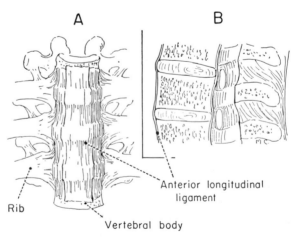

Figure 18–3. Anterior longitudinal ligament of the spine. *A,* Anterior view; *B,* sagittal section of vertebrae showing lateral view of ligament.

Posterior Longitudinal Ligament. (Fig. 18–4.) This extends from the occipital bone down the back of the vertebral bodies to the coccyx. It is a relatively narrow band with lateral expansions opposite each intervertebral fibrocartilage. It is thicker in the thoracic than in the cervical or lumbar region.

Articulations of the Vertebral Arches. (Fig. 18–5.) The articulations between the facets of the vertebral arches are non-axial diarthrodial joints. Each of these joints has an articular cavity and is enclosed within a capsule. A slight amount of gliding motion is permitted. The resultant movement of each vertebra is determined largely by the direction in which the articular facets face. The cervical spine appears to be somewhat of an exception, however. The facets in this region slant at about a 45 degree angle, lying halfway between the horizontal and the frontal planes (Fig. 18–6, *A*). Such a slant would seem to favor rotation and lateral flexion and to be unfavorable to flexion and hyperextension. Yet these latter movements occur as freely as does lateral flexion, whereas rotation, from the second cervical vertebra down, can be rated only as moderate. In the thoracic region they lie slightly more in the frontal and less in the horizontal plane than the cervical articulations, and they have a slight inward and outward slant (Fig. 18–6, *B*). The upper facets face backward, slightly upward and lateralward; the lower facets forward, slightly downward and medialward. They are adapted equally well to rotation and to lateral bending. In the lumbar region, except at the lumbosacral articulation, the articular facets lie more nearly in the sagittal plane (Fig. 18–6, *C*). The upper facets face inward and slightly backward; the lower facets face outward and slightly forward. Furthermore, the upper facets present slightly concave surfaces, and the lower facets

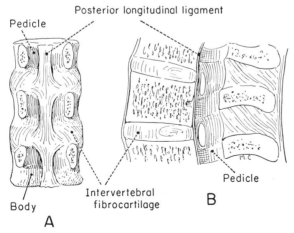

Figure 18–4. Posterior longitudinal ligament of spine. *A,* Frontal section of vertebrae showing posterior view of ligament. *B,* Sagittal section of vertebrae showing lateral view of ligament.

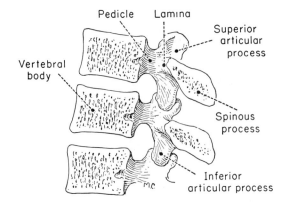

Figure 18–5. Sagittal section of vertebrae showing articulations of the vertebral arches.

convex. By this arrangement of the facets the lumbar vertebrae are virtually locked against rotation. The slight amount of rotation that does occur is made possible by the looseness of the capsules. At the lumbosacral articulation the facets lie somewhat more in the frontal plane than is true of the other lumbar joints.

Ligaments of the Vertebral Arches

LIGAMENTA FLAVA. (Fig. 18–7, *A* and *B*.) These are thick elastic plates which connect the laminae of adjacent vertebrae. They are thickest in the lumbar region, less thick but fairly strong in the thoracic region, and thin, broad and membranous in the cervical region.

INTERSPINOUS LIGAMENTS. (Fig. 18–7, *B*.) These are thin membranous ligaments, connecting the lower border of each spinous process with the upper border of the one below it. They are thickest and

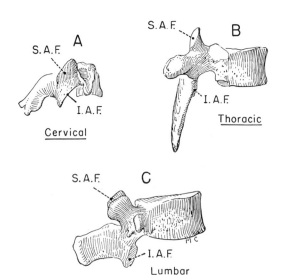

Figure 18–6. Articular facets of vertebrae. *A*, Cervical; *B*, thoracic; *C*, lumbar. *S.A.F.* = Superior articular facet. *I.A.F.* = Inferior articular facet.

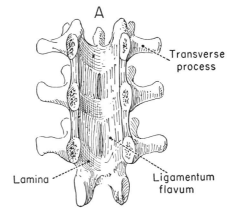

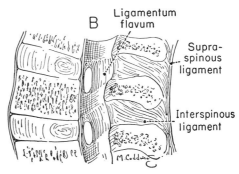

Figure 18–7. A, Frontal section of three lumbar vertebrae showing anterior view of vertebral arches and ligamenta flava. *B,* Sagittal view of lumbar vertebrae showing ligaments of vertebral arches.

broadest in the lumbar region and are but slightly developed in the cervical region.

SUPRASPINOUS LIGAMENT. (Fig. 18–7, *B.*) This is a strong fibrous cord which connects the tips of the spinous processes, extending from the seventh cervical vertebra to the sacrum. It is thicker and broader in the lumbar region than in the thoracic.

LIGAMENTUM NUCHAE. (Fig. 18–8.) This is the continuation of the supraspinous ligament in the cervical region. It extends from the seventh cervical vertebra upward to the occipital bone in the form of a thin fibrous membrane.

INTERTRANSVERSE LIGAMENTS. These rather poorly developed ligaments connect the transverse processes of adjacent vertebrae in the thoracic and lumbar regions. In the thoracic region they are round cords; in the lumbar, thin membranous bands.

Atlanto-occipital Articulation. (Fig. 18–9.) This is the articulation between the head and the neck. It consists of a pair of joints, one on each side. Each condyle of the occipital bone of the skull articulates with the corresponding superior articular fossa of the first vertebra, known as atlas. Each articulation by itself belongs to the ovoid (condyloid) classification, but the movement which occurs in the two joints together is more like that of a hinge joint. The rigid relation-

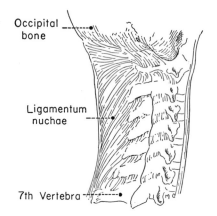

Occipital bone

Ligamentum nuchae

7th Vertebra

Figure 18–8. Side view of cervical spine showing ligamentum nuchae.

ship between the two joints results in a restriction of the lateral motion that would normally occur in an ovoid joint. The movements which take place at the atlanto-occipital articulation are chiefly flexion and extension, with a slight amount of lateral flexion. There is no rotation.

Atlantoaxial Articulation. (Fig. 18–10.) This is a perfect example of a pivot joint—a joint whose sole function is rotation. The

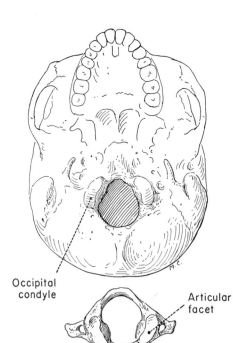

Occipital condyle

Articular facet

Atlas

Figure 18–9. Bones forming atlanto-occipital articulation.

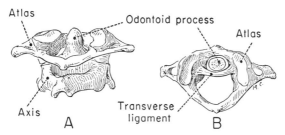

Figure 18–10. Atlantoaxial articulation. *A,* Posterior view; *B,* superior view.

toothlike peg (odontoid process) that projects upward from the second cervical vertebra, otherwise known as axis or epistropheus, fits into the ring formed by the inner surface of the anterior arch of atlas and the transverse ligament which bridges across the tips of the arch. Since no rotation occurs at the atlanto-occipital joint, rotation of atlas on axis will carry the head with it; thus the movement occurring at the atlantoaxial joint contributes to the movement of the head on the trunk.

Movements of the Spine as a Whole. The movements of the spinal column resemble those of a ball-and-socket joint.

FLEXION. (Fig. 18–11, A.) This is forward-downward bending in the sagittal plane about a frontal-horizontal axis. It involves a compression of the anterior parts of the intervertebral disks and a gliding motion of the articular processes. It occurs most freely in the cervical, upper thoracic and lumbar regions. The cervical curve may be reduced to a straight line, and the lumbar curve, in flexible individuals, may be reversed.

EXTENSION AND HYPEREXTENSION. (Fig. 18–11, B.) Extension is the return movement from flexion. Hyperextension is a backward-downward movement in the sagittal plane. It occurs most freely in the cervical and lumbar regions and particularly at the lumbosacral junction. In the thoracic region hyperextension is limited by the overlapping of the spinous processes.

LATERAL FLEXION. (Fig. 18–11, C.) This is a sideward bending in the frontal plane about a sagittal-horizontal axis. It is freest in the cervical region and quite free in the lumbar region and at the thoracolumbar junction. But it is limited in the thoracic region by the presence of the ribs. Each rib (except the first, tenth, eleventh and twelfth) articulates with two adjacent vertebrae and the intervening disk, and each rib (except the eleventh and twelfth) articulates with the transverse process of the lower of the two vertebrae (Fig. 18–12). Thus it is seen that the ribs serve as splints, restricting lateral flexion of the thoracic spine to a marked degree. It is amazing that any motion can take place there at all. For several reasons—the slant of the articular processes, the presence of the anteroposterior curves of the spine, and muscular and ligamentous tensions—lateral flexion is always accompanied by a certain amount of torsion.

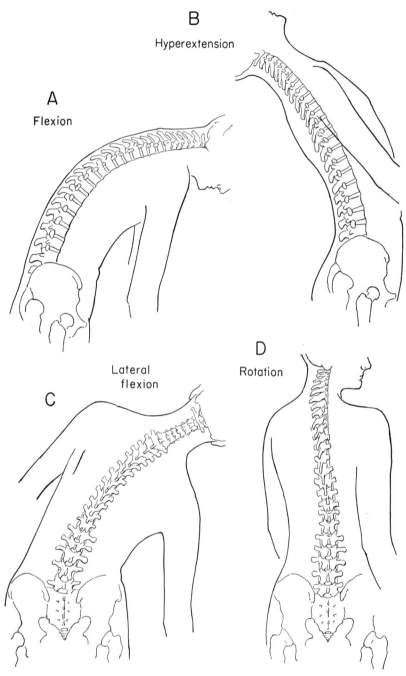

Figure 18–11.   Movements of the spinal column.

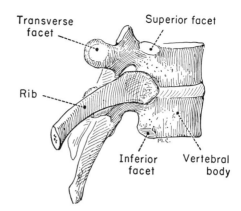

Transverse facet

Superior facet

Rib

Inferior facet

Vertebral body

Figure 18–12. Articulation of a rib with two adjacent vertebrae.

ROTATION. (Fig. 18–11, *D*.) This is a rotatory movement of the spine in the horizontal plane about a vertical axis. Spinal rotation is named by the way the front of the upper spine turns with reference to the lower part. Thus a turning of the head and shoulders to the right constitutes rotation to the right. A turning of the legs and pelvis to the left, without turning the upper part of the body, also constitutes rotation of the spine to the right since the anatomic relationships are the same as in the former example. The movement of rotation is most free in the cervical region, 90% of the movement being attributed to the atlantoaxial joint. It is next most free in the thoracic region and at the thoracolumbar junction.[8] Owing to the interlocking of the articular processes, it is extremely limited in the lumbar region, there being only about 5 degrees of rotation to each side. In the cervical region there is no rotation between atlas and the skull, but free rotation at the pivot joint between atlas and axis. Whenever rotation occurs in the spine, it is accompanied by a slight amount of unavoidable lateral flexion to the same side.

INFLUENCE OF THE STARTING POSITION ON LATERAL FLEXION AND THE TORSION ACCOMPANYING IT. When lateral flexion is performed from the erect position, the maximum movement occurs in the lumbar region and at the thoracolumbar junction, with only slight involvement of the lower thoracic spine. (The cervical spine is excluded from this discussion.) The torsion occurs in the same part of the spine and consists in a turning of the vertebral bodies toward the side of the lateral flexion. Thus if the spine bends to the right (forming a curve concave to the right), the vertebral bodies of the lumbar and lower thoracic vertebrae turn slightly to the right, the spinous processes, therefore, turning to the left.

If the lateral flexion is performed from a position of hyperextension, and the hyperextension is maintained throughout the movement, the lateral flexion moves lower in the spine, occurring almost entirely below the eleventh thoracic vertebra. The torsion occurs in this same region and in the same manner that it does when the lateral flexion is performed from the erect position. The position of hyperextension seems to lock the thoracic spine against lateral movements.

If the lateral flexion is performed from a position of forward flexion, the movement occurs higher in the spine than ordinarily, the greatest deviation being at the level of the eighth thoracic vertebra. The torsion in this case reverses itself. Thus in a side bend to the right the vertebral bodies turn to the *left*, and the spinous processes to the right. This reversal is not inconsistent. It is directly related to the anteroposterior curves of the spine. In the first two examples, that is, when the lateral flexion is performed either from the erect or from the hyperextended position, most of the movement takes place in the lower part of the spine, the part that is concave to the rear. The rotation that accompanies the side bend in these two cases is called concave-side rotation because the bodies turn in the direction of the concave or inner side of the laterally curved spine. When the side bend is performed from the flexed position, most of the movement takes place in the thoracic spine, the region that is convex to the rear. The rotation that accompanies the lateral flexion in this case is called convex-side rotation because the vertebral bodies turn in the direction of the convex or outer side of the laterally curved spine.

INFLUENCE OF THE STARTING POSITION ON ROTATION AND THE LATERAL FLEXION ACCOMPANYING IT. When performed from the erect position, rotation of the spine (below the seventh cervical vertebra) occurs almost entirely in the thoracic region. When performed from the position of hyperextension, the movement shifts lower in the spine, occurring in the vicinity of the thoracolumbar junction. When performed from the flexed position, the rotation is higher than usual, occurring in the upper thoracic spine. Regardless of the position in which the rotation is performed — whether erect, flexed or hyperextended — the slight lateral flexion which accompanies it is always to the same side as the rotation. Thus if the spine rotates to the left, it flexes slightly to the left. This movement is very slight, however, and can scarcely be detected.[14]

CIRCUMDUCTION. This is a circular movement of the upper trunk on the lower, being a combination of flexion, lateral flexion and hyperextension, but not including rotation.

Summary of Spinal Movements

    Flexion; extension; hyperextension

        Free in all three regions

        Cervical and thoracic curves may be reduced to straight lines

        Lumbar curve may be reversed in flexible subjects

    Lateral flexion

        Free in cervical and lumbar regions

        Limited in thoracic region by rib attachments

        Accompanied by torsion

    Rotation

        Freest at top, least free at bottom of spine

        Accompanied by slight lateral flexion

Circumduction
    Sequential combination of flexion, lateral flexion and hyper-
        extension

Regional Classification of Spinal Movements
Occipitoatlantal joint
    Flexion and extension
    Hyperextension
    Slight lateral flexion
Atlantoaxial joint
    Rotation
Remaining cervical joints
    Free flexion and extension
    Free hyperextension
    Free lateral flexion
    Free rotation
Thoracic region
    Moderate flexion
    Slight hyperextension
    Moderate lateral flexion
    Free rotation
Lumbar region
    Moderate to free flexion and extension
    Free hyperextension
    Free lateral flexion
    Slight rotation

Summary of Factors Which Influence the Stability and Mobility of the Spinal Column. Before considering the movements of the spine it is well to review some of the special characteristics which contribute to its stability and which modify its mobility in one way or another.

1. PRESSURE AND TENSION STRESSES. The tendency of the compressed intervertebral disks to push the vertebrae apart, combined with the tendency of the ligaments to press them together, is an important factor in the stability of the spinal column.

2. ANTEROPOSTERIOR CURVES. The alternating anteroposterior curves of the spinal column influence the nature and the degree of movements that occur in the different regions. Individual variations from the so-called normal curves cause variations in the movement patterns (see pages 343 to 346). The anteroposterior curves are said to serve as a safeguard against the development of abnormal lateral curves (curvature of the spine; scoliosis).

3. RELATIVE THICKNESS AND SHAPE OF THE INTERVERTEBRAL DISKS. There is a direct relationship between the thickness of the disks and the degree of movement permitted, there being greater freedom of motion where the disks are thicker.

4. THICKNESS AND STRENGTH OF THE LIGAMENTS. These differ in the different regions, and have a corresponding influence on the motions permitted in each region.

5. DIRECTION AND OBLIQUITY OF THE ARTICULAR FACETS. These are characteristic for each region and play an important part in determining the type of motion permitted in each.

6. SIZE AND OBLIQUITY OF THE SPINOUS PROCESSES. These overlap like shingles in the thoracic region, hence limit hyperextension. In the lumbar region they are horizontal, and, although they are wide, they do not restrict motion.

7. ARTICULATIONS OF THE RIBS WITH THE VERTEBRAE. These limit lateral flexion in the thoracic region.

Muscles. The muscles responsible for the movements of the spine include not only those which have one or both attachments on the vertebrae, but also the abdominal muscles and the hyoids. Both these groups are superficially located on the front of the body; nevertheless they are important muscles of the spinal column.

The muscles acting on the spine are as follows:

MUSCLES OF THE HEAD AND NECK
    Anterior:
        Prevertebral muscles
        Hyoid muscles
    Lateral:
        Three scaleni
        Sternocleidomastoid
        Levator scapulae
    Posterior:
        Splenius capitis and cervicis
        Suboccipitals
        Capitis and cervicis portions of posterior muscles of spine
MUSCLES OF THE THORACIC AND LUMBAR SPINE
    Anterior and anterolateral (abdominal muscles):
        Rectus abdominis
        External oblique
        Internal oblique
    Lateral:
        Quadratus lumborum
        Psoas
    Posterior:
        Erector spinae
        Semispinalis thoracis
        Deep posterior spinal muscles

In general, the muscles situated anterior to the spine, flex it; those posterior to it, extend it; and those lateral to it, when acting on one side only, flex it laterally. Because of the effect of gravity, however, the anterior muscles fulfill their function as flexors most successfully when the body is supine; the posterior muscles as extensors, when the body is prone; and the lateral muscles as lateral flexors, when the body is resting on its side (flexor action takes place on the side opposite to the side of support). This should be kept in mind when studying the actions of the following muscles.

PREVERTEBRAL MUSCLES. (Fig. 18–13.) This group of deep anterior muscles of the head and neck consists of longus capitis, longus colli, rectus capitis anterior and rectus capitis lateralis.

Lower attachments. (O) Anterior surfaces of various parts of cervical vertebrae and of upper three thoracic vertebrae.

Upper attachments. (I) Anterior portions of occipital bone and of cervical vertebrae.

Nerve supply. Cervical nerves.

Cannot be palpated.

Action

    Both: Flexion of head and neck.

    One: Lateral flexion of head and neck.

HYOID OR STRAP MUSCLES. (Fig. 18–14.) These include the suprahyoids and the infrahyoids, that is, the muscles above and below the hyoid bone.

Attachments. The suprahyoids are attached to the temporal bone and the mandible above (O) and to the hyoid bone below (I). The infrahyoids are attached to the hyoid bone above (I) and to the sternum and shoulder girdle below (O).

Nerve supply. Facial, inferior alveolar, hypoglossi and ansa hypoglossi.

Where to palpate. The suprahyoids may be palpated just below the jaw bone. The infrahyoids cannot be palpated.

Action (at cervical spine). Flexion.

Comments. These muscles are primarily muscles of some phase of the act of swallowing. They contract in cervical flexion, however, whenever the movement is performed against resistance. By neutralizing one another's pull on the hyoid bone their action is transferred to the skull, and thence to the cervical spine.

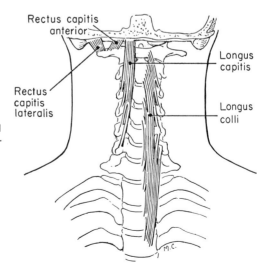

Figure 18–13. Prevertebral muscles of cervical spine. (Anterior view.)

Rectus capitis anterior

Rectus capitis lateralis

Longus capitis

Longus colli

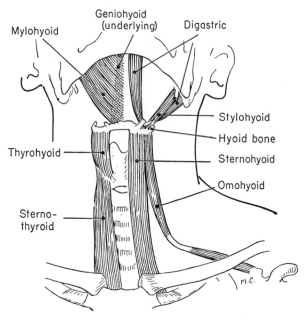

Figure 18–14.   Hyoid muscles. (Anterior view.)

THE THREE SCALENI (SCALENUS ANTERIOR, POSTERIOR AND MEDIUS) (Fig. 18–15.)

Lower attachments. (O)   First two ribs.

Upper attachments. (I)   Transverse processes of cervical vertebrae.

Nerve supply.   Branches from second to seventh cervical nerves, inclusive.

Where to palpate.   On the side of the neck between the sternocleidomastoid and upper trapezius. Difficult to identify.

Action

Both: Help to flex neck.

One: Lateral flexion of neck.

STERNOCLEIDOMASTOIDEUS (Fig. 18–16.)

Lower attachments. (O)   By two heads from top of sternum and medial third of clavicle.

Upper attachments. (I)   Mastoid process of temporal bone and adjacent portion of occipital bone.

Nerve supply.   Accessory and branches from the second and third cervical nerves.

Where to palpate.   On the side of the neck from just under the ear to the front of the neck at the junction of the clavicle and sternum. It may easily be seen.

Action

Both: Flexion of head and neck.

One: Lateral flexion; rotation to opposite side.

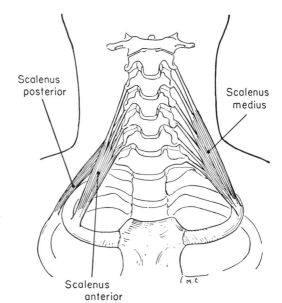

Scalenus
posterior

Scalenus
medius

Figure 18–15. The three
scaleni muscles. (Anterior
view.)

Scalenus
anterior

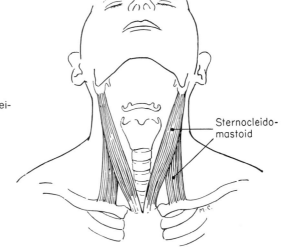

Figure 18–16. Sternocleidomastoid muscle.

Sternocleido-
mastoid

Comments. From the upper attachment of this muscle, one would expect it to hyperextend the head on atlas, regardless of the movement of the cervical vertebrae. In fact, some authors claim this movement for it. The writer, however, has not been able to detect contraction of the sternocleidomastoid when the head was being hyperextended unless the neck was being flexed at the same time. One can only conclude that the pull of the sternocleidomastoid is more nearly in line with the transverse axis of motion than it appears. Basmajian confirmed Campbell's observation that both the sternocleidomastoid and the three scaleni show marked activity as soon as a person in the supine position begins to raise his head.[1]

LEVATOR SCAPULAE (Fig. 18–17.) (See also muscles of the shoulder girdle.)

Upper or proximal attachments. (O) Transverse processes of upper four cervical vertebrae.

Lower or distal attachments. (I) Vertebral border of scapula between medial angle and root of spine.

Nerve supply. Dorsal scapular and branches from third and fourth cervical nerves.

Cannot be palpated.

Action (at cervical spine)
      Both: None
      One: Lateral flexion.

Comments. As the name indicates, the levator scapulae is primarily a muscle of the shoulder girdle. If one scapula is fixed, however, the levator scapulae muscle on that side will flex the cervical spine laterally. If both muscles contract at the same time when both scapulae are fixed, they neutralize each other without effecting any movement. They may possibly help to stabilize the neck, especially when the body is in the prone position, supported by the hands and feet, or by the hands and knees.

SPLENIUS, CAPITIS AND CERVICIS (Fig. 18–17.)

Lower attachments. (O) Lower half of ligamentum nuchae; spinous processes of seventh cervical and upper six thoracic vertebrae.

Upper attachments. (I) Mastoid process of temporal bone and adjacent part of occipital bone; transverse processes of upper three cervical vertebrae.

Nerve supply. Branches from the second, third and fourth cervical nerves.

Where to palpate. On the back of the neck just lateral to the trapezius and posterior to the sternocleidomastoid, above the levator scapulae, especially if the head is extended against resistance in the prone position and the shoulders are kept relaxed. It is difficult to identify, however.

Action
      Both: Extension and hyperextension; supports head in erect posture.
      One: Lateral flexion; rotation to the same side.

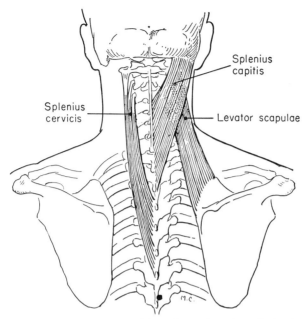

Figure 18–17.   Posterior and lateral muscles of cervical spine.

Comment.   This is an important posture muscle, one of its chief functions being to hold the head erect against the downward pull of gravity. In this it is aided by semispinalis capitis.

THE SUBOCCIPITALS (Fig. 18–18.)

Lower attachments. (O)   Posterior portions of atlas and axis.

Upper attachments. (I)   Occipital bone and transverse process of atlas.

Nerve supply.   Branches from first two cervical nerves.

Cannot be palpated.

Action

Both: Extension and hyperextension of head.

One: Lateral flexion; rotation to the same side.

Comments.   The suboccipitals consist of the rectus capitis posterior major and minor and the obliquus capitis superior and inferior. They are short muscles, situated deep under the skull.

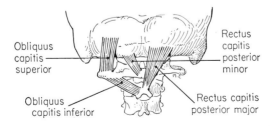

Figure 18–18. Suboccipital muscles. (Posterior view.)

The remaining posterior muscles of the head and neck consist of the capitis and cervicis portions of erector spinae, semispinalis and the deep posterior muscles of the spine.

ERECTOR SPINAE. (Fig. 18–19.) This extensive muscle of the back consists of three branches: namely, iliocostalis, the lateral branch; longissimus, the middle branch; and spinalis, the medial branch. The attachments given here are of necessity general, as they are for the muscle as a whole, not separate branches.

Lower attachments. (O) Thoracolumbar fascia; posterior portions of lumbar, thoracic and lower cervical vertebrae; angles of ribs.

Upper attachments. (I) Angles of ribs; posterior portions of cervical and thoracic vertebrae; mastoid process of the temporal bone.

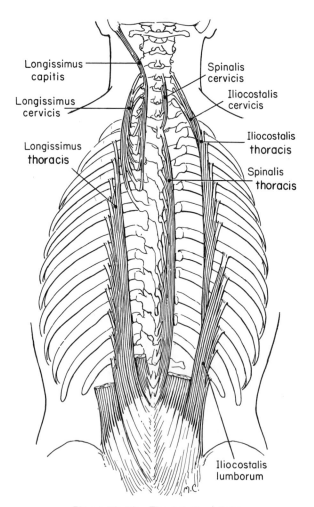

Figure 18–19.   The erector spinae.

Nerve supply. Posterior branches of spinal nerves.

Where to palpate. In the lumbar and lower thoracic regions of the back, in two broad ridges on either side of the spine.

Action

> Both: Extension and hyperextension of head and entire spine.
> One: Lateral flexion and rotation of head and spine to same side.

Comments. The muscle commences as a large mass in the lumbosacral region, but soon divides into three branches.

The iliocostalis branch consists of lumbar, thoracic and cervical portions which are named lumborum, thoracis and cervicis, respectively. It receives an additional tendon of origin from each rib throughout the thoracic region and gives off small slips to insert into the ribs in the thoracic region and into the transverse processes of the vertebrae in the cervical region.

The longissimus branch consists of three distinct portions which, in fact, appear to be three separate muscles (see Fig. 18–19). Longissimus thoracis is a broad band lying against the angles of the ribs; longissimus cervicis is narrower and lies slightly closer to the spine, connecting the transverse processes of the upper thoracic vertebrae with those of the lower cervical vertebrae; and longissimus capitis is a thin strand which lies against the vertebrae for its lower two thirds and then slants outward and upward to the mastoid process of the temporal bone.

The spinalis branch lies against the vertebrae and is attached by separate slips to the spinous processes. It is of significance in the thoracic region only.

Electromyographic studies have shown that the erector spinae contributes little to the maintenance of erect posture unless a deliberate effort is made to extend the thoracic spine more completely, or unless the weight is carried forward over the balls of the feet, in which case some static contraction of the muscle is required. In ordinary standing, however, the muscle is relaxed.[1]

In forward flexion from the standing position, the erector spinae undergoes eccentric contraction until the weight of the trunk is supported by the ligaments. When the trunk returns from this position the muscle contracts concentrically until the body is again erect and balanced.[1]

The muscle engages most forcefully in its functions of extension, hyperextension and lateral flexion when these movements are performed against gravity or other resistance. Hyperextension from the prone lying position is considered the best exercise for strengthening the erector spinae.[17]

SEMISPINALIS THORACIS, CERVICIS AND CAPITIS (Fig. 18–20.)

Lower attachments. (O) Transverse processes of all thoracic and seventh cervical vertebrae; articular processes of lower four cervical vertebrae.

Upper attachments. (I) Spinous processes of upper four thoracic and lower five cervical vertebrae; occipital bone.

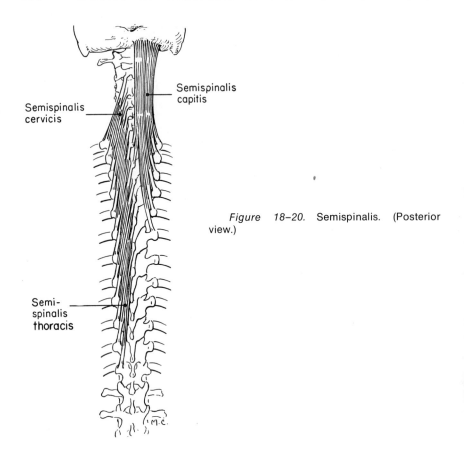

Semispinalis capitis

Semispinalis cervicis

Semi-spinalis thoracis

Figure 18–20. Semispinalis. (Posterior view.)

Nerve supply. Posterior branches of cervical and upper six thoracic nerves.

Cannot be palpated.

Action

Both: Extension and hyperextension of head, neck and thoracic spine.

One: Lateral flexion of head, neck and thoracic spine; rotation of thoracic spine to opposite side.

Comments. The thoracic and cervical portions consist of tendinous bands which extend obliquely upward and medialward from the transverse processes in the thoracic region and spinous processes in the cervical region to spinous processes of vertebrae above. These portions of the muscle lie beneath the erector spinae. Semispinalis capitis is constructed differently from thoracis and cervicis. It consists of a broad band of fibers extending vertically upward from the upper six thoracic and lower four cervical vertebrae to the occipital bone. It lies beneath the splenius capitis and the upper trapezius.

DEEP POSTERIOR MUSCLES OF THE SPINE. (Fig. 18–21.)   These

include the multifidus, the rotatores, the interspinales, the intertransversarii and the levatores costarum.

Lower attachments. (O)   Posterior surface of sacrum and posterior processes of all the vertebrae.

Upper attachments. (I)   Spinous and transverse processes and laminae of vertebrae slightly higher than lower attachments.

Nerve supply.   For first four muscles: Branches of spinal nerves.

For levatores costarum: Intercostal nerves and eighth cervical nerve.

Cannot be palpated.

Action

Both: Extension and hyperextension of spine.

One: Rotation to the opposite side; assistance in lateral flexion.

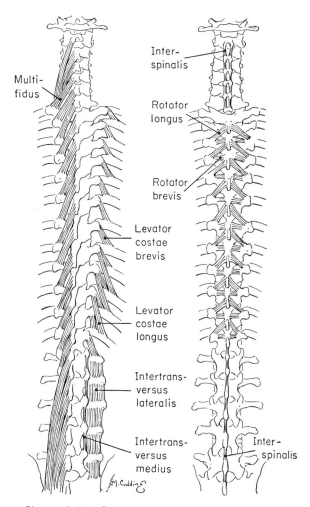

Figure 18–21.   Deep posterior muscles of the spine.

Comments. These muscles consist of small slips, in most cases inserting into the vertebrae immediately above their lower attachments. Some of the fibers run vertically, and some slant medially as they ascend. The former are best developed in the cervical and lumbar regions, where their action is that of extension. The latter are best developed in the thoracic region, where they either extend or rotate. It has been suggested that the muscles in this group are responsible for localized movements. It seems likely that they also help to stabilize the spine.

Thoracolumbar fascia. (Fig. 18–24.) The thoracolumbar fascia binds together the erector spinae and other deep muscles of the spine, holding them close to the skeletal structure and separating them from the more superficial muscles of the back. In the lumbar region it curves around the lateral margin of the erector spinae and folds in front of it to attach to the tips of the transverse processes of the vertebrae and to the intertransverse ligaments. Its lateral portion provides attachment for the transversus abdominis (Fig. 19–11), and its posterior portion blends with the aponeurosis of the latissimus dorsi (Fig. 12–6).

RECTUS ABDOMINIS (Fig. 18–22.) (See also muscles of the thorax.)

Lower attachment. (O)   Crest of pubis.

Upper attachments. (I)   Cartilages of fifth, sixth and seventh ribs.

Nerve supply.   Anterior branches of lower six intercostal nerves.

Where to palpate.   The front of the abdomen, from the pubis to the sternum.

Action (at spine)

Both: Flexion of thoracic and lumbar spine.

One: Lateral flexion of thoracic and lumbar spine.

Comments. The rectus abdominis is situated on the anterior surface of the abdomen on either side of the linea alba. It is a long flat band of muscle fibers extending vertically between the pubis and the lower part of the chest. At three different levels transverse fibrous bands, known as tendinous inscriptions, cross the muscle fibers. The muscle is enclosed in a sheath formed by the aponeuroses of the other muscles making up the abdominal wall.

Electromyographic studies have shown the rectus abdominis to be strongly active in head raising from the supine lying position[4, 7] and inclining the trunk backward from the erect position.[16, 18] The upper rectus was found to be more active in exercises involving the upper part of the body, e.g., spine flexion from the supine position.[18] In the latter movement it was also found to start contracting a moment before the lower rectus.[5] The lower rectus was found to be more active in movements involving a decrease in the pelvic tilt, e.g., in the supine position bending the knees and lifting them toward the face until the fifth lumbar vertebra is lifted approximately five inches above the supporting surface.[18]

OBLIQUUS EXTERNUS ABDOMINIS (Fig. 18–23.) (See also muscles of the thorax.)

Upper, lateral attachments. (O)   Lower border of lower eight

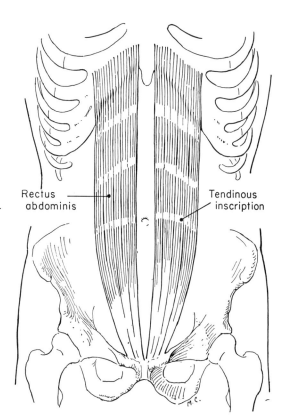

Figure 18–22. Rectus abdominis.

Rectus abdominis

Tendinous inscription

ribs by tendinous slips which interdigitate with those of the serratus anterior.

Lower, medial attachments. (1) Anterior half of crest of ilium; aponeurosis from ribs to crest of pubis.

Nerve supply. The lower seven intercostal nerves and the iliohypogastric nerve.

Where to palpate. At the side of the abdomen.

Action (at spine)

Both: Flexion of thoracic and lumbar spine.

One: Lateral flexion. Rotation to the opposite side.

Comments. The fibers of this muscle run diagonally upward and outward from the lower part of the abdomen, the two muscles together forming an incomplete V, as seen from the front. The external obliques have been found to show the greatest activity in movements performed in the supine position, e.g., forward and lateral flexion of the spine, decreased pelvic tilt, forward flexion combined with rotation, and double knee circling.[16, 18] In combination with the internal obliques, the external showed marked activity in two types of movements, namely straining and bearing down when the breath was held[1, 4] and forced exhalation.[1, 4, 7]

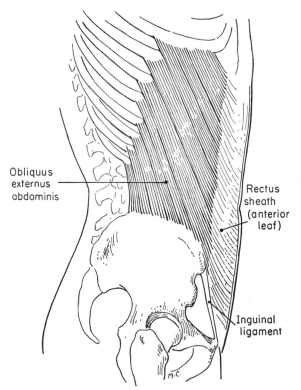

Obliquus externus abdominis

Rectus sheath (anterior leaf)

Inguinal ligament

Figure 18–23. External oblique abdominal muscle (obliquus externus abdominis).

OBLIQUUS INTERNUS ABDOMINIS (Fig. 18–24.) (See also muscles of the thorax.)

Lower, lateral attachments. (O) Inguinal ligament; crest of ilium; thoracolumbar fascia.

Upper, medial attachments. (I) Anterior and middle fibers into crest of pubis, linea alba and aponeurosis on front of body; posterior fibers, by three separate slips, into the cartilages of the lower three ribs.

Nerve supply. The lower three intercostal nerves, the iliohypogastric and the ilio-inguinal nerves.

Where to palpate. The side of the abdomen, beneath the external oblique. It may be palpated through the external oblique when the latter is relaxed, as in rotation.

Action

Both: Flexion of thoracic and lumbar spine.

One: Lateral flexion. Rotation to the same side.

Comments. This muscle lies beneath the external oblique. The fibers fan out from the crest of the ilium, most of them passing diagonally forward and upward toward the rib cartilages and sternum, some horizontally forward toward the linea alba, and some diagonally forward and downward toward the crest of the pubis.

The internal obliques have been found to be the most active of the abdominal muscles in rotation of the trunk. They were also found to show marked activity in the following movements: leaning backward, decreasing the pelvic tilt; in the supine position, raising the knees to the chest and lowering them together first to one side, then the other; also raising the knees still farther and lifting the buttocks off the supporting surface.[16]

The Abdominal Wall. The abdominal wall consists of the three abdominal muscles just described and the transversus abdominis (Fig. 19–11). The latter muscle is a broad sheet of horizontal fibers whose function is to compress the abdomen. It is primarily a muscle of respiration and other physiologic functions. Together, these four muscles form a strong anterior support for the abdominal viscera. They are subject to considerable stress from the pressure of the latter against their inner surface. The more stretched they become, as in the case of a protruding abdomen, the more heavily the organs rest upon the abdominal wall, subjecting it to direct gravitational stress. Thus a vicious circle is set in motion. The pressure against the lower abdominal wall stretches it still more, causing its protrusion to increase and subjecting it to ever increasing gravitational stress. As is so often the case, correction of this postural fault is much more difficult than its prevention. A strong abdominal wall is greatly to be desired.

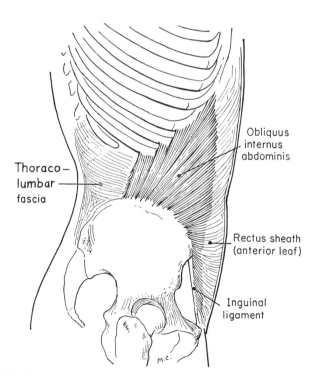

Figure 18–24. Internal oblique abdominal muscle (obliquus internus abdominis).

QUADRATUS LUMBORUM (Fig. 18–25.)

Lower attachments. (O)   Crest of ilium and iliolumbar ligament.

Upper attachments. (I)   Lower border of twelfth rib and tips of transverse processes of upper four lumbar vertebrae.

Nerve supply.   Branches from the upper three or four lumbar nerves.

Where to palpate.   Just lateral to the erector spinae in the lumbar region. It is difficult to palpate and can be felt only on thin, muscular subjects.

Action.   Acting unilaterally, it flexes the lumbar spine to the same side. Acting bilaterally, it stabilizes the pelvis and lumbar spine.

Comments.   This is a flat muscle, situated behind the abdominal cavity at the side of the lumbar spine. It probably helps to support the weight of the pelvis on the side of the swinging leg in walking.

Knapp, who made an extensive study of the muscle, objects to its being described as quadrate. He describes it as consisting of two layers, a rather thin anterior layer and a large, fan-shaped posterior layer. He defines three directions of force, one more or less vertical from the twelfth rib to the iliac crest, a second obliquely downward and outward and a third obliquely upward and outward. The vertical fibers, he states, cause lateral flexion of the trunk to the same side; and the oblique fibers, by pulling the vertebrae laterally, cause a lateral curve which is concave to the opposite side. He believes the chief function of the muscle as a whole to be stabilization of the lumbar spine.[12]

PSOAS (See also muscles of the hip; Fig. 15–7.)

Upper attachments. (O)   Lateral anterior margins of bodies of twelfth thoracic and all lumbar vertebrae, transverse processes of lumbar vertebrae, and intervertebral disks.

Lower attachments. (I)   Lesser trochanter of femur.

Nerve supply.   Upper three lumbar nerves.

Where to palpate.   See information about the psoas muscle in the chapter on the hip and pelvis. The psoas cannot be palpated when it acts on the spine because of the contraction of the abdominal muscles.

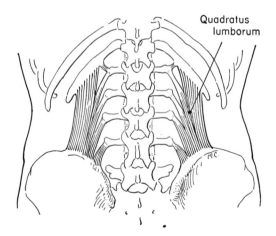

Figure 18–25.   Quadratus lumborum. (Posterior view.)

Action (at spine). When the distal attachment is fixed, contraction of the psoas muscle, in addition to flexing the entire trunk on the thighs, may contribute either to flexion or to hyperextension of the lumbar spine, depending upon various factors. Its more important role, however, would seem to be stabilization or balancing of the spine in response to other forces acting on the latter. Unilateral contraction contributes to lateral flexion of the lumbar spine.

Comments. Like the quadratus lumborum, the psoas is situated at the back of the abdominal cavity. Together, they form the posterior abdominal wall. Although the psoas is primarily a muscle of the hip joint, its action on the lower spine and pelvis is of interest. (See the section on The Psoas Major and the Lumbar Spine in the Supplementary Material.)

SUPPLEMENTARY MATERIAL

The Psoas Major and the Lumbar Spine. Because the psoas major muscle, at its proximal end, attaches to the sides of the bodies and to the front and lower borders of the transverse processes of all the lumbar vertebrae, it has been thought to be a mover of the lumbar portion of the spinal column. A review of textbooks of kinesiology and of corrective exercises shows that there are conflicting statements concerning such movements. Some say that when its distal attachment is fixed, it flexes the lumbar spine; some say that it hyperextends it; others say that sometimes it flexes and sometimes it hyperextends, according to the current relation of its line of pull to the lumbar joints. This relationship is thought to be affected by the position of the body, by the anteroposterior postural curve of the lumbar spine, and by its current status, whether in a position of flexion or hyperextension.

In the hope of having some light thrown on this subject, the writings of four experimental clinicians (physicians or physical therapists of known repute for their wide experience in observing the muscular action of patients)[3, 5, 11, 21] and the statements of four researchers (or teams of researchers) based on their electromyographic experimentation,[6, 10, 13, 15] were carefully examined. Unfortunately, this perusal served only to bring to light more conflicting statements.

What is the reader to conclude from this? Does it actually imply opposing points of view? It seems to this reviewer that there may be a number of logical explanations for the seeming disagreements. For instance, the writer may not have been explicit regarding techniques used or specific conditions at the time of examining or experimenting; he may use terminology that is subject to misinterpretation; variations in muscular action may have been caused by variations in anatomic structure or in habitual posture; and finally, for one reason or another, the reader may have simply misunderstood the writer's meaning.

When there appear to be diverse opinions regarding muscular actions, it seems likely that the differences are not of great importance. Frequently, when there is lack of agreement regarding movement, one may safely assume that the true function of the muscular contraction, with reference to the joints in question, is more likely to be stabilization or balance than purposeful movement. This, in fact, has been suggested as a function of the psoas muscle by two investigators, Keagy et al, and Nachemson. The latter's study of the stabilizing action of the psoas appeared in a Scandinavian journal and has been brought to our attention both by Basmajian and by Jonsson. Brunnstrom has described this type of action with unusual clarity. She likens the muscles that are situated close to the spinal column (erector spinae, psoas major, etc.) to guy ropes that support an upright pole. When the pole starts to tip, the tension of the ropes on the opposite side increases. In like manner, if a person starts to lean backward, possibly to favor weak posterior muscles, the muscles on the front of the spine spring into action. She told of a patient with paralysis of the psoas muscles who, when he sat on a stool, always inclined his trunk forward. When she gently pushed his trunk to the erect position he had to grasp the sides of the stool to keep from falling over backward. The other hip flexors, largely because of their poor leverage, were not equal to the task of holding the trunk erect. While this does not necessarily exemplify spinal action, it emphasizes an important function of the psoas muscle which is often overlooked.

Atypical Spinal Contours. Wells investigated the spinal contours of 100 college women as recorded in routine anteroposterior

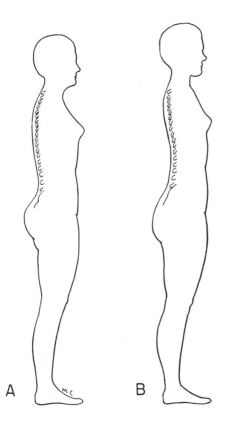

Figure 18–26. Lateral views of two female figures illustrating variations in spinal type. *A,* Convex or "anthropoid" type of spine. *B,* Concave or "humanoid" type of spine.

A   B

TABLE 18-1. Comparison of "Anthropoid" and "Humanoid" Types of Spines with Reference to the Depth and Length of the Anteroposterior Curves of the Thoracic and Lumbar Portions of the Spine (Wells)

(Mean values of measurements taken from the posture photographs of 100 college women, 50 representing the "anthropoid" type and 50 the "humanoid" type.)

Aspect of Spine Measured	"Anthropoid" Spine	"Humanoid" Spine
Total length of thoracic and lumbar portion of spine	3.54 cm.	3.54 cm.
Length of posterior convexity	2.79 cm. (79%)	1.48 cm. (42%)
Length of posterior concavity	0.75 cm. (21%)	2.06 cm. (58%)
Depth of posterior convexity	0.22 cm.	0.08 cm.
Depth of posterior concavity	0.06 cm.	0.16 cm.

posture photographs in which the MacEwan pointers were used to show the location of the tips of the spinous processes. These 100 photographs were selected from 1200, fifty of them on the basis of a predominantly convex spine, that is, a spine in which the thoracic convexity involves a portion, possibly all, of the lumbar region; and fifty on the basis of a predominantly concave spine, that is, a spine in which the lumbar concavity extends well up into the thoracic region. Because the convex spine is characteristic of the anthropoid apes, this group was called the "anthropoid spine" group; and because a lumbar curve is characteristic of the human spine, the second group was called the "humanoid spine" group (Fig. 18–26). Measurements made on the photographs revealed that significant measureable differences existed between the two types of spine. The mean values of these measurements are presented in Table 18–1.[19]

Patterns of Anteroposterior Spinal Flexibility. An interesting study of the flexibility of the spinal column of four individuals was made by Wiles. Two of the subjects were normally active women; two were acrobatic dancers, one of them a child and the other a man. While too small in scope to be of any real significance, this study is interesting because it suggests the wide variation in flexibility found in the human spine. In the light of Wells' study, it is interesting to note that the photograph of Miss P. showed a spine of "normal" contours; that of Miss R. showed a long convexity or "anthropoid type" of spine; that of the child showed a marked lordosis; and that of the man showed a shallow but long concavity or "humanoid type" of spine. The range of motion in each spine, as measured on x-rays, is recorded in Table 18–2. The relationship between the type of spine and the degree and pattern of flexibility should be noted. The Wiles study, although it involves only four individuals, two of whom were highly atypical from the point of view of agility, nevertheless suggests a relationship between structure and function. It is interesting to note that Miss R., whose spine seemed to be of the "anthropoid type," showed a marked limitation in hyperextension, whereas the adult male acrobat, who seemed to represent the extreme "humanoid type,"

TABLE 18–2. Anteroposterior Spinal Flexibility of Four Selected Cases (Wiles)

Subject	Flexion	Hyperextension	Total
Miss P...64°	35°	99°
Miss R...62°	19°	81°
Child ....76°	39°	115°
Man...50°	71°	121°

showed extreme hyperextension, but limited flexion.[20] A study of the flexibility of a large sampling of these two spinal types might prove to be of value to the physical educator and the athletic coach.

The significance of studies such as the two preceding ones lies in their implication for posture education and for recommendations regarding activity. Such studies are valuable to the degree that they give (1) a broad concept of the "normal," (2) an appreciation of the relatedness between structural type and physical skills and (3) an awareness of the limitations characteristic of each type. Physical educators and therapists should realize that identical goals of posture, flexibility and function cannot be laid down for all types of body build. Just what the specific abilities and limitations of each type are, and just what the goals for each type should be, are problems that are still wide open for investigation.

Comparison of Surface Measurements of Lumbosacral Portion of Spine with Similar Measurements Made on X-ray. In 1934 Boynton made a study of the pelvis and lumbar spine, using for her subjects fifty college women. Her data consisted both of anthropometric measurements and of measurements taken from lateral x-rays. She found considerable variation in the contour and position of the sacrum, and she observed a close relationship between these and the slope of the lower lumbar vertebrae. In her opinion the slope of the lower lumbar vertebrae is determined by the slope of the top of the sacrum and the position of the sacrum in the pelvis. She also observed that the angle of pelvic obliquity varies with these factors. Furthermore—and this is probably Boynton's most important contribution—she found that the correlation between the measurements on the surface of the body and those on the x-rays was so low that it was impossible to judge accurately the slope of the lower lumbar vertebrae and the angle of pelvic obliquity from the external measurements (Fig. 15–20). The coefficients of correlation which she computed give further emphasis to this revealing observation.[2]

Coefficients of Correlation between Measurements
Made on Surface of Body and Measurements
Made on X-ray

Position of sacrum... .0222
Slope of sacrum .... .2430
Slope of lower lumbar vertebrae....................... .0465

DEMONSTRATIONS AND LABORATORY EXERCISES

Joint Structure

1. Study the bones of the spinal column, then fill out an outline like the one in Appendix B for each of the following joints, including the articulations of both the bodies and the arches.
   a. Atlanto-occipital
   b. Atlantoaxial
   c. A middle cervical joint
   d. The joint between the seventh cervical and the first thoracic vertebra
   e. A middle thoracic joint
   f. The joint between the twelfth thoracic and the first lumbar vertebra
   g. A middle lumbar joint
   h. The lumbosacral joint

Joint Action

2. Have a subject sit tailor-fashion on a table and flex his spine as completely as possible. Observe the shape of the spine as seen from the side. Compare the three regions of the spine as to forward flexibility. Make a line drawing of the side view of the spine.

3. Have a subject sit astride a chair, facing its back, and hyperextend the spine as completely as possible. Observe and record the shape of the spine as in 2.

4. Have a subject sit astride a bench and bend sideward as far as possible, first to one side and then to the other. Observe from the rear and draw a line representing the spine in maximum lateral flexion, both left and right.

5. Have a subject sit astride a bench with the hands at the neck, then rotate the trunk as far as possible, first to one side, then to the other. Observe and compare the regions of the spine as to rotating ability.

6. Observe flexion, hyperextension, lateral flexion and rotation of the spine in several subjects, preferably subjects representing different body builds, and note individual differences.

7. Have a subject lie face down on a table with the legs and pelvis supported on the table, the trunk extending forward beyond the table, and the hands clasped behind the neck.
   a. Have the subject bend laterally. Compare the thoracic and lumbar regions. Note the torsion accompanying the lateral flexion.
   b. Have the subject flex the spine and then flex it laterally. Observe as in *a*.
   c. Have the subject hyperextend the spine (with someone helping to support the elbows) and then flex laterally. Observe as in *a*.
   d. Have the subject rotate the trunk to one side as far as possible. Compare the thoracic and lumbar regions. Is any lateral bending apparent in the spine?
   e. Have the subject flex the spine and then rotate it. Observe as in *d*.

f. Have the subject hyperextend the spine and then rotate it. Observe as in *d.*

Muscular Action

The purpose of these exercises is not to test the strength of the muscles, but to enable the observer to study the action of the muscles in simple movements of the body. The procedure, therefore, is quite different from that followed by the physical therapist in testing muscle strength. It is suggested that students work in groups of three, one acting as the subject, one as an assistant helping to support or steady the stationary part of the body and giving resistance to the moving part, and one palpating the muscles and recording the results. The check lists in Appendix F may be used for this purpose. They may also be used for the analysis of other movements.

8. FLEXION OF THE NECK

a. Subject: Lie on the back and lift the head, bringing the chin toward the chest.

Observer: Palpate and identify as many of the contracting muscles as possible.

b. Subject: Lie on the back and lift the head, leading with the chin.

Observer: Compare the action of the sternocleidomastoid in *b* with its action in *a.*

9. EXTENSION AND HYPEREXTENSION OF THE NECK

a. Subject: Lie face down on a table with the head over the edge. Raise the head as far as possible, hyperextending both the head and the neck.

Assistant: May resist the movement if stronger muscular action is desired.

Observer: Palpate and identify as many of the contracting muscles as possible.

b. Subject: Lie face down on a table with the head over the edge. Raise the head as far as possible with the chin tucked in.

Assistant: Resist the retraction of the chin.

Observer: Compare the muscular action in (*b*) with that in (*a*).

10. LATERAL FLEXION OF THE HEAD AND NECK

Subject: Lie on one side and raise the head toward the shoulder without turning the head or tensing the shoulder.

Assistant: Give slight resistance at the temple.

Observer: Palpate and identify as many muscles as possible.

11. ROTATION OF THE HEAD AND NECK

Subject: Sit erect and turn the head to the left as far as possible.

Assistant: Give fairly strong resistance to the side of the jaw.

Observer: Palpate the sternocleidomastoids. Which one contracts?

12. FLEXION OF THE THORACIC AND LUMBAR SPINE

Subject: Lie on the back with the arms folded across the chest. Raise the head, shoulders and upper back from the table, keeping the chin in. There is no need to come to a sitting position, since this is intended as a movement of spinal, not hip, flexion.

Assistant: Hold the thighs down.

Observer: Palpate the rectus abdominis and the external oblique abdominal muscle.

13. EXTENSION AND HYPEREXTENSION OF THE THORACIC AND LUMBAR SPINE

Subject: Lie face down with the hands on the hips. Raise the head and trunk as far as possible.

Assistant: Hold the feet down.

Observer: Palpate the erector spinae and the gluteus maximus (the large hip extensor muscle located in the buttocks). What is the function of the latter muscle in this movement?

14. LATERAL FLEXION OF THE THORACIC AND LUMBAR SPINE

Subject: Lie on one side with the under arm placed across the chest and the hand resting on the opposite shoulder, and with the hand of the top arm resting on the hip. Raise the trunk sideways.

Assistant: Hold the legs down. If necessary, help the subject by pulling at the elbow.

Observer: Palpate the rectus abdominis, external oblique abdominal muscle, erector spinae and latissimus dorsi (the large superficial muscle of the lower back whose tendon of insertion forms the posterior margin of the armpit).

15. ROTATION OF THE THORACIC AND LUMBAR SPINE

Subject: Sit astride a bench with the hands placed behind the neck. Twist to one side as far as possible without leaving the bench.

Assistant: Resist the movement by grasping the subject's arms close to his shoulders and pushing (or pulling) in the opposite direction.

Observer: Palpate as many of the spinal and abdominal muscles as possible. Disregard the muscles of the scapula and arm.

Action of the Muscles Other Than the Movers

16. THE SIT-UP

Subject: Lie on the back and come to a sitting position, keeping the spine as rigid as possible.

Assistant: Hold the feet down.

Observer: Palpate the abdominal muscles, the erector spinae and the sternocleidomastoid. Explain the function of each.

17. DOUBLE LEG LOWERING

Subject: Lie on the back. Raise both legs, then slowly lower them half way.

Observer: Palpate the abdominal muscles and the erector spinae. Explain the function of each.

18. TRUNK BENDING FORWARD

Subject: Stand with the feet slightly separated. Bend forward from the hips, keeping the back flat.

Observer: Palpate the erector spinae. Explain its function.

19. PUSH-UP

Subject: Assume a front-leaning-rest position on the hands and toes with the body straight. Let the elbows bend until the chest almost touches the floor, then push up again, keeping the body straight the entire time. Do not let it sag or hump.

Observer: Palpate the abdominal muscles. Explain their function.

REFERENCES

1. Basmajian, J. V.: Muscles Alive, 2nd ed. Baltimore, The Williams & Wilkins Company, 1967.
2. Boynton, B.: Individual differences in the Structure of Pelvis and Lumbar Spine as a Factor in Body Mechanics. Thesis, State University of Iowa, 1934.
3. Brunnstrom, S.: Clinical Kinesiology, 2nd ed. Philadelphia, F. A. Davis Company, 1966.
4. Campbell, E. J. M.: An electromyographic study of the role of the abdominal muscles in breathing. J. Physiol., 117:222–233, 1952.
5. Crowe, P., O'Connell, A. L., and Gardner, E. B.: An electromyographic study of the abdominal muscles and certain hip flexors during selected sit-ups. Report presented at National Convention of the American Association for Health, Physical Education, and Recreation, 1963.
6. Flint, M. M.: An electromyographic comparison of the function of the iliacus and the rectus abdominis muscles. J. Am. Phys. Ther. Assn., 45:248–252, 1965.
7. Floyd, W. F., and Silver, P. H. S.: Electromyographic study of patterns of activity of the anterior abdominal wall muscles in man. J. Anat., 84:132–145, 1950.
8. Hollinshead, W. H.: Anatomy of the spine. J. Bone & Joint Surg., 47A:209–215, 1965.
9. Jonsson, B.: Morphology, innervation, and electromyographic study of the erector spinae. Arch. Phys. Med. & Rehab., 50:638–641, 1969.
10. Keagy, R. D., Brumlik, J. B., and Bergan, J. J.: Direct electromyography of the psoas major muscle in man. J. Bone & Joint Surg., 48A:1377–1382, 1966.
11. Kendall, H. O., and Kendall, F. P.: The role of abdominal exercises in a program of physical fitness. J. Health & Phys. Ed., 14:480, 481, 504–506, 1943.
12. Knapp, M. E.: Function of the quadratus lumborum. Arch. Phys. Med., 32:505–507, 1951.
13. LaBan, M. M., Raptou, A. D., and Johnson, E. W.: Electromyographic study of function of iliopsoas muscle. Arch. Phys. Med. & Rehab., 46:676–679, 1965.
14. Lovett, R. W.: Lateral Curvature of the Spine and Round Shoulders, 5th ed. Philadelphia, P. Blakiston's Son and Co., Inc., 1931, Chapter 3.
15. Nachemson, A. Quoted in Jonsson, B.: Morphology, innervation, and electromyographic study of the erector spinae. Arch. Phys. Med. & Rehab., 50:638–641, 1969.
16. Partridge, M. J., and Walters, C. E.: Participation of the abdominal muscles in various movements of the trunk in man. Phys. Ther. Rev., 39:791–800, 1959.
17. Pauly, J. E.: An electromyographic analysis of certain movements and exercises. I. Some deep muscles of the back. Anat. Rec., 155:223–234, 1966.
18. Walters, C. E., and Partridge, M. J.: Electromyographic study of the differential action of the abdominal muscles during exercise. Am. J. Phys. Med., 36:259–268, 1957.
19. Wells, K. F.: An investigation of certain evolutionary tendencies in the female human structure, Res. Quart. Am. Assn. Health, Phys. Ed. & Recrn., 18:260–270, 1947.
20. Wiles, P.: Movements of the lumbar vertebrae during flexion and extension. Proc. Roy. Soc. Med., 28:647–651, 1935.
21. Wright, W. G.: Muscle Function. New York, Hafner Publishing Company, 1962.

RECOMMENDED READINGS

Jonsson, B.: Morphology, innervation and electromyographic study of the erector spinae. Arch. Phys. Med. & Rehab., 50:638–641, 1969.
Morris, J. M., Lucas, D. B., and Bresler, B.: Role of the trunk in stability of the spine. J. Bone & Joint Surg., 43A:327–351, 1961.

CHAPTER 19

The Movements of the
Thorax in Respiration

The thorax is a bony-cartilaginous cage, shaped like a beehive, with an inverted V shaped doorway in the front (Fig. 19–1). It is formed mainly by the ribs and their cartilages, but also includes the sternum, which constitutes the anterior base of attachment for the ribs, and the thoracic portion of the spine, which constitutes the posterior base of attachment. The upper seven ribs are called true ribs because their cartilages articulate directly with the sternum. The remaining five ribs are called false ribs; a misleading term, the only difference

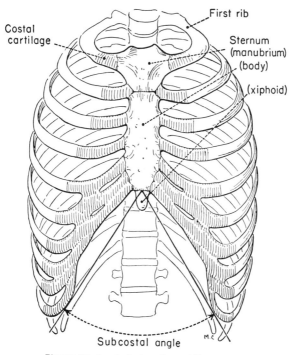

Figure 19–1. Anterior view of thorax.

between "true" and "false" ribs being that the latter do not articulate directly with the sternum. The cartilages of the eighth, ninth and tenth ribs, in each case, unite with the cartilage above; the eleventh and twelfth ribs, known as the "floating ribs," have no anterior attachment. These ribs, shorter than those immediately above, have only short tips of cartilages and, except for their muscular attachments, are free at their anterior ends.

The angle formed between the margins of the lower rib cartilages at the front of the chest (the "door" to the "beehive") is called the subcostal angle. This is characteristically wider in individuals of stocky build than in those of slender build. The thorax is wider from side to side than it is from front to back, and is slightly flattened in front. An infant or young child has a more "barrel-shaped" chest than does an adult, that is, a thorax whose anteroposterior diameter more nearly approaches its transverse diameter than it does in the adult.

Before studying the articulations and the movements of the thorax the student should review the ribs by observing them on a skeleton, noting particularly their shape and the way in which they twist. If no skeleton is available, he should look carefully at pictures of the ribs such as those shown in Figure 19–2.

Articulations and Ligaments.   The majority of the articulations of the thorax belong to the non-axial, diarthrodial classification. They permit a very slight amount of gliding.

COSTOVERTEBRAL

Capitular (costocentral).   The head of the rib articulates with the costal facets of two adjacent vertebrae and the intervertebral disk between them (Fig. 18–12). The first, tenth, eleventh and twelfth ribs each articulate with a single vertebra. The joint is a non-axial, diarthrodial one and permits only a slight gliding motion. It is enclosed in a capsule and is strengthened by a radiate ligament and an interarticular ligament (Fig. 19–3).

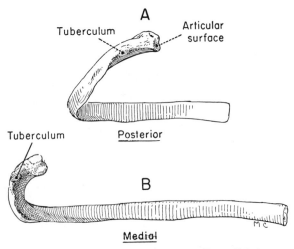

Figure 19–2.   Rib. *A,* Posterior view; *B,* medial view.

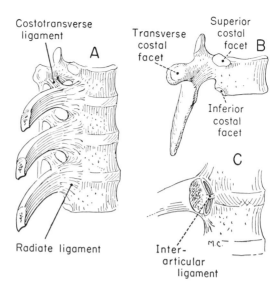

Figure 19–3. Anterior and lateral views of costovertebral articulations.

Costotransverse. (Fig. 19–4.) The tubercle on the under side of each rib (Figs. 19–2 and 19–4), with the exception of the eleventh and twelfth, articulates with the adjacent transverse process. This is a non-axial, diarthrodial joint. The articular capsule, which is thin and membranous, is reinforced by the anterior and posterior costotransverse ligaments (Figs. 19–3 and 19–4) and the strong little ligaments of the neck and tubercle of the rib, respectively.

STERNOCOSTAL ARTICULATIONS. (Fig. 19–5.) There are four groups of articulations in the sternocostal region: (1) the sternocostal joints between the costal cartilages and the sternum; (2) the joints between each rib and its cartilage, known as the costochondral joints; (3) the joints between one costal cartilage and another, called the interchondral joints; and (4) the two intersternal joints, one between the manubrium and body of the sternum, the other between the body and the xiphoid process. The reinforcing ligaments in this region include the radiate sternocostal, the interarticular sternocostal and the costoxiphoid.

Figure 19–4. Superior view of costovertebral articulations.

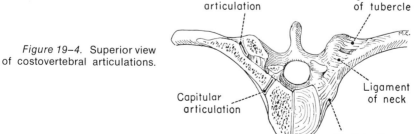

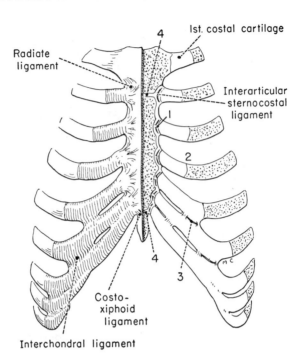

Figure 19–5. Sternocostal articulations. Key: *1,* Sternocostal; *2,* costochondral; *3,* interchondral; *4,* intersternal.

Movements. Because most of the ribs are attached both posteriorly and anteriorly, their movement is extremely limited. In the thoracic expansion associated with inhalation the anterior ends of the ribs are elevated in a flexion type of movement. This is accompanied by a slight eversion in which the lower margin of the central portion of the rib turns upward and lateralward, the inner surface being made to face somewhat downward. As the anterior ends of the upper ribs move upward they also push forward, carrying the sternum forward and upward with them. In the case of the lower ribs, the anterior ends move laterally, thus "opening" the chest and widening the subcostal angle.

The expansion of the thorax is associated not only with inhalation, but also with all movements of the body requiring effort. If one were to push or lift a heavy piece of furniture, for instance, he would first inhale, then hold his breath while making the effort to move the object. The inhalation that occurs may be considered a secondary function of the thorax in this case. The primary function is the stabilization of the ribs and sternum for the purpose of providing firm anchorage for the muscles which attach to them, namely, the abdominal muscles, the pectoralis major and minor, and the serratus anterior.

In inhalation the thorax is enlarged in three diameters — transverse, anteroposterior and vertical.

INCREASE IN THE TRANSVERSE DIAMETER. (Fig. 19–6.) This is due to the elevation and eversion of the lateral portion of the ribs. The shape and twist of the ribs, together with their anterior and posterior attachments, are responsible for what has so aptly been called "bucket-handle inspiratory movement." The elevation of the lower ribs is accompanied by a lateral movement of their anterior ends. This widening of the lower part of the thorax increases the power of the diaphragm by putting it on a stretch.

INCREASE IN THE ANTEROPOSTERIOR DIAMETER. (Fig. 19–6.) This is due to elevation of the anterior ends of the obliquely placed ribs and to elevation of the body of the sternum, caused by the elevation of the ribs. The elevation of the anterior ends of the ribs causes the ribs to assume a more horizontal position and results in a straightening of the costal cartilages. The movements of the thorax in the anteroposterior and transverse diameters are inseparable. The expansion in both directions when the ribs are elevated is the natural result of their shape and of the oblique direction of their axes of motion.

INCREASE IN THE VERTICAL DIAMETER. This is due partly to the elevation of the first two ribs, but even more to the depression of the central tendon of the diaphragm. If inhalation is forced, expansion of the thorax is aided by complete extension of the thoracic spine.

Muscles. Muscular action is required for all inhalation, no matter how shallow, but ordinary exhalation is brought about by the recoil of the elastic structures of the thorax and by the weight of the chest. In vigorous or resisted exhalation, however, and in all forms of vocalization, muscular action is required.

Muscles of normal inhalation
   Diaphragm
   External intercostals
   Internal intercostals, anterior cartilaginous region
Additional muscles of vigorous inhalation
   Sternocleidomastoid*
   The three scaleni*
   Levatores costarum
   Serratus posterior superior
   Pectoralis minor*
   Trapezius I*
   Levator scapulae*
   The thoracic spine extensors*
Muscles of vigorous exhalation
   Internal intercostals, posterior and lateral portions
   Transversus abdominis
   Rectus abdominis*
   Oblique abdominal muscles*
   Transversus thoracis
   Serratus posterior inferior

---

*These are primarily muscles of either the spine or the shoulder girdle.

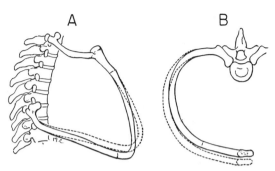

Figure 19–6. Expansion of thorax during inhalation. *A,* Lateral view; *B,* superior view.

DIAPHRAGM (Fig. 19–7.)

Peripheral attachment. (o)   Circumference of thoracic outlet.

Central attachment. (i)   Central tendon, a clover leaf-shaped aponeurosis.

Nerve supply.   Phrenic nerve.

Cannot be palpated.

Action.   Depression of the central tendon, hence an increase in the vertical diameter of the thorax. Also has a tendency to lift the lower ribs, which is probably resisted by the quadratus lumborum and iliocostalis lumborum.

Comments.   The diaphragm is a dome-shaped muscular sheet which separates the thoracic and abdominal cavities. When it contracts, it pulls down at its central tendon, thus increasing the vertical diameter of the thorax. In doing this, it presses against the abdominal organs, which in turn push forward against the relaxed abdominal wall. By increasing the intra-abdominal pressure it helps in defecation, vomiting and other forms of expulsion. Although primarily a muscle of inhalation, it assists indirectly in exhalation by means of its elastic recoil when it relaxes.

INTERCOSTALES EXTERNI (Fig. 19–8.)

Attachments.   Lower border of one rib and upper border of rib beneath.

Nerve supply.   Branches from corresponding intercostal nerves.

Where to palpate.   On thin subjects, between the ribs anterior to the serratus anterior.

Action.   Elevation of the ribs.

Comments.   These muscles lie between the ribs, from the spine in back to the costal cartilages in front. They consist of short parallel fibers which slant downward and forward in the same direction as the fibers of the external oblique abdominal muscle. They lift the ribs, thus increasing the thoracic cavity in both the transverse and anteroposterior diameters.

INTERCOSTALES INTERNI (Fig. 19–8.)

Attachments.   Inner surface and costal cartilage of one rib and upper border of rib immediately below.

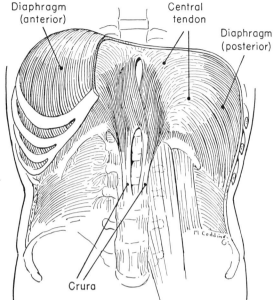

Figure 19-7. The diaphragm.

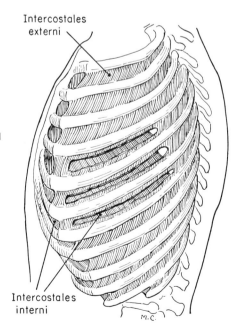

Figure 19-8. The intercostal muscles.

Nerve supply. Branches from corresponding intercostal nerves. Cannot be palpated.

Action

Anterior portion: Elevation of ribs.

Lateral and posterior portions: Depression of ribs.

Comments. Like the external intercostals, these consist of short parallel fibers which lie between the ribs, but, unlike them, the fibers of the internal intercostals slant downward and backward. This is the same direction as that taken by the fibers of the internal oblique abdominal muscle. They extend from the sternum in front to the angles of the ribs in back. Since the external intercostals extend only as far forward as the costal cartilages, the anterior portion of the internal intercostals is not covered by the external.

STERNOCLEIDOMASTOIDEUS (Fig. 18–16.)   (See also muscles of the spine.)

Lower attachments. (O)   By two heads from top of sternum and medial third of clavicle.

Upper attachments. (I)   Mastoid process of temporal bone and adjacent portion of occipital bone.

Nerve supply. Accessory and branches from the second and third cervical nerves.

Where to palpate. On the side of the neck just under the ear and on the front of the neck at the junction of the clavicle and sternum.

Action (on thorax). Helps to elevate the sternum and clavicle.

Comments. In vigorous inhalation the head is held firmly erect and the sternocleidomastoid, instead of flexing the head and neck, pulls up on the sternum and sternal end of the clavicles, lifting them slightly.

THE THREE SCALENI (Fig. 18–15.)   (See also muscles of the spine.)

Upper attachments. (O)   Transverse processes of cervical vertebrae.

Lower attachments. (I)   First two ribs.

Nerve supply. Branches from second to seventh cervical nerves, inclusive.

Where to palpate. On the side of the neck between the sternocleidomastoid and the upper trapezius. They are difficult to identify.

Action (at thorax). Help to elevate first two ribs.

Comments. In vigorous inhalation the head and neck are held firmly erect. This makes it possible for the scaleni muscles to lift the first two ribs.

LEVATORES COSTARUM (LEVATOR COSTAE) (Fig. 19–9.)

Upper attachments. (O)   Ends of transverse processes of seventh cervical and upper eleven thoracic vertebrae.

Lower attachments (I)

Upper eight muscles: In each case, to the rib immediately below, between the tubercle and the angle.

Lower four muscles: By two bands each, one to the rib immediately below and the other to the second rib below.

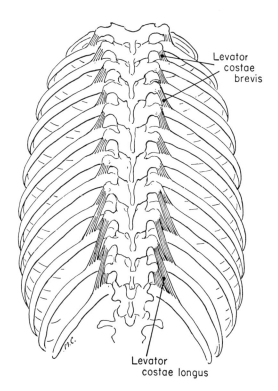

Levator
costae
brevis

Levator
costae longus

Figure 19-9. Levatores
costarum (levator costae).

Nerve supply. Branches from corresponding intercostal nerves. Cannot be palpated.

Action (at thorax). Elevation of ribs.

Comments. The levatores costarum are sometimes called the posterior portions of the external intercostals. Although they are in a position to elevate the ribs, their leverage for this action is poor.

SERRATUS POSTERIOR SUPERIOR (Fig. 19-10.)

Upper attachments. (O) Spinous processes and ligaments of lower two or three cervical and upper two thoracic vertebrae.

Lower attachments. (I) Upper borders of second, third, fourth and fifth ribs.

Nerve supply. Branches from the first four intercostal nerves. Cannot be palpated.

Action. Elevation of second, third, fourth and fifth ribs.

Comments. This is a flat quadrilateral muscle whose parallel fibers slant upward and medialward from the upper ribs to the spine.

PECTORALIS MINOR (See also muscles of the shoulder girdle; Fig. 12-12.)

Lower attachments. (O) Anterior surface of third, fourth and fifth ribs near their cartilages.

Upper attachment. (I) Tip of coracoid process of scapula.

Nerve supply. Medial anterior thoracic nerve.

Where to palpate. Halfway between the clavicle and the nipple, or between this point and the tip of the shoulder.

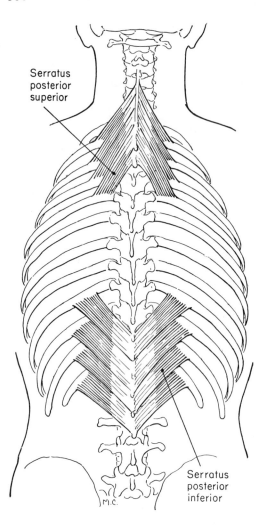

Serratus
posterior
superior

Serratus
posterior
inferior

Figure 19–10. Serratus posterior superior and inferior.

Action (at thorax). Elevation of third, fourth and fifth ribs.

Comments. The pectoralis minor can reverse the direction of its pull and lift the ribs only if the thoracic spine is extended and the scapula is stabilized. The most favorable position for the latter is one of elevation and adduction.

TRANSVERSUS ABDOMINIS (Fig. 19–11.)

Lateral attachments. (O) Inguinal ligament, crest of ilium, thoracolumbar fascia and cartilages of lower six ribs.

Medial attachments. (I)   Linea alba and crest of pubis.

Nerve supply. Branches of lower six intercostal nerves, ilio-hypogastric and ilio-inguinal nerves.

Cannot be palpated.

Action. Compression of the abdomen and depression of the lower ribs.

Comments. This is one of the four muscles forming the abdominal wall. Its fibers run horizontally from the thoracolumbar fascia and cartilages of the lower ribs forward to the linea alba. Its pull is inward against the abdominal viscera; hence it is a strong muscle of exhalation and expulsion. It also helps to stabilize the trunk when acts requiring great effort are performed. Together with the other muscles of the abdominal wall, it is credited with compressing the abdominal contents into a semi-rigid cylinder.

RECTUS ABDOMINIS, EXTERNAL AND INTERNAL OBLIQUES (Figs. 18–22, 18–23 and 18–24.)   (See also muscles of the spine.)

Attachments. Lower ribs and rib cartilages, thoracolumbar fascia, upper portions of pelvis, and linea alba. (For exact attachments, see muscles of the spine.)

Nerve supply. Intercostal iliohypogastric and ilio-inguinal nerves.

Where to palpate. Front and sides of the abdomen.

Action (at thorax). Depression of the lower ribs and sternum; compression of the abdomen.

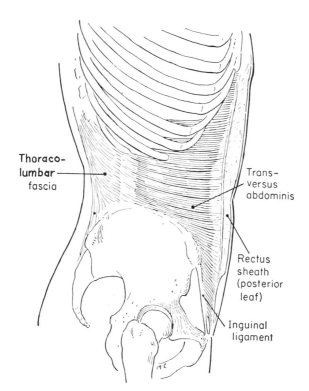

Figure 19–11. Transversus abdominis.

Comments. When the spine is fixed in extension, these muscles contract in vigorous exhalation. By compressing the abdominal viscera they indirectly exert an upward pressure against the diaphragm, causing it to be pushed up into the thorax.

TRANSVERSUS THORACIS (Fig. 19–12.)

Medial attachments. (O) Lower half of inner surface of sternum and adjoining costal cartilages.

Lateral attachments. (I) Lower borders and inner surfaces of costal cartilages of second, third, fourth, fifth and sixth ribs.

Nerve supply. Branches from upper six thoracic intercostal nerves.

Cannot be palpated.

Action. Depression of the ribs to which it is attached.

Comments. This muscle consists of flat bands and is located on the inner surface of the front wall of the thorax. The bands radiate upward and outward from the sternum to the ribs, the lowest fibers being continuous with those of the transversus abdominis.

SERRATUS POSTERIOR INFERIOR (Fig. 19–10.)

Lower, medial attachments. (O) Spinous processes and ligaments of lower two thoracic and upper two or three lumbar vertebrae.

Upper lateral attachments. (I) Lower borders of lower four ribs.

Nerve supply. Branches from ninth, tenth and eleventh intercostal nerves.

Cannot be palpated.

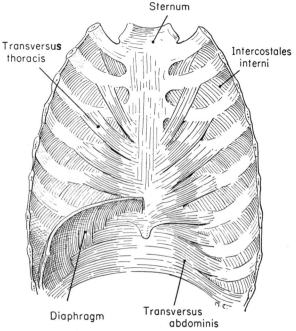

Figure 19–12. Posterior (inner) view of anterior wall of thorax.

Action. Depression of the lower four ribs.

Comments. Like the superior, this is a flat quadrilateral muscle. The fibers slant downward and medialward from the lower ribs to the spine.

Muscles, Other Than the Principal or Assistant Movers, Acting in Respiration. Since the muscles which act as the movers in inhalation and exhalation have already been listed (p. 355), it seems unnecessary to repeat them here. The principal movers are the muscles which belong primarily to the thorax; the assistant movers, those which are primarily muscles of the spine or shoulder girdle. Some of the latter muscles also serve as stabilizers in respiration.

STABILIZERS IN INHALATION

Quadratus lumborum. This anchors the last rib against the pull of the diaphragm.

The three scaleni. These hold the upper two ribs against the pull of the external intercostals.

Cervical and thoracic extensors. These stabilize the head and neck against the pull of the sternocleidomastoid and scaleni.

Abdominal muscles. By their normal tension these muscles stabilize the lower ribs against the pull of the diaphragm.

Upper trapezius and levator scapulae. These stabilize the scapula against the pull of the pectoralis minor.

STABILIZERS IN EXHALATION

Erector spinae. Stabilizes the spine and pelvis against the pull of the abdominal muscles.

DEMONSTRATIONS AND LABORATORY EXERCISES

1. MOVEMENT OF THE THORAX IN RESPIRATION

Subject: Breathe naturally for a while, then as deeply as possible.

Observer: (*a*) Place the hands on the sides of the thorax and note the movement in the lateral diameter. (*b*) Place one hand on the ribs at the subcostal angle (just below the sternum) and the other hand against the back at the same level. Note the movement in the anteroposterior diameter. (*c*) Place the fingers on the sternum. Can you detect any movement in normal respiration? In deep respiration?

2. MUSCULAR ACTION IN FORCED INHALATION

a. Subject: Inhale through a small rubber tube, pinching it slightly in order to furnish resistance.

Observer: Note the action of the sternocleidomastoid, cervical and thoracic extensors, and upper trapezius. Can any other muscular action be detected? If so, explain.

b. Subject: Run in place or around the room until short of breath. Hang from a horizontal bar.

Observer: Can you detect any action of the pectoralis major accompanying inhalation? (By stabilizing the arms, the hanging position causes the pectoralis major to act on the ribs.)

3. MUSCULAR ACTION IN VIGOROUS EXHALATION

Subject: Blow through a small rubber tube, pinching it slightly or holding a finger loosely over the end. (Or blow into a spirometer, flarimeter or toy balloon.)

Observer: Note the action of the abdominal muscles and of the erector spinae.

REFERENCE

1. Morris, J. M., Lucas, D. B., and Bresler, B.: Role of the trunk in stability of the spine. J. Bone & Joint Surg., *43A*:327–351, 1961.

RECOMMENDED READING

Steindler, A.: Kinesiology of the Human Body. Springfield, Ill., Charles C Thomas, Publisher, 1955, Lecture 13. (For advanced students.)

PART THREE

Applications of Kinesiology

INTRODUCTION TO PART THREE

The application of kinesiology to physical education activities has gone through several different eras of emphasis during the twentieth century. For the first twenty or twenty-five years anatomic, especially muscular, analysis was emphasized. This coincided with the period when high school and college physical education curriculums consisted largely of calisthenics, gymnastics, field and track, stunts and tumbling, some sports (team sports at first but later individual sports as facilities became available), folk dance and clog dance (later known as tap).

As the curricular emphasis gradually shifted to sports, the emphasis in kinesiology shifted to athletic skills. Yet the emphasis on gymnastic activities did not diminish. In fact, during the forties there was an upsurge of interest in the application of mechanical principles to these activities. This was due in large part to the influence of C. H. McCloy who toured the country in the late thirties and early forties giving lectures with demonstrations showing specific ways in which performance could be improved by the application of appropriate mechanical principles. He was one of the first to develop a course in the Mechanical Analysis of Motor Skills. The current literature reflects the growing and continued interest in the mechanical aspects of athletic skills. Examples of this are *Scientific Principles of Coaching* by John W. Bunn (1954), *The Mechanics of Athletics* by Geoffrey Dyson (1965), and *Science of Swimming* by James Counsilman (1968).

Since the mid-forties there has been a renewal of interest in muscular analysis. This was the direct result of the development of the electromyographic technique for studying the actions of muscles. For the first time it was possible to provide objective evidence of muscular action in various movement patterns, showing not just the *fact* of participation, but the duration and relative intensity of contraction in a given movement. This technique started a rash of research studies in physical education graduate programs and had a tremendous impact on course content in kinesiology. Since World War II the emphasis on both anatomic and mechanical analysis has continued hand in hand, but it has gradually come to be recognized that whereas joint and muscular analysis is of prime concern in programs of physical fitness and conditioning exercises, it is of little more than academic interest in the sports program, except possibly as it may relate to the prevention of injury.

On the other hand, mechanical analysis has proved to be extremely pertinent to sports by pointing the way to greater skill in (1) moving one's own body with reference to its environment, in (2) solving problems of equilibrium, water resistance, suspension, and so on, and in (3) the giving and receiving of impetus of balls and other objects. Up until the present time it may well be said that kinesiology has been synonymous with the analysis of human motion. Joint and muscular analysis, and mechanical analysis between them, have contributed a volume of essential information concerning musculoskeletal movements.

Some other areas deserving of attention are newer methods of collecting kinesiologic data as, for instance, the method described by Plagenhoef in the March 1966 issue of the Research Quarterly, and the use of computers in processing kinesiologic data as described by Garrett, Widule and Garrett in *Kinesiology Review 1968*. There is also a growing interest in the psychological aspects of physical education, especially in relation to motor learning. It behooves kinesiology instructors and students to keep abreast of this field of study and research and to be aware of its significance.

How are these new kinesiologic materials and techniques to be used by the kinesiology instructor? To answer this, one must first answer the question, "What are the objectives of kinesiology?" One seemingly logical answer to this question is, "To improve performance." Unfortunately some instructors, and especially coaches, have a tendency to apply this only to the already highly skilled athlete who desires to excel. This is not an unworthy goal, yet the average teacher deals with many more beginners and students of average ability than he does with potential athletic stars. His chief concern should be for this large group and his goal for them should be to help them develop sufficient skill to derive genuine enjoyment from participating in a variety of recreational sports and activities. The initial steps in attaining such a goal are to inspire interest and to increase understanding. This the teacher can do by using his imagination and teaching skill to select the aspects most needing emphasis and by devising simple demonstrations which will help the student to understand the reason for performing in a certain way.

Part Three consists of seven chapters, each treating a particular area of physical education to which the principles of kinesiology are pertinent. The first three of these are concerned with fundamental concepts and activities: the postures of the human structure as they relate to mechanical and organic efficiency; the selection and evaluation of exercises from the standpoint of their contribution to physical fitness and conditioning; and the basic locomotor activities — walking and running. The next chapter, twenty-three, deals with the very core of the physical education program — namely, sports and gymnastic activities. Following this is a chapter on the motor skills common to normal, daily living. In Chapter Twenty-Five the kinesiologic principles relating to the avoidance of injury are summarized.

The concluding chapter is addressed particularly to the student majoring in physical education who will soon be joining the ranks of physical education teachers. It discusses the implications of kinesiology for effective instruction in the activity program. It presents different views concerning the value of teaching mechanical principles to students as an aid to learning motor skills. Some investigators have found this practice beneficial, others have not. As to the value of a sound knowledge of mechanical principles to the instructor himself, there is no disagreement. The increased understanding which this gives him provides a scientific basis for selecting one particular technique in preference to another; it enables him to diagnose individual needs and difficulties; it reveals basic similarities between motor skills in the same category and thus enables him to present more clearly new sports that involve the same movement patterns as a sport with which the class is already familiar; it enables him to make pertinent suggestions with true insight. A thorough grasp of this subject adds immeasurably to the instructor's background. In short, the intelligent use of one's knowledge of kinesiology could make all the difference between effective and ineffective teaching.

CHAPTER 20

Postural Concepts and Principles

There are innumerable concepts of human posture, and innumerable interpretations of its significance. Posture may well claim to be "all things to all men." To the physical anthropologist posture may be a racial characteristic, or it may be an indication of phylogenetic development; to the orthopedic surgeon it may be an indication of the soundness of the skeletal framework and muscular system; to an artist it may be an expression of the personality and the emotions; to the actor it serves as a tool for expressing mood or character; to the physician, the biologist, the fashion model, the employer, the sculptor, the dancer, the psychologist—to each of these, posture has a different significance. Each sees posture within the framework of his own profession and interest. This is no less true of the kinesiologically oriented physical educator. To him, posture is a gauge of mechanical efficiency, of kinesthetic sense, of muscle balance and of neuromuscular coordination.

Part of the difficulty in identifying postural principles lies in the fact that no individual's posture can be adequately described. Posture means position, and a multisegmented organism such as the human body cannot be said to have a single posture. It assumes many postures and rarely holds any of them for an appreciable time. To be sure, certain characteristic patterns become apparent as we have the opportunity to observe an individual over an extended period, but it is difficult, if not well nigh impossible, to measure, or even record, characteristic postural patterns. It would take a series of candid camera motion pictures to do so.

Another difficulty in identifying postural principles is the many varieties of human physique. The importance of considering these individual differences of build when evaluating posture has been emphasized by Frost.[9]

Thus we see the dual fallacy upon which so-called posture norms are based. Posture norms are appropriate only for the mythical average figure, and apply only to the static standing position, which may or may not represent habitual postural patterns. Nevertheless an attempt is made here to present specific postural principles whenever there is objective justification for so doing. When specific principles cannot be stated, tentative ones are suggested if the clinical evidence or common experience seems to warrant their inclusion. In some instances ideas which are commonly accepted as principles are mentioned for the sole purpose of pointing out that there is no evidence to support them. This does not preclude the possibility of such evidence being presented some time in the future, however.

In view of the fact that activity postures should be of greater concern to the physical educator than static postures, it may be well to say a word in defense of the common practice of examining and photographing the posture of subjects in the erect standing position. It is admitted that the posture in such a position is of little importance in itself. It becomes significant, however, when it is taken as the point of departure for the many postural patterns assumed by the individual, both at rest and in motion (Fig. 20–1). Since there is an almost endless variety of activity postures, and since these are extremely difficult to judge, it is a convenient custom to accept the standing posture as the individual's basic posture from which all his other postures stem. Hence, as a reflection of the individual's characteristic postural patterns, the standing posture takes on an importance it would not otherwise have. It should be kept in mind, however, that *its importance is in direct proportion to the extent to which it represents the individual's habitual carriage.*

Principles Related to the Mechanism for Maintaining and Adjusting Erect Posture. Posture is regulated in part by reflex action and in part by volitional effort. Since these have both been discussed elsewhere (pp. 171 and 172), they are but briefly mentioned here.

1. Stimuli arising from vision, from the semicircular canals, from the stretching of antigravity muscles and from pressure on the soles of the feet elicit an increase in the tonus of the antigravity muscles and thus provide the body with a means of remaining upright without the necessity for conscious control.

2. Temporary postural adjustments can be made volitionally by means of the same mechanism by which all volitional movements are made (p. 172). These adjustments are necessarily within the structural limitations of the individual.

3. The gradual changing of habitual postural patterns can be brought about by the same means by which any neuromuscular habits are changed. This is a slow process of reconditioning the neuromuscular pathways. The specific methods for accomplishing this form the basis for the different schools of thought in the field of posture education and corrective exercise. Some believe that it can be accomplished by the frequent repetition of carefully selected exercises performed with control and with constant attention to correct form.[10, 12, 20, 22, 25] Others believe that the rebuilding of the necessary neuromuscular pathways can be accomplished only by the indirect method, that is, by influencing the individual's neuromuscular response by means of his thought processes. Mental concepts are

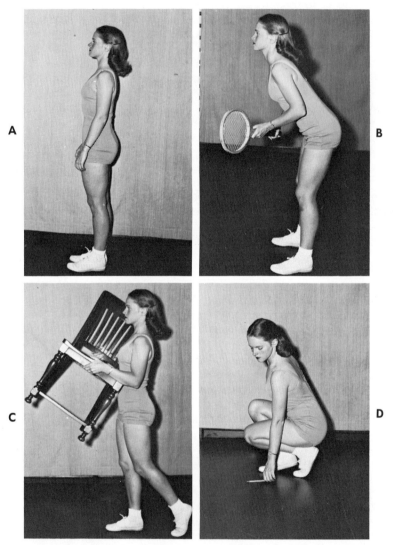

Figure 20-1. The erect standing posture is the point of reference for other postural patterns. *A,* Erect standing posture; *B,* adaptation of posture to a sport activity; *C,* adaptation of posture to carrying a large object; *D,* adaptation of posture to picking up a small object from the floor. (Photos by MacLaurin.)

utilized for this purpose.[27, 28] Still others seek to establish new postural habits by practicing movements which are believed to develop the natural postural reflexes.[11, 13] All groups recognize that the establishing of new postural patterns can take place only within the limits of the individual's structural heritage.

4. The kinesthetic sense would seem to be a vital factor in the mechanism for establishing and adjusting postural patterns, but this has not yet been demonstrated. It is believed that if valid tests could be found for habitual carriage and for kinesthetic awareness of head and trunk positions, a relationship between posture and kinesthesis could be established.

Principles Related to Stability

1. Hellebrandt demonstrated that even the erect standing posture is not literally static. "Standing," she concluded, "is, in reality, *movement upon a stationary base.*"[14] Her experiments revealed that the center of gravity did not remain motionless above the base of support no matter how still the subject attempted to stand, but moved forward, backward and sideward. This motion indicated that the subjects were constantly swaying. When the swaying was prevented by artificial means, there was a tendency to faint. Hence the involuntary swaying was seen to serve the purpose of a pump, aiding the venous return and assuring the brain of adequate circulation for retaining consciousness.

2. In the same experiments Hellebrandt found that the oscillations of each individual were balanced so exactly that the average position of the line of gravity, relative to the base of support, was remarkably constant. From this it would seem that we can assume the presence of a controlling factor in our tendency to sway. Apparently the stretch reflex, the kinesthetic sense and vision all operate here to confine the oscillations to a limited area, an area well within the boundaries of the base of support.

3. Some experimenters have investigated the possibility of a relationship between the position of the line of gravity, relative to the base of support, and the quality of posture. The findings of the different investigators do not agree, however. Hence there would seem to be insufficient evidence to support a claim for such a relationship. (See the summary of investigations by Cureton and Wickens, Crowley, and Johnston in the Supplementary Material for Chapter 1.)

4. In informal class experiments the author found that the relation of the line of gravity to the base of support was not affected significantly or consistently when the subject assumed different positions of the upper extremities or held external objects such as books, a suitcase or a tray. This would seem to provide evidence of the body's tendency to compensate for deviations of some of its parts from the fundamental standing position. The principle would appear to be established that, under ordinary circumstances, the disalignment of one segment of the body, whether anteroposteriorly or laterally, is accompanied by a compensatory disalignment of another segment or segments. If the disalignment is not exactly balanced, excessive tension in certain

muscle groups results. This is particularly apparent when external loads are not adequately compensated. To the best of the author's knowledge there has been no large-scale investigation of this matter of compensatory alignment. Objective evidence is suggested, but is as yet inconclusive.

Principles Related to the Alignment of Body Segments

1. In much of the literature on posture, statements are made that in the ideal standing posture, as viewed from the side, the line of gravity bears a definite relation to certain anatomic landmarks, such as the mastoid process, the acromion process, the junctions of the antero-posterior curves of the spine, the hip joint (greater trochanter of the femur), the knee joint and the lateral malleolus.* In a class study made on only six subjects at Wellesley College the relation of the line of gravity to some of these landmarks was investigated. The variation among these six subjects is shown by the following measurements:

Distance from Line of Gravity to:		Total Range
Ankle joint	3.80 cm. in front to 6.65 cm. in front	2.85 cm.
Knee joint	0.46 cm. behind to 2.85 cm. in front	3.31 cm.
Hip joint	6.65 cm. behind to 0.95 cm. in front	7.60 cm.
Shoulder joint	1.80 cm. behind to 6.65 cm. in front	8.45 cm.
Mastoid process	0.95 cm. behind to 5.23 cm. in front	6.18 cm.

In evaluating this and similar studies the reader should be aware of the influence of body sway on the relation of the anatomic landmarks to a vertical line and should appreciate the difficulty of locating some of these landmarks. The students who conducted the study found it particularly difficult to locate the surface point which corresponds to the midpoint of the hip joint. It might be of interest to repeat an investigation of this sort, using a large number of subjects, representing both sexes and a variety of physique types. In determining the location of the line of gravity it would be well to take the mean of several measurements on each subject in order to minimize the influence of sway. The results of such a study might reveal what could be accepted as a "normal zone" of the line of gravity in the erect standing position. It might help also in analyzing the alignment of the body segments and thus lend itself to diagnostic purposes.

2. It has been stated that a standing posture in which each weight-bearing segment was balanced vertically upon the segment beneath it made less demand on the muscles than a posture in which the segments formed a zigzag alignment.[2, 20] Good posture, they say, takes less muscular effort to maintain than poor. They offer the explanation that when a segment is not in vertical alignment, the force of gravity is not parallel with its long axis, and hence exerts a rotatory component of force. This reasoning seems entirely logical,

---

*According to Brunnstrom this belief is the result of an incorrect translation and interpretation of Braune and Fischer's discussion of "Normalstellung."[3]

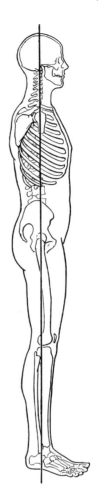

Figure 20-2. Vertical alignment of the body.

but overlooks the fact that even in the most ideal posture rotatory components of force are present, owing to (1) the supporting column of the trunk (i.e., the spine) not being centrally located anteroposteriorly, (2) the supporting base (the feet) being projected forward from the lower extremities instead of centered beneath them, (3) the spinal column being curved anteroposteriorly, and (4) the chest forming an anterior load upon which gravity is constantly exerting a rotatory force. The weight of the breasts in women constitutes an additional anterior weight, causing an even greater rotatory component of gravitational force.

The question of the energy cost of standing posture has been investigated by both Hellebrandt[16] and McCormick.[21] Both concluded that the increase of metabolic rate in standing over the basal rate was so small, compared with the metabolic cost of moving and exercising, that it was negligible. McCormick included both anteroposterior and lateral measurements of body alignment. From these she concluded that the type of posture which involved a minimum of metabolic increase appeared to be one in which the knees are hyperextended as completely as the joints permit, the hips are pushed forward to the limit of extension, the thoracic curve is increased, the head is projected forward and the upper trunk is inclined slightly backward in a posterior list (see Fig. 20–5, B). As one might expect, this is a typical picture of fatigue posture. A common variation of it is a shift of the weight to one foot with accompanying asymmetric adjustments in the spine and lower extremities.

From these two studies and from the writings of other investigators, such as Basmajian, Evans, Joseph, Steindler and others, it is seen that there is a lack of agreement concerning the degree of muscular activity required for maintaining upright posture. Doubtless this is partly due to confusion in what is meant by "upright posture." To some, it may mean merely the ability to stay on one's feet and resist the downward pull of gravity. To others, it may mean "good" alignment as opposed to a "zigzag" alignment. The studies based on energy cost appear to indicate that although it takes little more energy to stand erect than to sit, minimum energy expenditure cannot be accepted as a criterion of posture. Metabolic economy is desirable up to a point, as it implies the absence of hypertonicity, but from the physical educator's point of view good alignment should not be sacrificed for it.

It is the author's opinion that the energy requirement for maintaining erect posture in reasonably good alignment bears a direct relationship to the individual's habitual carriage. It is a matter of common observation that there is a wide range of body alignments seen in "upright posture." Any physical educator who has had the task of evaluating the posture of large groups of students and of giving help to those with "poor posture" is impressed with the variation in effort it takes for a student to stand in "good posture." Whereas one individual apparently has no difficulty in assuming this posture because it is his natural posture, another cannot assume it even momentarily without the instructor's help and without becoming overtense. It is obvious that the second student is using much more muscular energy than is the first. The physical education teacher who is concerned with posture instruction would like to see these individual variations more thoroughly explored. The combination of metabolic determination and electromyography should prove a good tool for such research. It would be of particular interest to the posture and corrective exercise instructor to learn whether such instruction over a specified period would reveal a relationship between posture improvement and the amount of muscular energy required for assuming an "acceptable posture" and maintaining it while participating in selected activities for a specified period of time.

There appears to be a definite relationship between the alignment of the body segments and the integrity of the joint structures. It is

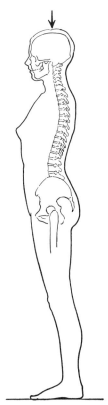

Figure 20–3. When the body is in good standing posture, the rotatory effect of the force of gravity is minimized.

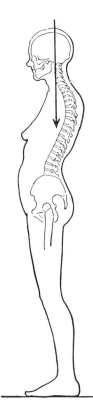

Figure 20–4. When the body is in a poor standing posture, the force of gravity has an exaggerated rotatory effect on the weight-bearing segments.

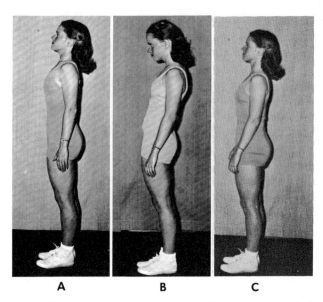

Figure 20–5. The relation of posture to metabolic economy. *A,* An overtense posture is more costly. *B,* An overrelaxed posture is economical, but it subjects the ligaments to strain. *C,* An easily erect posture, which involves no unnecessary tension, is best from all points of view. (Photo by MacLaurin.)

generally accepted that prolonged postural strain is injurious to these structures. Ligaments that are repeatedly subjected to stretch become permanently stretched, and cartilages that are subjected to uneven pressures and to abnormal friction become damaged. There is adequate clinical evidence to support the contention that prolonged postural strain is a factor in the arthritic changes which take place in the weight-bearing joints. Objective evidence may be lacking, but it might not be difficult to secure if postural records and x-rays of the weight-bearing joints could be obtained for an adequate number of subjects over a ten- or twenty-year period. Such an investigation might prove or disprove the claim that the human machine functions more efficiently when the weight-bearing segments are in "proper" alignment, with a minimum of stress and strain on them.

Principles Related to Evolutionary and Hereditary Influences
    1. In tracing the evolution of the human structure and its posture, Morton[24] has shown the influence that the force of gravity has had on the morphologic development, first of the terrestrial quadrupeds, then of the arboreal primates and finally of man. The evolution from horizontal to vertical posture was achieved, he claimed, by the force of gravity pulling on the suspended body of the arboreal primates when they engaged in brachial locomotion. The changes which developed in man's structure, he stated, were the direct result of the shift from a vertically suspended position to a vertically supported one. This shift was responsible not only for the changes in the weight-

bearing parts of the musculoskeletal structure, but also for changes in the upper extremities, which were now freed for the development of a great variety of manipulative skills. While no specific principle is derived from this explanation of the role played by the force of gravity in the evolution of man's structure, an awareness of it might be of help in the analysis of individual postures.

2. Attention has already been called to individual variations in posture. In attempting to correct a person's posture one must be realistic and accept the limits imposed by a possible hereditary factor. Improvement can doubtless be made, but one must not expect to effect a radical change in the basic shape of the spine.

3. Certain pathologic conditions, such as congenitally dislocated hips, tuberculosis of the spine, cerebral palsy and poliomyelitis with resultant paralysis of trunk muscles, may cause such changes in an individual's posture that the usual hereditary and environmental influences are obscured.

Principles Related to Organic Function. One frequently mentioned criterion of good posture is the relationship of the alignment of the body to organic function.[10, 20] Postural patterns are not thought to be good unless they both permit and encourage normal function of the vital physiologic processes, particularly those of respiration, circulation, digestion and elimination. Considerable clinical evidence has been presented to substantiate this belief, but experimental evidence is scarce.[6, 15, 19]

In this regard, Hellebrandt commented that the concept of the harmful effect of poor posture on visceral function was "based on more or less tenuous evidence without regard for the wide margin of safety under which all organ systems function and the paucity of proof that the anatomical position of a viscus is a valid criterion of the adequacy of its physiologic behavior."[15] And Karpovich has remarked, ". . . .except for the fact that lordosis may be associated with orthostatic albuminuria, there is no scientific proof that improvement of slight irregularities in posture leads to definite improvements in the physiologic functions of the body."[19] There is, however, some evidence of a relationship between menstrual function and posture. Hoffman studied the findings of the routine orthopedic examination for two groups of college women, one group known as the "dysmenorrhea group," the other as the "no-pain group." The two groups were found to differ significantly with respect to two postural traits, namely anteroposterior pelvic tilt and bilateral hip asymmetry.[17]

Fox also studied the relation of certain aspects of posture to dysmenorrhea.[8] She investigated the incidence of dysmenorrhea in three groups of young women, one a control group, one a group characterized by sway back (posterior list of the trunk), and one group characterized by faulty pelvic tilt (increased inclination). She found that dysmenorrhea occurred with greater severity among the sway back group than among the control group. Unlike Hoffman, however, she did not find a significant relationship between pelvic tilt and dysmenorrhea.

Principles Related to Strength and Flexibility. That strength and flexibility are factors in posture would seem to be a universally accepted thesis, judging by the preponderance of strength and flexibility exercises included in the majority of corrective programs, also by the strength and flexibility measurements included in posture tests. Interest has been shown particularly in the strength of the abdominals, scapular adductors and thoracic spinal extensors, and in the flexibility of the pectorals and the hamstrings. There seems to have been little scientific investigation of the relation of these strengths and flexibilities to posture. It would seem that the widespread assumption of such a relationship may have been responsible for the attitude that there was no need for such investigation. Yet nowhere in the literature can the author find a clear statement as to what constitutes optimal strength or optimal flexibility for the maintenance of good posture. Possibly it is a matter of balance between opposing muscle groups, rather than of strength or flexibility *per se*, or it may be a matter of relative muscle length. These aspects would seem to bear investigation.

In comparing the abdominal strength of a control group with that of two faulty posture groups — one characterized by sway back and the other by faulty pelvic tilt — Fox did not find that abdominal strength was a differentiating factor. She recommended that further study be made of this problem, especially as her sway back group was much smaller than the others.[8]

Principles Related to Psychological Aspects of Posture. There are several psychological aspects of postural problems with which the instructor should be prepared to deal. For instance, not all posture problems can be explained in terms of physical causes, either musculoskeletal or environmental. Atypical postures may be symptoms of personality problems or emotional disturbances. The hanging head and drooping shoulders of some adolescent girls are often not physical in origin but are symptoms of their shyness and lack of self-confidence. Postural exercises will do little to help such girls unless they are used in conjunction with psychological help. The same is true of the small man whose bantam-cock posture is merely an overcompensation for his feelings of inferiority. Proficiency in some sport in which physical size is not important (e.g., swimming or diving) might be much more effective for correcting his lordosis than hours of posture exercises in the corrective gym.

One pernicious psychological cause of undesirable posture among girls is the example set by dress models. This influence on certain girls is more difficult to combat than almost any other cause of poor posture.

Another type of psychological problem is demonstrated by the emotional reaction of an overly sensitive individual to a conspicuously abnormal posture. As is true of other physical handicaps, it may interfere with the individual's personal and social development unless he learns to see it in its right perspective. The abnormal posture may be impossible to correct, in which case the problem is to achieve as much improvement as possible and then to discover ways of standing, sitting and walking that will minimize the conspicuousness of what cannot be corrected. As in the case of the undersized man, proficiency in some sport can be effective in providing a healthy type of compensation. The instructor's role here is to offer suggestions and to present opportunities. He should be matter-of-fact and should avoid over-persistence.

In the types of problems described above, the chief principles to follow are (1) to learn as much as possible about the psychology of behavior and adjustment and (2) when feasible, to work with or at least to seek the advice of a psychiatrist or psychologist who is treating the student in question.

An important role of psychology in posture education is that of motivation. No matter how well the teacher or the therapist has selected the exercises, and no matter how conscientiously the student or the patient practices them, they will have little effect in improving the individual's habitual postural patterns unless he is motivated to *want* to improve them.

And finally, psychology is used as a technique of treatment by those who like the method of using mental concepts to change neuromuscular pathways (see p. 371). For success in this method they depend completely upon the cooperation of the individual in mental participation, for it is by this means that the changes in the neuromuscular pathways are effected.

SUMMARY

A summary of this chapter emphasizes the dearth of actual objective support for specific principles relating to posture. The following areas appear to be the only ones for which there is such support:

1. Postural reflex action
2. Stability of the erect standing position as evidenced by the relationship of the line of gravity to the base of support
3. The influence of heredity and environment on posture
4. The relationship between certain postural faults and two manifestations of faulty organic function, namely orthostatic albuminuria and dysmenorrhea.

Since so much emphasis is placed on posture, it is indeed unfortunate that there is so little objective evidence that our efforts are being made in the right direction. The author is inclined to be sympathetic toward Miller's conclusions:

. . . although orthopedists and physical educators have been working actively for the past fifty years with the problems involved in posture, there is still a seemingly unwarranted lack of agreement among practitioners of both fields. Three basic differences of opinion are implicated in this bewildering lack of unanimity: (1) whether any particular posture is more advantageous physiologically than any other posture; (2) whether prescribed physical activity can actually modify posture; and (3) whether it is possible to agree upon a definition of "good" posture and upon a method of accurately measuring such a concept. Eminent authorities in both physical education and medical circles can be found to support either side of any of these questions.[23]

In view of this lack of evidence and these differences of opinion, what stand shall the kinesiologist take in regard to posture? Shall he ignore it, or shall he formulate tentative principles to guide him in posture education and correction, and shall he adhere to these until they are definitely disproved and indications for other principles have become apparent? The author believes that, either consciously or unconsciously, the physical educator is bound to be guided by *some* principles of posture, whether they are founded on fact or conjecture. In view of the difficulty of devising an accurate measure of habitual posture the formulation of some guiding principles, based on the best knowledge available, incomplete though it may be, would seem to be justifiable, even imperative, if we are to continue to teach body mechanics in our schools and clinics. In full recognition of their limitations, and knowing that they may be superseded as new evidence is revealed by further research or by clinical evidence, the following postural principles are suggested:

1. The weight-bearing segments of the body are so aligned in good standing posture that the line of gravity passes through these segments within certain "normal" limits, yet to be defined. Such a definition should either be applicable to all physiques, or else indicate to what types of physique it is, or is not, applicable.

2. Inasmuch as Hellebrandt found that in every individual she had observed, the average location of the center of gravity was close to the geometric center of the supporting base, it would seem that the relation of the line of gravity to the base of support is not indicative of body alignment and therefore does not serve as a measure of posture.

3. Good standing posture is a position of extension of the weight-bearing joints. This should be an easy extension and should not be accompanied by strain or tension.

4. From the point of view of energy expenditure, good posture would seem to be a position which requires a minimum expenditure of energy *for the maintenance of good alignment.* Excess energy expenditure indicates hypertonicity or poor neuromuscular coordination, or both. A posture requiring an absolute minimal energy expenditure does not fulfill the requirements of good posture because it is characterized by "hanging on the ligaments," that is, a dependence upon the ligaments of the weight-bearing joints, rather than upon muscle tonus, for resisting the downward pull of gravity.

5. Good posture, in repose and in activity, permits mechanically efficient function of the joints. In other words, friction in the joints is minimized, tensions of opposing ligaments are balanced and pressures within the joints are equalized. Hence the skeletal structure is architecturally and mechanically sound and there is a minimum of wear and tear on the joints.

6. Good posture, both static and dynamic, requires normal muscle tonus. This implies adequate development of the antigravity muscles to resist the pull of gravity successfully and to maintain good alignment without excessive effort or tension. It also implies a balance between antagonistic muscle groups. There is no indication, however, that "the stronger the muscles the better the posture."

7. Good posture, both static and dynamic, requires sufficient flexibility in the structures of the weight-bearing joints to permit good alignment without interference or strain. Poor flexibility may be caused by tight ligaments or fasciae, by short muscles or by hypertrophied muscles. The flexibility should not be so great, however, that excessive muscular effort is needed to keep the weight-bearing joints in alignment.

8. Good posture requires good coordination. This implies good neuromuscular control and well developed postural reflexes.

9. Adjustments in posture can be made more readily by individuals who have a good kinesthetic awareness of the postures they assume and of the degree of tension in their muscles.

10. Good posture, both static and dynamic, is favorable, or at least not detrimental, to organic function.

11. A relationship exists between habitual posture and personality, also between habitual posture and emotional states.

12. In view of the great variety of human physiques and individual differences in structure, due either to heredity or to early environmental influence, there can be no single detailed description of good posture.

13. In the last analysis, both the static and the dynamic posture of any individual should be judged on the basis of how well it meets the demands made upon it throughout his lifetime.

DEMONSTRATIONS AND LABORATORY EXERCISES

1. To demonstrate the alignment of the body segments take from five to seven large wooden blocks, each having a vertical line painted in the center of one side. A layer of thick felt should be glued to the top and bottom of each block and a small hook screwed into each of two opposite sides.

   a. Arrange the blocks in a straight column with the painted lines in front. Connect the hooks on the sides with elastic bands. The elastic "ligaments" will be under equal tension and the felt "cartilages" under equal pressure when the column is in perfect alignment.

   b. Now insert wedges between the blocks in such a way that every other block tips to the left and the alternate blocks tip to the right. The elastic "ligaments" will now be under unequal tension and the felt "cartilages" under unequal pressure. The zigzag alignment of the painted lines illustrates graphically the poor alignment of the segments.

2. To demonstrate good and poor alignment of a single weight-bearing joint, such as the knee, two blocks arranged like those described above may be used in a similar manner.

3. Demonstration and practice of the postural reflexes described by Haynes:[13]

   a. Lying face down, contract the gluteal muscles by pinching the buttocks together. Note the involuntary extension of the spine, knees and ankles, the supination of the feet and the increased tension in the abdominal muscles.

b. Lying face down, raise one leg slightly and extend it completely. Note the increased tension in the extensor muscles of the other leg.

4. Using the method described in Chapter 1 (pp. 16 ff.), take anteroposterior line of gravity photographs of several subjects representing various postures. After drawing the line of gravity on each photograph observe them carefully and note the relation of the line to the head, shoulders, upper trunk, lower trunk, pelvis, knees and ankles.

5. Take ten anteroposterior line of gravity photographs of one subject within a period of one week. Compare these.

6. Take anteroposterior line of gravity photographs of several subjects representing different physique types. Can you make any generalizations about the relation of physique to posture?

7. Do an original posture study using a small number of subjects.

REFERENCES

1. Basmajian, J. V.: Muscles Alive, 2nd ed., Baltimore, The Williams & Wilkins Company, 1967.
2. Bowen, W. P., and Stone, H. A.: Applied Anatomy and Kinesiology, 7th ed. Philadelphia, Lea & Febiger, 1953.
3. Brunnstrom, S.: Clinical Kinesiology, 2nd ed. Philadelphia, F. A. Davis Company, 1966.
4. Campbell, D. G.: Posture: A gesture toward life. Physiother. Rev., *15*:43–47, 1935.
5. Cowell, C. C.: Bodily posture as a mental attitude. J. Health & Phys. Ed., *1*:14–15, 56, 1930.
6. Deaver, G. G.: Posture and its relation to mental and physical health. Res. Quart. Am. Assn. Health, & Phys. Ed., *4*:221–228, 1933.
7. Evans, F. G., (Ed.): Biomechanical Studies of the Musculo-Skeletal System. Springfield, Ill., Charles C Thomas, Publisher, 1961.
8. Fox, M. G.: The relationship of abdominal strength to selected posture faults. Res. Quart. Am. Assn. Health, Phys. Ed. & Recrn., *22*:141–144, 1951.
9. Frost, L. H.: Individual structural differences in the orthopedic examination. J. Health & Phys. Ed., *9*:90–93, 122, 1938.
10. Goldthwait, J. E., Brown, L. T., Swaim, L. T., and Kuhns, J. G.: Essentials of Body Mechanics in Health and Disease, 5th ed. Philadelphia, J. B. Lippincott Company, 1952.
11. Haller, J. S., and Gurewitsch, A. D.: An approach to dynamic posture based on primitive motion patterns. Arch. Phys. Med., *31*:632–640, 1950.
12. Hawley, G.: Kinesiology of Corrective Exercise, 2nd ed. Philadelphia, Lea & Febiger, 1949.
13. Haynes, R. S.: Postural reflexes in relation to the correction of improper body position. Am. J. Dis. Child., *36*:1095–1107, 1928.
14. Hellebrandt, F. A.: Physiology and the physical educator. Res. Quart. Am. Assn. Health, Phys. Ed. & Recrn., *11*:12–29, 1940.
15. Hellebrandt, F. A.: Postural adjustments in convalescence and rehabilitation. Fed. Proc., *3*:243–246, 1944.
16. Hellebrandt, F. A., and Franseen, E. B.: Physiological study of the vertical stance of man. Physiol. Rev., *23*:220–255, 1943.
17. Hoffman, E.: Certain Physical and Physiological Characteristics as Related to the

Incidence of Severe Dysmenorrhea. Unpublished M.S. thesis. Wellesley College, 1942.

18. Joseph, J.: Man's Posture; Electromyographic Studies. Springfield, Ill., Charles C Thomas, Publisher, 1960.
19. Karpovich, P. V.: Physiology of Muscular Activity, 4th ed. Philadelphia, W. B. Saunders Company, 1953, p. 279.
20. Kelly, E. D.: Adapted and Corrective Physical Education, 4th ed. New York, Ronald Press Company, 1965.
21. McCormick, H. G.: The Metabolic Cost of Maintaining a Standing Position, with Special Reference to Body Alignment. New York, King's Crown Press, 1942.
22. Mensendieck, B.: Mensendieck System of Functional Exercises. Portland, Me., Southworth-Anthoensen Press, 1937.
23. Miller, K. D.: A physical educator looks at posture. J. Sch. Health, *21*:89–94, 1951.
24. Morton, D. J.: Human Locomotion and Body Form. Baltimore, The Williams & Wilkins Company, 1952.
25. Rathbone, J. L., and Hunt, V. V.: Corrective Physical Education, 7th ed. Philadelphia, W. B. Saunders Company, 1965.
26. Steindler, A.: Kinesiology of the Human Body. Springfield, Ill., Charles C Thomas, Publisher, 1955, Lecture XIV.
27. Sweigard, L. E.: Body mechanics and posture in modern life. Symposium on Posture, printed by Phi Delta Pi, 1938.
28. Todd, M. E.: The Thinking Body. Boston, Charles T. Branford Company, 1949.

RECOMMENDED READINGS

Kendall, H. O., and Kendall, F. P.: Developing and maintaining good posture. J. Am. Phys. Ther. Assn., *48*:319–336, 1968.
Metheny, E. R.: Body Dynamics. McGraw-Hill, Inc., 1952, Chap. 7.
Wells, K. F.: What we don't know about posture. J. Health, Phys. Ed. & Recrn., *29*: 31–32, 1958.

CHAPTER 21

Exercises for Physical Fitness, Conditioning and Posture Improvement

A complete physical fitness program goes far beyond the performance of special exercises. It embraces all aspects of physical fitness — adequate endurance, strength, flexibility, agility, balance, coordination, and the habit of practicing efficient body mechanics in all physical activities, work skills and sport skills alike. Exercises, nevertheless, do play an important part in many of these objectives, the chief exception probably being the development of cardiovascular endurance. For this purpose it has been fairly well established that a program of aerobics is more effective than exercises, as such.[2]

The role of exercises in the total program of physical fitness would appear to be (1) developing specific strengths and flexibilities, (2) improving posture in general and correcting specific faults, and (3) building habits of good body mechanics. Group exercises are beneficial for all of these purposes but individually prescribed ones are by far the most effective. It is in this area that kinesiology makes its greatest contribution. Initial physical examinations and motor skill tests will reveal the strengths and weaknesses of the students, as well as the postural and health conditions that need correction. A thorough kinesiologic background enables the instructor to know what conditions can be helped by exercises and to select the exercises best fitted to the individual's needs. It also enables him to recognize the kinesiologic requirements of certain sport skills and dance techniques and to select the exercises best suited to preparing the students for these.

The general category of exercises which are used for these purposes is the one known by the old-fashioned and not-so-popular term, "calisthenics." In actuality, this term represents the goals of physical fitness surprisingly well, for in Webster's New Collegiate Dictionary we find it defined as, "the science of bodily exercise without apparatus, or with light hand apparatus, to promote strength and gracefulness." The Greek origins of the word are indeed apropos — kallos, meaning beauty, and sthenos, meaning strength. A balance between the two is an appropriate expression of the objectives of physical fitness, conditioning and good posture.

386

Flexibility. From the kinesiologic point of view there are three main factors to consider regarding the flexibility of any region, namely (1) the normal range of motion, (2) the causes of restricted motion, and (3) methods of increasing motion. Methods of measuring individual joint motion will not be discussed here. For this, the reader is referred to Chapter 2 and to the recommended readings at the end of that chapter. A physical educator should not attempt to diagnose the cause of exaggerated restrictions of motion, nor should he attempt to increase flexibility in such cases if there is the slightest suspicion of pathology. Unless prescribed or approved by a physician, flexibility exercises should be taught only to young adults or children who are considered to have slight or moderate degrees of restriction.

The various kinesiologic forces which can be used to increase flexibility should be taken into consideration. The ones commonly employed are: (1) the force of gravity, (2) momentum (the force of motion) and (3) the force provided either by another person or by some part of one's own body, e.g., a pushing or pulling force, either self-administered or applied by another person, either manually or through the use of special equipment.

The use of gravity as a force for stretching the pectoral muscles and anterior shoulder ligaments can easily be graded from mild to relatively severe. Merely lying on the back with the hands behind the neck and with a narrow pillow placed crosswise under the midthoracic region of the back, provides a mild stretch; lying on a narrow plinth with the arms extended obliquely sideward, somewhat above shoulder level, with a five pound dumbbell in each hand, gives a relatively strong stretch. In the latter type of exercise the instructor needs to be aware of the possibility that the return movement from the position of stretch may encourage further shortening of the tight muscles. For instance, if the subject raises his arms vertically before returning them to the bent arm position at his sides, he would be contracting his pectoral muscles and this would defeat the primary purpose of the exercise. It takes an alert instructor, thoroughly conversant with muscular actions, to prevent the subject from working at cross purposes in this way.

Another example of using gravity as a stretching force is passive hanging from a horizontal bar; still another is standing facing an open doorway with the arms extended obliquely upward, the palms against the door frame and the entire body inclined forward from the ankles. Momentum is the force used in the Danish type of flexibility exercises, such as double arm flinging, sideward, upward and somewhat backward in a vigorous ballistic movement repeated rhythmically. There has been some criticism of this method of increasing flexibility because of the supposed danger of stimulating the stretch reflex and causing contraction of the muscles that were being stretched, thus defeating the purpose of the exercise. The author's experience with the Niels Bukh Danish exercises has not borne this out. Furthermore, as Holland has indicated, there are (or were in 1967) insufficient data for comparing the efficacy of ballistic and static methods of increasing joint mobility.[10]

A good example of stretching by using the force of another person is seen in the passive chest lifting exercise, described on page 401. A Danish hamstring-stretching exercise is an example of the subject using his own force for stretching. In this exercise he lies on his back with one knee bent to the chest. He grasps his instep with the opposite hand and, maintaining this hold, pushes his other hand against his knee in an attempt to straighten his leg forcibly in a vertically upward direction.

An important factor in some manual stretching exercises is the leverage employed. In the passive chest lifting exercise, for instance, the operator can conserve his own strength and give a more forceful stretch by grasping the subject's elbows rather than his upper arms. The force arm of the lever is then the entire length of the subject's upper arm, instead of only part of it.

Whatever the method of stretching used, the instructor needs to be thoroughly familiar with the structure and function of the joint in question. He must know not only the degree of limitation of motion, but also what tissues are responsible for the limitation. He should also know under what conditions the stretch reflex is likely to defeat his purposes. In the analysis of the passive chest lifting exercise it is shown how, by having the subject cooperate actively in the movement and by the operator's taking care to pull the elbows back gradually, reflex contraction of the pectorals may be prevented.

Strength. Strength is increased by observing the overload principle. This means exercising against maximal, or near maximal, resistance. Progressive resistance exercise, advocated in the early fifties by DeLorme and others, is based on the use of progressively increasing resistances.[4] This method has been used extensively in both therapy and conditioning programs. The resistance is usually provided by weights, or combinations of weights and pulleys as in the specially designed DeLorme table, or frequently by more modest home-made equipment; however, progressive resistance can also be given manually. Physical therapists who have used the latter method have noticed — sometimes to their pleasure, but more often to their dismay — the increased strength and bulk of their own muscles.

In the same decade when progressive resistance exercise was so widely publicized, the use of isometric exercise for rapid strengthening of muscles was introduced by a German physiologist.[17] The exaggerated popularity of this technique is well known to physical educators. Because of the misleading publicity it received in newspapers and popular magazines, the public tends to have a distorted interpretation of its value, as well as a total lack of appreciation of its potential harmfulness. For the definitions of isometric and isotonic exercise, the reader should turn back to page 39. One common misconception of the value of isometric exercise is that it is an effective method for building physical fitness, whereas its *only* function is increasing muscular strength. It does not increase cardiovascular endurance or flexibility, nor does it contribute to any objectives of physical fitness other than those related to strength. It should be mentioned, however, that there is some slight evidence, not yet corroborated, that isometric exercises are effective in weight reduction and in reduction of waistline girth measurements.[16]

Inasmuch as the extreme effort exerted in isometric exercises causes considerable internal pressure, especially if the breath is held, it is not wise for persons out of condition, such as the middle aged or the elderly, to engage in them. The strain might be injurious to anyone with a cardiovascular impairment, or with a weakness in the abdominal wall. For persons in good health and good cardiovascular condition, isometric exercises, when given under proper supervision, have proved to be an effective and relatively quick method of increasing muscular strength. They appear to be particularly useful for strengthening muscle groups that have been weakened as the result of injuries to joints. A comparative study of isometric and isotonic exercises for strengthening the quadriceps muscles is summarized in the Supplementary Material at the end of this chapter. A similar study showed that a positive relationship existed between the two methods when used for strengthening the elbow flexor muscles and that the absolute values of a test of isometric strength were significantly higher than those of a test of isotonic strength.[1]

Still another exercise system has been receiving attention in the past few years, especially in the field of physical therapy. This is known as isokinetic exercise and is characterized by holding the speed of the movement of the body segment to constant rates and at the same time permitting maximum force to be exerted throughout the range of motion.[9, 15] Thus it appears to embrace the best features of isometric and isotonic exercises as it increases muscular torque throughout the range of motion and, in addition, increases the work performance of a muscle more rapidly than either isometric or isotonic exercises (using pulleys). Its drawback, for widespread use, is that it requires special equipment which can be used for only one muscle group at a time. For physical therapy treatments, however, and for research purposes it appears to be unsurpassed.

EXERCISES FOR PHYSICAL FITNESS

The exercises selected for kinesiologic analysis are the push-up, the pull-up and the partial curl-up—all strengthening exercises. For each of these, following the analysis of the basic exercise, a progressive sequence of similar exercises is suggested. It should be noted that there are two methods of increasing the difficulty of an exercise for developing strength, namely, (1) increasing the magnitude of the resistance, and (2) increasing the length of the resistance arm of the anatomic lever. The reader should note which method is used for each exercise in the three progressive sequences. In some instances both methods are used.

THE PUSH-UP

Starting Position. The front-leaning-rest position, i.e., semi-prone with the body extended, the arms extended vertically toward the floor, and the weight supported by the hands and toes. The body is in a straight line from head to heels; there is no sag at the spine nor hump at the hips. The hands are approximately shoulder width apart with the palms flat on the floor.

Movement. With the body kept straight, the elbows are allowed to bend, and the body is lowered until the chest almost touches the floor. By pushing the hands vigorously against the floor, the body is raised until it is in the starting position. This movement is repeated slowly or rapidly, either a given number of times or as many times as the subject is able to repeat it *in correct form.*

Essential Joint and Muscle Analysis

THE DIP. (Fig. 21–1, *B*.)   Flexion at the elbow joints accompanied by a lowering of the body until it almost touches the floor.

Shoulder joints

  Horizontal extension: Pectoralis major, anterior deltoid, coracobrachialis and subscapularis in eccentric contraction

Shoulder girdle

  Adduction: Pectoralis minor and serratus anterior in eccentric contraction

Elbows

  Flexion: Triceps and anconeus in eccentric contraction

Wrists

  Reduction of hyperextension: Extensor carpi radialis longus and brevis and extensor carpi ulnaris in eccentric contraction

Maintenance of straight alignment from head to heels against the pull of gravity

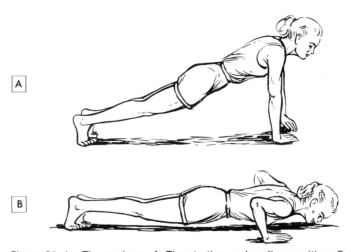

Figure 21–1.   The push-up. *A,* The starting and ending position; *B,* the dip.

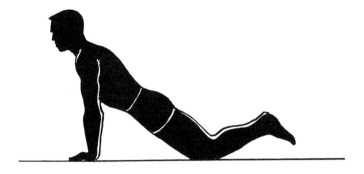

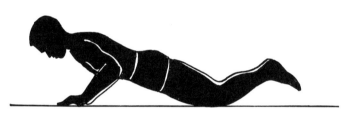

Figure 21–2. Push-up series for arm strength: Exercise 2, half dip and push-up from knees.

Head and Neck: Cervical extensors in static contraction

Lumbar spine: Rectus abdominis and external and internal obliques in static contraction

Hips: Flexors in static contraction

THE PUSH-UP. Extension at the elbow joints until the body is again in the position shown in Figure 21–1, A.

Shoulder joints

Horizontal flexion: Pectoralis major, anterior deltoid, coraco-brachialis and subscapularis

Shoulder girdle

Abduction: Serratus anterior and pectoralis minor

Elbows

Extension: Triceps and anconeus

Wrists

Hyperextension: Extensor carpi radialis longus and brevis and extensor carpi ulnaris

Maintenance of straight alignment from head to heels: Same as above

Progressive Sequence. In the case of the push-up, the familiar exercise represents the most difficult level in the series. Starting at what might be considered the lowest level and working up, the following push-up exercises are suggested.

1. Standing on hands and knees with hip and knee joints bent at right angles, dip and push up.

2. In semi-prone position with hips straight and weight supported by hands and knees, perform a half dip and push-up (Fig. 21–2).

3. Same position as for 2, but complete the full dip and push-up.

4. Front-leaning-rest position, facing stairs with feet on floor and hands on fourth or fifth step, body in a straight line from head to heels, dip and push up (Fig. 21–3).

5. Continue, placing hands on lower step until able to perform regulation push-up from floor (Fig. 21–4).

Discussion.   Before a student is ready to try a full push-up in any of the elementary or intermediate positions, he may practice a reverse push-up (a slow full or half dip) or a half push-up, i.e., a push-up from a half dip position. An easy return from a reverse push-up may be achieved by first bringing one or both feet forward and perhaps assuming a kneeling position on one knee. Whatever type of push-up is practiced, the student should repeat it several times in good form before being permitted to try the more advanced type.

There are two common faults that must be guarded against in the

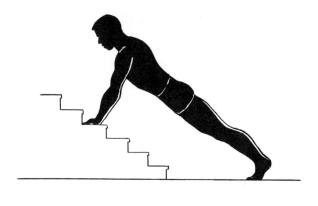

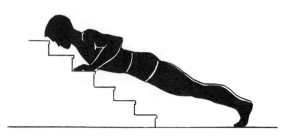

Figure 21–3. Push-up series for arm strength: Exercise 4, push-up from stairs with hands on fourth step.

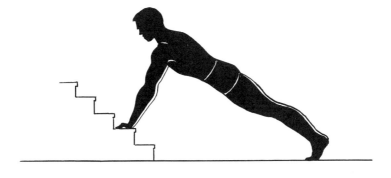

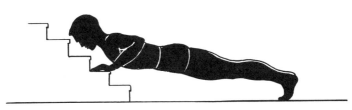

Figure 21–4. Push-up series for arm strength: Exercise 5, push-up from stairs with hands on second step.

push-up. These are (1) a sagging back and (2) humped-up hips. The latter fault is usually caused by an "overcorrection" of the first one, namely maintaining a flexed position at the hips in order to prevent the back from sagging. The correction of both of these faults lies in strengthening the abdominal muscles and training them to prevent hyperextension of the lumbar spine when the body is in the extended position. Until the subject is kinesthetically aware of his position, the use of a mirror may be helpful.

The progressive lowering of the position of the hands in the staircase series of push-ups increases the strength requirement because the upper extremities are called upon to bear an increasingly larger proportion of the body weight. This can be demonstrated by placing a bathroom scales under each hand. The push-up from a half dip is easier than the push-up from a full dip in any given position because the weight of the body is lifted through a shorter distance, and also because the joint positions permit the muscles of the elbows and shoulders to work to better advantage. The reverse dip is easier to execute than the push-up, from any given level, because the muscles are performing negative rather than positive work, that is, they are engaging in eccentric (lengthening) rather than concentric (shortening) contraction.

THE PULL-UP

Starting Position. Straight arm hanging from a horizontal bar with the hands approximately shoulder width apart, the palms facing the body, and the thumb in opposition to the fingers (Fig. 21–5, *C*).

Movement. From a "dead hang" and with a minimum of movement of the trunk and lower extremities, the subject pulls himself steadily upward until his chin is level with the bar.

Joint and Muscle Analysis

Shoulder joints

    Extension: Pectoralis major (sternal portion), latissimus dorsi, teres major, posterior deltoid

Shoulder girdle

    Downward rotation combined with some adduction toward end: Rhomboids, trapezius III and IV, probably pectoralis minor

Elbows

    Flexion: Biceps, brachialis, brachioradialis

Radioulnar

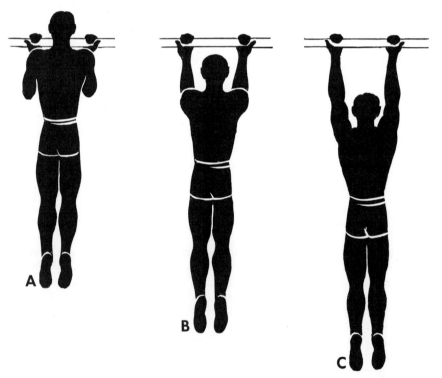

Figure 21–5. Pull-up series for arm strength. Exercise 1, reverse pull-up: *A,* bent arm hanging; *B,* half way position; *C,* straight arm hanging. (For pull-up, start with *C* and end with *A.*)

Maintained in supination by fixed position of hands.

Wrists

Possibly slight flexion. Muscles probably stabilize wrist for action of finger and thumb muscles.

Fingers and Thumb

Flexion: Static contraction of all flexors

Thumb adduction of carpometacarpal joint: Static contraction of adductor pollicis

Return movement: Reverse joint action of shoulder joints and girdle and elbows. Same muscles but contracting eccentrically instead of concentrically. Finger and thumb muscles remain in static contraction.

Progressive Sequence

EASIER PULL-UPS

1. Reverse pull-up, that is, slow let-down from bent arm hanging position which can be reached by stepping up or jumping (Fig. 21–5).

2. Modified pull-up from low boom or bar with body in semi-supine hanging position, arms straight, heels on floor, and body straight from heels to head.

3. Standing on bench high enough to permit subject to grasp bar (or rings) with elbows partially flexed, pull up the rest of the way.

MORE DIFFICULT PULL-UPS

Basic pull-up with weights attached to waist or ankles.

Discussion. Pull-ups are frequently taught with the forearms in pronated position, that is, with the palms facing away from the face. From the kinesiologist's point of view there is no justification for this as it is the least favorable position for both the biceps and the sternal portion of the pectoralis major muscles. The only justification appears to be the military one of developing the ability to climb over high walls. (See discussion in Supplementary Material at end of Chapter 13.)

THE PARTIAL CURL-UP

Starting Position. Supine lying position with hands resting on front of thighs, elbows straight.

MOVEMENT. The subject pulls in the chin and lifts the head and shoulders until the shoulder blades are clear of the floor. He holds the position for at least six seconds. (See Figs. 21–6 and 21–7, A.)

Essential Joint and Muscle Analysis

Head and cervical spine

Flexion: Sternocleidomastoid, prevertebral muscles

Thoracic spine (possibly some lumbar involvement)

Flexion: Rectus abdominis; external oblique; internal oblique (upper fibers)

Hip joints

Stabilization: Iliopsoas and probably other hip flexors

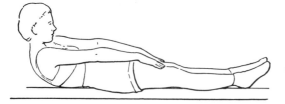

Figure 21–6. The partial
curl-up.

Progressive Sequence
EASIER CURL-UPS

1. Hands clasped low in front of body. Assistant holds legs down
with one hand or forearm and with other helps pull subject to partial
curl-up position.

2. Same as basic partial curl-up but with feet supported.

3. Feet unsupported, subject's arms and hands on floor at sides
of body. Subject gives slight push from elbows and hands to reach
position, then with palms on thighs, holds position for one to three
seconds.

4. Reverse curl-up from long sitting position. Start by flexing
lumbar spine and slowly assume lying position on back with lumbar
region touching floor before thoracic region. Hands may be in any
of the positions suggested for the partial curl-up.

MORE DIFFICULT PARTIAL CURL-UPS (feet unsupported)

1. Fingertips on shoulders and elbows reaching forward.
2. Holding 3 lb. weight against chest.
3. Hands clasped on top of head.
4. Holding 5 lb. weight against chest.
5. Holding 7 lb. weight against chest.
6. Holding 5 lb. weight on top of head.
7. Holding 10 lb. weight against chest.
8. Holding 7 lb. weight on top of head.
9. Holding 10 lb. weight on top of head.

Discussion. The most common fault in the curl-up (also found in
the sit-up) is coming up or at least starting too quickly, using momentum rather than gradual muscular contraction. This nullifies the value
of the exercise. Beginners are sometimes tempted to push off with the
elbows, but this can be prevented if care is taken to see that the arms
are in the correct position.

A fault which is common in the sit-up, but less so in the curl-up, is
arching the lower back (hyperextending the lumbar spine) at the
beginning of the movement. Strong retraction of the abdomen before
and during the lifting of the head will help to prevent this fault. If
this is ineffective, easier forms of the exercise are indicated.

In the initial stage of the curl-up (also of the sit-up if the head is
lifted first) the rectus abdominis and external oblique muscles are
acting as movers to flex the spine; the iliopsoas and other hip flexors
act as stabilizers to fix the pelvis against the pull of the abdominal

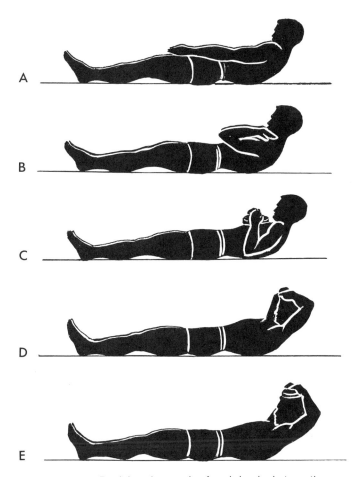

Figure 21–7. Partial curl-up series for abdominal strength.

muscles. In the last half or two-thirds of a full sit-up or curl-up the hip flexors are acting as movers to flex the trunk as a whole on the thighs. If no further spinal flexion occurs, the abdominal muscles serve as stabilizers to fix the pelvis against the pull of the hip flexors.

ABDOMINAL EXERCISES

Interesting electromyographic studies of various forms of abdominal sit-up and curl-up exercises were made during the 1955–1965 decade. Although they cannot be compared item for item because of lack of uniformity in the methods of performing the exercise and because of different points of emphasis, the following conclusions, culled from their findings, appear to be justified.

1. Sit-ups and curl-ups elicit stronger abdominal than iliopsoas action:

a. When the feet are not held down;

b. When the legs are either straight, or flexed at the knees to an angle not smaller than 110 degrees;

c. During the first 30 to 45 degrees of motion, especially if the legs are straight.

2. The lower rectus abdominis is more active than the upper when the feet are supported, and the upper rectus more active when the feet are not supported.

3. The greatest abdominal action occurs during the first 45 degrees of trunk movement. (LaBan et al. found no iliopsoas action during the first 30 degrees of trunk movement when the legs were straight.[13] Flint found the iliopsoas to be unaffected by extension or flexion of the knees.[5]

4. The sit-up requires more total muscular effort than the curl-up (because the curl-up shortens the lever arm),[3] but the initial stage of the curl-up, until the shoulder-blades are off the floor, is more effective for strengthening the abdominal muscles (especially if the position is held for several seconds) than the complete sit-up or curl-up movement. When the position is held the exercise is isometric in nature.

One important aspect of abdominal exercises which, to the best of the author's knowledge, has not been investigated electromyographically, is the tendency to arch (i.e., hyperextend) the lumbar spine in exercises performed from the supine lying position. When this occurs, as it frequently does in sit-ups, trunk curls and slow leg raising and lowering, it indicates that the abdominal muscles do not have enough strength to prevent the hip flexors from increasing the pelvic tilt. This weakness reveals the need for a milder abdominal exercise. As Kendall has warned, this kind of exercise may cause harmful strain; it may even cause a hernia.[12]

It is for this reason that double leg raising and slow leg lowering from the supine position are not recommended as abdominal strengthening exercises. Only those who already have strong abdominal muscles are able to do them without hyperextending the lumbar spine (Fig. 21–8).

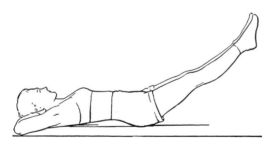

Figure 21–8. Slow leg lowering. Note the increased curve of the lumbar spine.

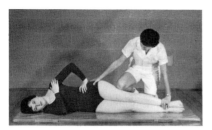 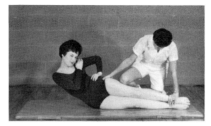

Figure 21–9. Lying on side with feet supported, trunk lifting sideward. (From Wells, K. F.: Posture Exercise Handbook – A Progressive Sequence Approach. Copyright © 1963, The Ronald Press Company, New York.)

Recommended Abdominal Exercises. The following exercises have been suggested by various investigators as effective ones for strengthening the abdominal muscles.[3, 5, 6, 7, 18]

1. Partial curl position (supine lying or hook lying with knees at 110 degree angle) held for two to three seconds.

2. Curl-up with a twist (touching hand to outer surface of opposite knee).

3. Basket hang (double knee bending to chest from hanging position).

4. Side lying with legs supported, trunk lifting sideward (Fig. 21–9).

5. Kneeling with hips and spine extended, i.e., with trunk and thighs vertical, leaning backward to a 60–45 degree angle.

6. The "V" sit-up (from hook lying, trunk raising and double leg extending upward at same time).

Principles for Selecting Abdominal Exercises

1. The criterion for an abdominal exercise performed in the supine position is the performer's ability to prevent the tilting of the pelvis and the hyperextension of the lumbar spine. If the pelvic tilt and lumbar curve increase, it would seem to indicate the failure of the abdominal muscles to stabilize the pelvis and spine against the pull of the iliopsoas. Since the task is too great for them, there is danger of straining them.

2. An objective in building a strong abdominal wall is to strengthen all four of the abdominal muscles: rectus abdominis, external oblique, internal oblique and transversus abdominis. To do this successfully requires a knowledge of the exercises in which these muscles participate and of the relative intensity of their action.

3. It seems reasonable to assume that a protruding abdomen indicates that the abdominal muscles have been stretched. It would seem to be a function of abdominal exercises, therefore, to shorten as well as to strengthen these muscles. This suggests that exercises like back bends that put the abdominal wall in a stretched position are not a desirable method for strengthening them.

CONDITIONING EXERCISES

For general purposes, conditioning exercises are the same as physical fitness exercises. They tend to be called conditioning exercises when they are used as preparation for particular sports or for specific purposes such as (1) increasing plantar flexion of the ankle for modern or ballet dance techniques or for the flutter kick in swimming, (2) strengthening the knee and hip extensor muscles for skiing, or (3) strengthening the wrist muscles for racket games. Conditioning exercises for swimming, dancing, skiing, and similar activities are best found in books for those particular activities as they are written by specialists in those areas.

EXERCISES FOR POSTURE IMPROVEMENT

The problem of posture improvement and correction is such an individual one that exercises for this purpose should be selected on an individual basis if at all possible. This presupposes a postural examination or inspection for analyzing the student's present posture and identifying his particular needs.

The following section represents one small sample from the field of posture improvement. Its purpose is merely to demonstrate how kinesiology may be applied to the corrective uses of exercises. No attempt is made to demonstrate its application to all the problems associated with the corrective aspects of posture education. These are far too extensive and complex to be discussed adequately in a general kinesiology text. The appropriate sources for such information are textbooks in corrective physical education. Furthermore, in addition to anatomic and mechanical principles, there are physiologic, psychologic and pedagogic principles of posture correction of equal importance but not ordinarily covered in kinesiology texts.

In order to illustrate the application of kinesiology to posture problems, one common fault and two exercises for its correction have been selected for analysis. The postural fault is the condition commonly referred to as "round shoulders." It includes a forward head and low chest as well as protracted scapulae.

Anatomic Analysis of "Round Shoulders" (Fig. 21–10.)

HEAD AND NECK.   Hyperextended. The head is tipped back with the chin lifted.

THORACIC SPINE.   Convexity increased. The increased thoracic curve causes a forward head. Owing to the forward head, the sternocleidomastoid and scaleni muscles, which have their upper attachments on the head and neck, no longer exert their normal tension on the sternum and upper ribs. The thoracic portions of the erector spinae and other extensors are elongated because of the increased convexity.

SHOULDER GIRDLE.   Abducted and tilted laterally. The rhomboids and middle trapezius are elongated, and the pectoralis minor and serratus anterior shortened. The pectoralis minor fails to exert its

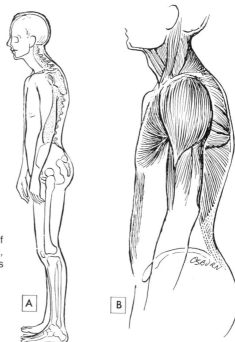

Figure 21–10. Anatomic views of forward head and round shoulders. *A,* Skeletal alignment; *B,* chief muscles affected.

usual tension on the third, fourth and fifth ribs. The pectoral fascia is likely to be tight.

SHOULDER JOINTS. Inward rotation. The abduction of the scapulae causes the arms to hang farther forward than usual and to turn slightly inward so that the palms face to the rear. Since the pectoralis major attaches to the upper part of the arm it no longer exerts its usual tension on the ribs.

CHEST. Depressed. The failure of the sternocleidomastoid, scaleni and pectoral muscles to exert their usual lifting effect on the sternum and ribs results in a lowered position of the chest. This in turn lowers the diaphragm, making it impossible for it to travel through as large an excursion as usual during respiration.

This picture does not end here, because compensatory adjustments take place through the entire body. The joints mentioned, however, are the ones most directly concerned in the posture defect of round shoulders. Two typical corrective exercises have been selected for analysis, one which has for its purpose the stretching of the shortened muscles and fascia; and the other, the strengthening and shortening of the muscles which have become unduly stretched.

PASSIVE CHEST LIFTING

Description. The subject sits on a low stool with the hands behind the neck (not clasped) and the elbows well back. The operator stands behind the subject with the toes of one foot on the edge of the stool and the knee against the subject's spine between the shoulder blades. A small pillow may be used to pad the knee, if desired. The operator grasps the subject's elbows, lifts them slightly and pulls them back with a strong steady pull. He holds the pull for several seconds, then gradually releases the tension. This is repeated from six to fifteen times. It is essential that the pull be applied with gradually increasing intensity, never with a jerk. Care must be taken to see that the subject avoids excessive hollowing of the back. This he can do by contracting the abdominal muscles. (See Fig. 21–11.)

Purpose.   To stretch the pectoral muscles and fasciae.

Anatomic Analysis.   The upward and backward pull of the arms puts the pectoralis major and minor muscles and the pectoral fascia on a stretch. The tension on the muscles produces a pull on their attachments to the ribs and sternum and results in a lifting of the chest, expansion of the thorax, and hyperextension of the thoracic spine. If the pull is applied with a quick jerk, a strong stretch reflex is likely to occur. This is an involuntary protective contraction of the pectoral muscles. It defeats the purpose of the exercise, since the muscles cannot be stretched when they are contracted. When the pull is applied slowly and gradually, the reflex action is either avoided or overcome. It is also less likely to occur if the subject is told to pinch the shoulder blades together just as the operator is pulling the elbows back. According to the law of reciprocal innervation, the scapular

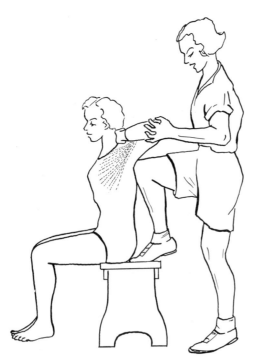

Figure 21–11. Passive chest lifting for stretching the pectoral muscles. (The dotted lines indicate the position of the pectoralis major. Pectoralis minor is beneath it.)

abductors relax when their antagonists, the adductors, are contracting. Experience has shown that an appreciably wider range of motion is possible when the movement is performed slowly and when the subject contracts the scapular adductors (see p. 175).

Mechanical Analysis.   The subject is in a stable position because of the relatively wide base of support and low position of the center of gravity.

The operator uses the subject's arms as levers. They serve as second class levers, the fulcrum being at the shoulder joint, the force point at the elbow, and the resistance point at the upper arm where the pectoralis major inserts. If the operator holds the arms at a point nearer the body, he loses leverage by shortening the length of the force arm and either has to use more force to compensate or else be content to give a less forceful stretch.

The stretching of the pectoralis minor is caused by the transmission of the force applied to the arm through the shoulder joint (due to the ligamentous attachments) to the coracoid process of the scapula, to which the pectoralis minor is attached.

It is important to note that if the trunk were free to move, the operator's pull on the elbows would simply result in a backward inclination of the trunk. But because of the resistance afforded by the pressure of his knee against the subject's back, movement at the hip joints is prevented. Likewise, if the spine were completely free to move, the backward pull on the arms would produce hyperextension of the entire spine. The subject himself must prevent this by contracting his abdominal muscles.

Common Faults

OF OPERATOR

1. Pulling so suddenly that a strong reflex action of the pectoral muscles results
2. Pulling so hard that the subject hyperextends the lumbar spine rather than endure the discomfort
3. Pulling so gently that no stretch results
4. Placing the knee too low. This encourages hyperextension of the lumbar spine and detracts from the pull on the pectorals.

OF SUBJECT

1. Failure to contract the abdominal muscles
2. Failure to hold the head in good position
3. Failure to contract the rhomboids and middle trapezius
4. Failure to relax the pectoral muscles

FRONT LYING, HEAD RAISING WITH PALMS TURNING OUTWARD

Description.   The subject lies face downward with the arms at the sides, palms down. He raises the head from 3 to 6 inches, looking at the floor directly beneath the nose. He should attempt to stretch the top of the head forward, making the body feel as long as possible.

As he raises his head, he lifts the hands from the floor, turning the thumbs up and the palms outward. At the same time that he is raising and turning his arms he should pull his shoulder blades together vigorously. After holding the position for at least five seconds he returns to the starting position and relaxes. The exercise should be repeated ten to twenty times. (See Fig. 21–12.)

A more effective but more difficult form of this exercise is to precede the head and arm movement with contraction of the abdominal and gluteal muscles, and to hold this contraction throughout the movement of the head and arms.

Purpose. To correct a forward head and round shoulders by strengthening the extensors of the thoracic spine, the adductors of the scapulae and the outward rotators of the arms.

Joint and Muscle Analysis

> HEAD AND NECK. Holding in extension (but not hyperextension) against the pull of gravity
>
>> Splenius cervicis and capitis, upper portions of erector spinae, semispinalis, etc. (static contraction)
>
> THORACIC AND LUMBAR SPINE. Extension and slight hyperextension; maintaining position against the pull of gravity
>
>> Erector spinae, semispinalis, multifidus, rotatores (concentric, followed by static contraction)

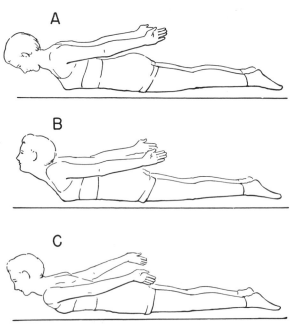

Figure 21–12. Front lying, head raising with palms turning outward. *A,* Correct form; *B,* incorrect; the head and neck are hyperextended; *C,* incorrect; the arms are rotating inward instead of outward.

SHOULDER JOINTS. Outward rotation and hyperextension
    Infraspinatus, teres minor, posterior deltoid, latissimus dorsi,
      teres major
SHOULDER GIRDLE. Adduction and reduction of lateral tilt
    Rhomboids, middle trapezius
ELBOWS AND FOREARMS. Extension and supination
    Triceps, anconeus, supinator
STABILIZATION OF PELVIS
    Gluteus maximus, hamstrings

Common Faults and Their Correction

1. Hyperextending the head and neck. This can be prevented by insisting that the subject look at a spot beneath his nose.

2. Lifting the body too high, thereby hyperextending the lumbar spine. This can be prevented by telling the subject to lift his head not more than 3 inches off the floor. (Although he will probably lift his head more than this, it is not likely that he will exceed the 6-inch limit.)

3. Rotating the arms inward instead of outward. This is more likely to occur if the subject is not told to start with the palms down. If he continues to have trouble after the movement of the hands has been carefully explained, he should try turning the arms both ways several times and learn to recognize the kinesthetic "feel" of the movements of the shoulder joints and shoulder girdle. Once he can distinguish these movements, he will know when he has turned his arms the wrong way. He should aim at "pinching the shoulder blades together."

Evaluation. This is one of the best exercises for correcting a forward head and round shoulders when it is done correctly. Unless the subject can be carefully supervised, however, it might be wise not to give it to anyone who has a tendency toward lordosis (hollow back). In such cases the exercise should be done with abdominal and gluteal contraction and the amount of lifting should be carefully regulated. Placing a small pillow beneath the abdomen is also helpful.

The exercise is more strenuous than those involving the same movements in a sitting or standing position, because in the horizontal position the movements are performed against the resistance of gravitational force.

THE PRACTICAL KINESIOLOGIST

If the discussions and applications of exercises which have been presented in this chapter have helped to give the student a sound basis for developing an effective program in physical fitness or in posture correction the chapter will have served its purpose. The physical educator who has a good kinesiologic background should be able to analyze and evaluate exercises, not only those with which he is already familiar, but also those that are brought to his attention by his students or seen on television or in popular magazines. He should be able to tell whether an exercise is suitable for the inexperienced performer, a performer of moderate experience and ability, or an advanced performer. He should know whether it has undesirable features such as the danger of straining ligaments, encouraging posture faults, or causing excessive tension. He should also recognize the mechanical problems that may be involved, such as problems of balance, leverage or momentum. In brief, his evaluation of an exercise should be based on the answers to the following questions:

1. What is the purpose of the exercise?
2. How effectively does it accomplish its purpose?
3. Does it violate any principles of good body mechanics?
4. What are the chief joint and muscular actions involved in it?
5. What are its intensity and difficulty? (Is it suitable for a beginner, a moderately experienced performer, or an advanced performer?)
6. Are there any elements of danger, injury or strain against which precautions should be taken?
7. Is it likely to call forth any undesirable or harmful responses against which the performer should be on his guard?
8. If the exercise is a difficult one, what preliminary exercise would serve to prepare the performer for it?

When the physical educator has acquired skill in answering such questions as these and in analyzing the individual needs of his students, he will have become what Huelster so aptly calls a "practical kinesiologist."[11]

SUPPLEMENTARY MATERIAL

Comparisons of Effectiveness of Isometric and Isotonic Exercises

Leach, Stryker and Zohn compared the two methods in a program of rehabilitation for men who were hospitalized for knee injuries requiring surgery.[14] They divided the 169 patients into two groups which were comparable with respect to age and type of injury. One group was given DeLorme type isotonic exercises, and the other was given isometric exercises. It took an average of 14.9 treatments for the men in the isotonic exercise group to be returned to naval duty as compared to an average of 11.7 treatments for the isometric exercise group—a difference of 3.2 treatments. The authors pointed out that this difference was "statistically and clinically significant." Incidentally, neither method caused hypertrophy of the muscles exercised.

Ward and Fisk investigated the difference in response of the quadriceps femoris and the biceps brachii to isometric and isotonic exercises.[19] The isotonic exercises were based on the overload principle with a 1.5 lb. increment at each session. The isometric exercises were held for six seconds each, this time corresponding to the time it took to lift and lower the weight through the range of motion in the isotonic exercises. Thus the muscles were contracting for approximately the same length of time for the two methods of exercise. As in the study by Leach et al., they found that the isometric exercises resulted in a more rapid increase of strength than the isotonic. They also noted that there was no significant muscle hypertrophy.

An Electromyographic Study of the Push-up for Women

In 1969 Hinson completed a study the purpose of which was to investigate electromyographically the muscular activity in the performance of four types of the push-up exercise and to determine the existence of patterns of muscular contraction among them.[8] The types of push-up used were (1) the full push-up, (2) the full push-up from a 13-inch bench, (3) the knee push-up, and (4) the full let-down (reverse full push-up). The subjects were divided into two groups, Group I consisting of ten women who could perform 10 or more full push-ups, and Group II of ten women who were able to perform no more than 5 knee push-ups. The muscles that were found to be the most involved in the push-up exercises were the anterior deltoid, followed by the triceps, trapezius, and clavicular portion of the pectoralis major. A similar muscular pattern was found in both groups, but Group II consistently showed greater muscular activity during the knee push-ups than the subjects in Group I. The muscular activity was essentially the same for the bench and full push-ups, and the let-down muscle action was similar but to a lesser extent than for the knee push-up.

Hinson concluded that the bench push-up did not justify the use of special equipment as the results were so similar to those of the full push-up from the floor. She also concluded that the let-down (reverse push-up) appeared to be a valid exercise for subjects whose upper arm and shoulder strength was inadequate for performing knee push-ups. A general observation was that the subjects in Group II showed greater muscular involvement than the subjects in Group I for the same task. This she interpreted as indicating a lack of efficiency or coordination on the part of those with lesser ability.

ASSIGNMENTS AND PROJECTS

1. Turn to Appendix G. State the purpose and give the essential joint and muscle analysis for as many of the exercises as possible.

2. Find a subject who has an increased lumbar curve and increased pelvic tilt. Analyze his posture, select two or three appropriate exercises, and suggest a sport which might be beneficial, also one which might be harmful to his posture.

3. Do the same for a subject who has weak lower back muscles.

4. Do the same for a subject who has severely pronated feet.

5. Select from three to ten exercises seen in popular magazines, newspapers, or television. Using the examples in this chapter as guides, analyze and evaluate these exercises and answer the eight questions on p. 406.

6. Observe someone doing a conditioning exercise. Analyze the exercise, using the examples in this chapter as guides.

7. Originate an exercise for stretching the hamstring muscles which will not tend to accentuate a round upper back.

8. In the straight leg lowering exercise from supine lying, identify the true resistance arm of the lever; also the rotatory component of the resistance. (See pages 96ff. and 101ff.)

9. Devise an exercise for a swimmer who wants to increase his ankle flexibility, especially his plantar flexion. (Note: Merely plantar flexing the feet volitionally is not forceful enough to increase the range of motion.)

10. Devise an exercise for a girl who is unable to lift herself onto the deck at the deep end of a pool.

REFERENCES

1. Carlson, B. R.: Relationship between isometric and isotonic strength. Arch. Phys. Med. & Rehab., 51:176–179, 1970.
2. Cooper, K. H.: Aerobics. New York, Bantam Books, Inc., 1968.
3. Crowe, P., O'Connell, A. L., and Gardner, E. B.: An Electromyographic Study of the Abdominal Muscles and Certain Hip Flexors during Selected Sit-ups. Part I. Report presented at National Convention of the American Association for Health, Physical Education and Recreation, 1963.
4. DeLorme, T. L., and Watkins, A. L.: Progressive Resistance Exercise. New York, Appleton-Century-Crofts, Inc., 1951.
5. Flint, M. M.: An electromyographic comparison of the function of the iliacus and the rectus abdominis muscles. J. Am. Phys. Ther. Assn., 45:248–253, 1965.
6. _____. Abdominal muscle involvement during the performance of various forms of sit-up exercises. Am. J. Phys. Med., 44:224–234, 1965.
7. Flint, M. M., and Gudgell, J.: Electromyographic study of abdominal muscular activity during exercise. Res. Quart. Am. Assn. Health, Phys. Ed. & Recrn., 36: 29–37, 1965.
8. Hinson, M. M.: An electromyographic study of the push-up for women. Res. Quart. Am. Assn. Health, Phys. Ed. & Recrn., 40:305–311, 1969.
9. Hislop, H. J., and Perrine, J. J.: The isokinetic concept of exercise. J. Am. Phys. Ther. Assn., 47:114–117, 1967.
10. Holland, G. J.: The physiology of flexibility; a review of the literature. In Kinesiology Review 1968. Washington, D.C., Am. Assn. Health, Phys. Ed. & Recrn., 1968, pp. 49–62.
11. Huelster, L. J.: Learning to analyze performance. J. Health & Phys. Ed., 10:84, 120–121, 1939.
12. Kendall, F. P.: A criticism of current tests and exercises for physical fitness. J. Am. Phys. Ther. Assn., 45:187–197, 1965.
13. LaBan, M. M., Raptou, A. D., and Johnson, E. W.: Electromyographic study of function of iliopsoas muscle. Arch. Phys. Med. & Rehab., 46:676–679, 1965.
14. Leach, R. E., Stryker, W. S., and Zohn, D. A.: A comparative study of isometric and isotonic quadriceps exercise programs. J. Bone & Joint Surg., 47A:1421–1426, 1965.
15. Moffroid, M., Whipple, R., Hofkosh, J., Lowman, E., and Thistle, H.: A study of isokinetic exercise. J. Am. Phys. Ther. Assn., 49:735–746, 1969.
16. Mohr, D. R.: Changes in waistline and abdominal girth and subcutaneous fat following isometric exercises. Res. Quart. Am. Assn. Health, Phys. Ed. & Recrn., 36:168–173, 1965.
17. Müller, E. A., and Hettinger, T. W.: Die Bedeutung des Trainingerlaufes für die Trainingsfestigkeit von Muskeln. Arbeitsphysiol., 15:452, 1954.

18. Partridge, M. J., and Walters, C. E.: Participation of the abdominal muscles in various movements of the trunk in man; an electromyographic study. Phys. Ther. Rev., 39:791–800, 1959.
19. Ward, J., and Fisk, G. H.: The difference in response of the quadriceps and the biceps brachii muscles to isometric and isotonic exercise. Arch. Phys. Med. & Rehab., 45:614–620, 1964.

RECOMMENDED READINGS

Kendall, F. P.: A criticism of current tests and exercises for physical fitness. J. Am. Phys. Ther. Assn., 45:187–197, 1965.
Mott, J. A.: Conditioning and Basic Movement Concepts. Dubuque, Wm. C. Brown Company Publishers, 1968.
Ricci, B.: Physical and Physiological Conditioning for Men. Dubuque, Wm. C. Brown Company Publishers, 1966.

CHAPTER 22

Locomotion: Walking and Running

Locomotion means the progressive movement of the entire body from one place to another by means of self-propulsion. Ordinarily the propulsion is provided by the lower extremities, but it is occasionally provided by all four extremities, as in creeping, or by the upper extremities alone, as in walking on the hands and hand traveling on a horizontal ladder. Locomotion may involve the use of wheels, blades, skis or other equipment attached to the feet, or it may involve a vehicle such as a bicycle or wheel chair, or a small craft such as a boat, canoe or surfboard propelled by means of the arms or legs, with or without the use of a propelling implement (e.g., oars, paddles, poles). Locomotion by self-propulsion may be on the ground or in the water, but, at the present writing, not in the air except when suspended.

Aside from the locomotor skills which are used for utilitarian purposes, there are the skills in which man indulges for sport and pleasure. These include walking, running, swimming and dancing. For purposes of systematizing the study of locomotor skills the following classification is suggested.

FORMS OF LOCOMOTION BY SELF-PROPULSION

1. On Foot
Walking
Running
Climbing (inclined plane, stairs, ladder, etc.)
Descending (inclined plane, stairs, ladder, etc.)
Jumping, leaping, hurdling
Skipping, hopping, sliding, side-stepping, etc.
Progressive dance steps, e.g., polka, mazurka, etc.
Snow shoeing
Skiing on level or up hill
Walking on stilts

2. **On Wheels and Blades**
   Bicycling*
   Roller skating
   Ice skating
   Propelling self in wheel chair*
3. **On Hands**
   Walking on hands
   Hand traveling on boom, horizontal ladder, traveling rings, etc.
4. **On Hands and Knees or Hands and Feet**
   Creeping
   Crutch walking*
   Stunts, e.g., dog running, rabbit hopping, etc.
5. **Rotatory Locomotion**
   Cartwheels
   Forward, backward and sideward rolls
6. **Aquatic Locomotion**
   Swimming
   Boating (rowing, paddling, punting, etc.)*
   Hand paddling on a board, air mattress or other floating device

Only two forms of locomotion are considered in this chapter, walking and running. These are examples of terrestrial locomotion. Swimming, a form of aquatic locomotion, is analyzed in Chapter 23.

WALKING

To the casual observer the movements involved in walking appear to be relatively simple, yet kinesiologic analysis shows them to be exceedingly complex. The dovetailing of muscular action and the synchronization of joint movements illustrate beautifully the team-work present in all bodily movements. Not even the most complex piece of machinery designed by the most skillful engineers of our time exceeds the movements of the human machine in perfection of detail or in smoothness of function.

Research on the gait, such as that conducted at the University of California as part of the Prosthetic Devices Research Project and that of Dr. Patricia Murray and others, has served to emphasize the complexity of human locomotion and the magnitude and difficulty of the task of synthesizing its various elements.[11, 12, 13, 14]

Neuromuscular Considerations. Walking is a reflex action; no conscious control is necessary. On the contrary, if attention is focused on any part of the gait, tension is likely to develop and the natural rhythm and coordination are disturbed. Reflexes control not only the movements of the limbs, but also the extension of both the supporting leg and the trunk in resisting the downward pull of gravity. This extension serves to give stability to the body in the

---

*These activities are also forms of manipulative skills.

supporting phases of locomotion, a stability which provides for effective muscular action in producing the necessary movements. Thus in walking, as in all the motions of the body, smooth, coordinated movement requires properly functioning reflexes, normal flexibility of the joints and optimum stability of the body as a whole in the weight-bearing phases of the act.

Mechanical Analysis of Walking. Walking is accomplished by the alternating action of the two lower extremities. (See Fig. 22–1.) It is an example of translatory motion of the body as a whole brought about by means of the angular motion of some of its parts. It is also an example of a periodic or pendulum-like movement in which the moving segment (in this case, the lower extremity) may be said to start at zero, pass through its arc of motion, and fall to zero again at the end of each stroke. In walking, each lower extremity undergoes two phases, the swinging or recovery phase and the supporting phase. The supporting phase is further divided into a restraining phase (from the moment the foot touches the ground until it is directly under the center of the body) and the propulsion phase (from the moment when the foot is under the center of gravity until it leaves the ground). The beginning of the restraining phase of one leg overlaps with the end of the propulsive phase of the other leg. Thus it constitutes a brief phase of double support when both feet are on the ground. This is characteristic of the walk and serves to differentiate it from the run. In the swinging phase of the walk the action of the lower extremity may be

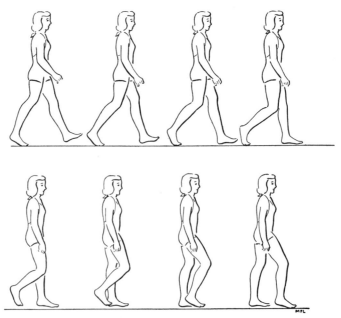

Figure 22–1. A normal gait at moderate speed. (Traced from a motion picture film.)

likened to that of the pendulum of a clock; in the supporting phase, to that of the inverted pendulum of a metronome. Gravity and momentum are the chief sources of motion for the swinging phase; hence this phase represents a ballistic type of movement (p. 42), particularly when the individual is walking at his natural pace. The source of motion for the supporting phase is, for the first half, the momentum of the forward-moving trunk (provided by the propulsive action of the other leg) and, for the second half, the contraction of the extensor muscles of the supporting leg. Whether the supporting phase can also be classed as ballistic movement is open to question. Even the swinging phase varies in its ballistic quality according to the speed of the gait, the skill, flexibility and build of the walker. A tense individual will tend to substitute muscular action for the pendulum swing of the lower extremity, and an individual with tight hamstrings will have to exert additional muscular force to overcome the restraining action of the short hamstrings. An individual who has knock-knees or fat thighs will also have difficulty in achieving a natural, pendulum swing because of friction and interference between the two limbs. In order to avoid this interference he must increase the lateral distance between his limbs, and thus introduce an undesirable lateral component of motion.

Walking and other similar forms of locomotion involve a balancing of forces. Only the most obvious of these are mentioned here.

1. The inertia of the stationary body is overcome by the horizontal component of force. Since periodic movement is characterized by an alternating increase and decrease of speed, inertia must be overcome at every step. As the center of gravity moves forward, it momentarily passes beyond the anterior margin of the base of support and a temporary loss of balance results. At this point the downward pull of gravity threatens a complete loss of equilibrium. A timely recovery of balance is brought about, however, as the foot is placed on the ground. Thus a new base of support is established and a new supporting phase is begun.

2. When forward motion has been imparted to the trunk by means of the backward thrust of the leg and foot, it tends to continue unless restrained by another force. Once the center of gravity passes beyond the base of support, it is essential to restrain the action of the trunk until a new base of support is established. Hence, as the foot is brought to the ground in front of the body at the close of its recovery phase, a restraining phase is constituted. This diminishes as the leg approaches a vertical position. During the period that the foot is in front of the center of gravity, there is a *forward* component of force in the thrust of the foot against the ground. This results in a *backward* counterpressure of the ground against the foot which is transmitted to the leg and thence to the trunk.

3. In the same phase of the step as that discussed above in section 2, the trunk is acted upon by the downward pull of gravity as well as by momentum. This downward force is counteracted by the vertical component of force of the supporting leg. During the phase of double

support each leg exerts some vertical force. If the vertical force exceeds that needed to balance the gravitational force, it results in an exaggerated lift of the body, causing a gait characterized by a bounce or unusual spring.

4. The forward-moving trunk meets with air resistance which tends to push it backward. By inclining the body forward, the pull of gravity is utilized to balance the force of the air resistance. When walking against a strong wind, it is necessary to incline the body farther forward in order to maintain balance. If the air resistance is not balanced by the force of gravity, it must be balanced by the contraction of the abdominal and other anterior muscles of the neck and trunk. If the body is inclined too far forward, however, the force of gravity acts too strongly on it and must be counteracted by tension of the posterior muscles. Thus the proper degree of forward inclination is a factor in muscular economy.

5. The degree to which the pressure of the foot actually imparts motion to the body in the propulsive phase, and restrains it in the restraining phase, is in direct proportion to the counterpressure of the supporting surface. If the surface lacks solidity, as in the case of mud, soft snow and sand, it offers too little resistance to give the needed counterpressure. The pressure of the foot results in slipping or sinking, and more pressure must be applied in order to achieve even a slow forward progress. Hence the efficiency of the gait depends upon the right balance between the pressure of the foot and the counterpressure of the supporting surface (Fig. 22–2).

6. Like counterpressure, friction is also an essential factor in the effective application of the forces needed in walking. Because of the diagonal thrust of the leg at the beginning and end of the supporting phase, friction between the foot and the ground is essential in order that the counterpressure of the ground may be transmitted to the body. For efficient walking, friction must be sufficient to balance the horizontal component of force. If it is insufficient, the thrust of the foot results in a slipping of the foot itself, rather than in the desired pro-

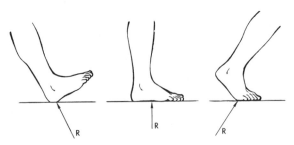

Figure 22–2. The ground reaction force R is equal in action line and magnitude to the downward thrust of the foot during walking, but opposite in direction. The force is greater at heel-strike than at mid-stance because of the body's momentum, and greater at push-off due to the plantar flexion thrust of the calf muscles driving the body forward. (From Williams, M., and Lissner, H. R., Biomechanics of Human Motion. Philadelphia, W. B. Saunders Company, 1962.)

pulsion of the body. The greater the horizontal component of force (as when walking with a long stride), the greater the dependence upon friction for efficient locomotion.

Anatomic Analysis of Walking. The action taking place in the joints of the lower extremity is essentially that of flexion and extension. But in much the same way that the shoulder girdle cooperates with the arm in movements of the upper extremity, the pelvic girdle cooperates in movements of the lower extremities. The pelvis has the double task of transmitting the weight of the body alternately first over one limb, then over the other, and of putting each acetabulum in a favorable position for the action of the corresponding femur. The adaptations of pelvic position are made in the joints of the thoracic and lumbar spine as well as in the hip joints. Thus as first one foot and then the other is put forward, the flexion and extension movements of the thigh are accompanied by slight movements of rotation and of abduction and adduction at the hip joints, and by slight lateral flexion and rotation of the spine.

The joint analysis, as presented below, is systematic rather than chronologic; that is, the action of each joint is analyzed separately, without regard for the chronologic sequences or the timing of the various movements in walking as they relate to one another.

The muscular analysis was originally based on the author's own investigations (using palpation and inspection), supplemented by the literature available in 1950. It was later revised to incorporate the findings of two electromyographic studies, the Prosthetic Devices Research Project at the University of California in Berkeley,[1] and the study made by Sheffield, Gersten and Mastellone.[16] Some revisions have since been made to incorporate findings from subsequent electromyographic investigations, but this has become increasingly difficult because of the vast amount of research in this area in recent years. The student should make every effort to keep abreast of such research, but at the same time should take into account the number of subjects used in each study, and should remember that the muscular analysis of walking, like that of any activity, is influenced by individual differences in movement patterns and by variations in speed.

Joint Analysis

SWINGING PHASE

Hip. Flexion; outward rotation (due to rotation of pelvis toward other limb); adduction at beginning and abduction at end of phase, especially if long stride is taken (due to rotation of pelvis and length of stride).

Knee. Flexion during first half; extension during second half.

Ankle and foot. Dorsal flexion; prevention of plantar flexion.

Pelvis and spine. Rotation toward opposite side; prevention of dropping of pelvis toward unsupported side.

Upper extremities. Unless restrained, the arms tend to swing in opposition to the legs, the left arm swinging forward as the right leg swings forward and vice versa. This is usually accomplished without obvious muscular action and serves to balance the rotation of the pelvis. It is a reflex action. When the arm swing is prevented, the upper trunk tends to rotate in the same direction as the pelvis, causing a tense, awkward gait.

SUPPORTING PHASE

Hip. Extension; reduction of outward rotation, followed by slight inward rotation; prevention of adduction of thigh and dropping of pelvis to opposite side.

Knee. Slight flexion at moment of contact, followed immediately by extension.

Ankle and foot. Slight plantar flexion, followed by slight dorsal flexion; prevention of further dorsal flexion which weight of body tends to cause. Plantar flexion at end of propulsive phase, especially in vigorous walking.

Pelvis and spine. See comments under Swinging Phase.

Upper extremities. See comments under Swinging Phase.

Toes. Hyperextension at metatarsophalangeal joints at end of propulsive phase, especially in vigorous walking.

Muscular Analysis (Fig. 22–3.)

SWINGING PHASE

Muscles of the spine and pelvis. Semispinalis, rotatores, multifidus and external oblique abdominal muscle on side toward which the pelvis rotates. Erector spinae and internal oblique abdominal muscle on opposite side. (Note: Rotation of the pelvis to the right constitutes rotation of the spine to the left. See p. 272.) The psoas and quadratus lumborum help to support the pelvis on the side of the swinging limb.

Muscles of hip joint. The tensor fasciae latae, sartorius, pectineus and iliopsoas contract during the first part of the swinging phase. The rectus femoris also contracts slightly at the very beginning, but soon relaxes. Whether it is acting chiefly at the hip joint or at the knee joint in this phase is difficult to say, but it seems likely that its action is primarily at the knee joint, since it roughly parallels the action of the vastus intermedius. In the latter part of this phase there is no appreciable action of the flexors of the thigh in normal walking on level ground. Since this is a ballistic movement, none would be expected. In rapid walking the actions of the sartorius and rectus femoris are noticeably increased and that of the tensor fasciae latae slightly so.

During the latter part of the swinging phase the hamstrings, particularly the long head of the biceps femoris, contract with moderate intensity, and the gluteus maximus and medius contract slightly at the very end of the swing. The adductors longus and magnus, and presumably brevis, contract slightly after the swinging limb has passed the halfway mark. Just what the function of the adductor magnus is, is not clear. It may help to steady and guide the forward-swinging limb. In any event its action is extremely slight, even in rapid walking.

It is assumed that the six deep outward rotators are responsible for the slight outward rotation of the thigh which compensates for

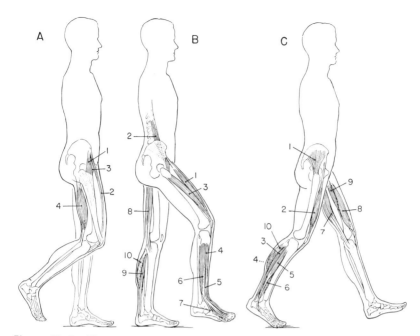

Figure 22–3. The muscles of the lower extremity used in walking. *Key: A:1,* Tensor fasciae latae; *2,* sartorius; *3,* pectineus; *4,* biceps femoris. *B: 1,* Rectus femoris; *2,* iliopsoas; *3,* vastus lateralis (medius and intermedius are not shown); *4,* tibialis anterior; *5,* extensor hallucis longus; *6,* extensor digitorum longus; *7,* peroneus tertius; *8,* semitendinosus and semimembranosus; *9,* soleus; *10,* gastrocnemius. *C: 1,* Gluteus medius; *2,* gluteus maximus; *3,* rectus femoris; *4,* gastrocnemius; *5,* soleus; *6,* peroneus longus; *7,* peroneus brevis; *8,* vastus medialis and intermedius (lateralis not shown); *9,* adductor longus; *10,* semitendinosus and semimembranosus; (tibialis posterior on right leg is not shown.)

the rotation of the pelvis in the opposite direction. These muscles are too deeply located, however, for our present methods of testing.

If the pelvis were allowed to drop on the unsupported side, abduction would occur on that side. That this does not occur in normal walking is due to the action of the abductors on the supported side and to that of the quadratus lumborum on the unsupported side. Action of the adductors on the swinging side appears to be negligible. The abduction which occurs at the end of a long stride is apparently produced by the gluteus medius and upper gluteus maximus.

Muscles of knee joint. At the beginning of the swinging phase when the foot is lifted from the ground, the action of the flexors is surprisingly slight in normal walking. The short head of the biceps femoris and the sartorius appear to be responsible for this action. Contraction of the popliteus is assumed, but cannot be tested. The rectus femoris and the vastus intermedius contract briefly at the very beginning of the swinging phase. Their contraction, which began toward the end of the supporting phase, appears to be tapering off during the beginning of the swinging phase. Since the leg is flexing at the knee joint at this time, their action must be eccentric contraction. Although the gastrocnemius is in a position to help flex the leg, it is not found to contract during this phase.

As the leg extends during the second half of the swinging phase, the short head of the biceps femoris increases its action and is joined by the long head, and later by the semimembranosus and semitendinosus. Since these are flexors of the leg and extensors of the thigh, it is assumed that they are contracting eccentrically. Their function here may be to prevent hyperextension of the knee at the end of the swinging phase.

In normal walking the quadriceps extensors contract slightly at the end of the swinging phase. The action of these muscles, as well as that of the medial hamstrings, increases in rapid walking. In an easy gait the movement appears to be initiated by gravitational force and continued by momentum. This force is sufficient to extend the leg at the knee, but in more vigorous walking the quadriceps femoris provides the force for leg extension.

Muscles of the ankle and foot. The tibialis anterior, extensor digitorum longus, extensor hallucis longus and probably the peroneus tertius contract with slight to moderate intensity at the beginning of the swinging phase, taper off during the middle portion of this phase but contract again with considerable force toward the end of it. The plantar flexors are completely relaxed throughout this phase.

SUPPORTING PHASE

Muscles of the hip joint. During the first part of the supporting phase all three gluteal muscles contract with moderate intensity; then the contractions of maximus and medius taper off during the middle part. Gluteus minimus continues to contract moderately during the middle portion. The only muscles of the hip which contract appreciably during the last part of the supporting phase are the adductors magnus and longus. In rapid walking the gluteus maximus and minimus contract with appreciable intensity during the first part of the supporting phase, and the adductor longus contracts with appreciable intensity during the last part. The hamstrings apparently have but a small part in the supporting phase of normal walking. Only the long head of the biceps contracts at all, and it contracts only slightly at the very beginning of this phase. In rapid walking both the long head of the biceps and the semitendinosus contract with moderate intensity during the first half of the supporting phase.

In considering the function of these muscles which act at the hip joint during the supporting phase of walking it would seem that the gluteus maximus, adductor longus and the long head of the biceps femoris are responsible for extending the thigh; gluteus medius and minimus for reducing outward rotation and producing slight inward rotation, also for preventing a tilt of the pelvis to the opposite side during the middle portion of the supporting phase. In this function they are aided by the quadratus lumborum on the opposite side. Just what the function of the adductor longus is, is not clear. It may be steadying the femur against the pull of the abductors, thus enabling them to act on the pelvis rather than on the femur.

Muscles of the knee joint. The quadriceps extensors contract moderately in the early part of the supporting phase, then gradually relax. They appear to control the slight flexion which occurs in the knee at the moment of contact. The vastus intermedius continues to contract throughout the first half of this phase. As the leg reaches the vertical position, the knee apparently locks and makes contraction of the extensors unnecessary. The tension of the stretched hamstrings at the end of the swinging phase, especially when a long stride has been taken, may well be the factor which initiates the slight flexion at the moment of contact. The rectus femoris and vastus intermedius contract slightly again at the end of the supporting phase. In rapid walking all these muscles contract more strongly and for a longer duration. There is an abrupt increase in their action in the second half of the supporting phase which would seem to indicate that the extension of the leg at the knee is much more forceful in rapid walking than in normal walking.

Muscles of the ankle and foot. Action current studies show that there is considerable action of the tibialis anterior in the early part of the supporting phase. It seems likely that this is related to the controlled lowering of the foot by eccentric contraction in order to prevent the foot from slapping down too hard. Its action during weight-bearing probably serves to prevent pronation. The extensors digitorum longus and hallucis longus follow a similar pattern. They reach their peak of contraction almost at the moment of transition between the swinging and the supporting phases, and then relax early in the supporting phase, and commence to contract slightly at the end of this phase.

Carlin[6] has emphasized the importance of recognizing the influence of the weight-bearing position on the action of the dorsiflexors of the ankle joint. In the stance or support phase of walking the leverage of the leg is reversed because the foot is fixed on the ground. The dorsiflexors, instead of acting on the foot, act on the tibia to pull the upper end forward over the foot. This is an important point and it is well to have it brought to our attention. But it is also suggested here that the relative force which these muscles have to exert is probably strongly influenced by individual variations in walking patterns. The tibialis anterior, extensor digitorum longus and extensor hallucis longus doubtless have to exert more force in a person who habitually walks with a backward list than in a person who tends to keep his weight over his forward foot. It would also seem that the length of the stride might be a factor, as it is related to the slant of the forward leg at the moment of contact with the ground.

The gastrocnemius, soleus and tibialis posterior contract slightly in the early part of the supporting phase and moderately in the middle and late parts. In rapid walking this contraction is strong. The peroneus longus follows a similar pattern, but does not seem to contract quite so strongly as the others, except in rapid walking. The peroneus brevis does not start to contract until about the middle of the supporting phase, but contracts more strongly than the longus.

In rapid walking it starts earlier and contracts with intensity soon after the halfway mark has been reached.

The flexor digitorum longus contracts slightly during the middle portion of the supporting phase and increases abruptly to moderate contraction in the last portion. In rapid walking the contraction becomes strong. The flexor hallucis longus follows the same pattern, except that it does not start to contract until the middle of the supporting phase.

Lateral balance is maintained by an interplay between the tibialis posterior, flexor hallucis longus and flexor digitorum longus on the one hand, and the peroneus longus and brevis on the other. The supinators are probably contracting almost constantly in order to combat the common tendency of the foot to pronate whenever it is bearing weight.

Muscles of the toes. The flexor hallucis longus, flexor digitorum longus, and the short flexors of the toes contract in response to the pressure of the ground against the toes. In the propulsive phase, especially in a vigorous walk, this contraction is intensified. In all parts of the supporting phase the contraction of the toe flexors is greater in barefoot walking than it is when shoes are worn. This is especially noticeable when walking on sand or grass.

Action of Upper Extremities in Walking. Murray and her co-workers, using the technique of interrupted light photography, investigated the action of the upper extremities in walking. They noted "patterns of sagittal rotation of the shoulder and elbow," or flexion and extension of both joints. They found that although the amplitudes of the arm swing pattern varied considerably from one subject to another, each individual had a similar pattern in all trials, even at higher speeds. Furthermore, they noted that the increased amplitude accompanying the faster speeds was due mainly to increased shoulder (hyper)extension in the backward swing and increased elbow flexion in the forward swing. Maximum flexion of both the shoulder and elbow joints occurred at the moment of heel-strike of the opposite foot and maximum extension at the moment of heel-strike of the foot on the same side.[13]

In an investigation of the muscular action of the arms, Hogue found that although they appear to swing without muscular effort in walking at a normal pace on level ground, actually their pendular action was caused by a combination of muscular activity and gravity. The mid and posterior deltoid and the teres major were the muscles that he found to be most concerned, the latter two being active mainly during the backward swing. The posterior deltoid also contracted toward the end of the forward swing. This would lead one to suspect that it was serving as a brake to check the movement. The middle deltoid was found to be active during both flexion and extension of the arm at the shoulder joint. As this muscle is primarily an abductor it seems that its function might be to keep the arms from brushing the sides of the body as they swing past it.[7]

Summary of Mechanical Principles Which Apply to Walking

1. Translatory movement of a lever is achieved by the repeated

alternation of two rotatory movements, the lever turning first about one end, then about the other end.[18]

2. A body at rest will remain at rest unless acted upon by a force. Since walking is produced by a pendulum-like motion of the limbs, the inertia of the body must be overcome at every step.

3. A body in motion will continue in motion unless acted upon by a force. Since motion is imparted to the trunk by the backward thrust of the leg, the trunk has a tendency to continue moving forward, even beyond the base of support. A brief restraining action of the forward limb acts as a check on the momentum of the trunk.

4. Force applied diagonally consists of two components, horizontal and vertical. The vertical component in walking serves to counteract the downward pull of gravity. The horizontal component serves (1) in the restraining phase, to check forward motion, and (2) in the propulsive phase, to produce it. The horizontal component of force in the propulsive phase must exceed that in the restraining phase if the end result is to be progressive forward motion.

5. The speed of the gait is directly related to the magnitude of the pushing force and to the direction of its application. This force is provided by the extensor muscles of the hip, knee and ankle joints, and the direction of application is determined by the slant of the lower extremity when the force is being applied.

6. The economy of the gait is related to its timing with reference to the length of the limbs. The most economical gait is one which is so timed as to permit pendular motion of the lower extremities.

7. Walking has been described as an alternating loss and recovery of balance.[18] This being so, a new base of support must be established at every step.

8. Since propulsion of the body is effected by the diagonal pressure of the foot against the supporting surface, the efficiency of locomotion depends upon the counterpressure and friction provided by this surface.

9. Stability of the body is directly related to the size of the base of support. In walking, the lateral distance between the feet is a factor in balance.

   a. Too narrow a lateral distance between the feet, such as occurs when one foot is placed directly in front of the other, increases the difficulty of maintaining balance as it decreases the width of the base of support.

   b. Too wide a lateral distance between the feet increases stability, but tends to cause a weaving gait and to make the body sway from side to side.

   c. The optimum position of the feet seems to be one in which the inner borders fall approximately along a single straight line.

Summary of Anatomic Principles Which Apply to Walking

1. Good alignment of the lower extremities reduces friction in the joints and eliminates the likelihood of strain and injury.

2. Normal flexibility of the joints (i.e., sufficiently long and flexible muscles, ligaments and fasciae) reduces internal resistance, and hence reduces the amount of force required for walking.

3. Speed of walking is increased by increasing both the length of the stride and the tempo of the gait.

4. The longer the stride, the greater the up and down movements of the body, unless the knee is kept slightly flexed during the middle portion of the supporting phase.

5. Unnecessary lateral movements result in an ungainly and uneconomical gait.

   a. Failure to keep the gluteus medius contracted when the weight is on the foot results in an exaggerated hip sway caused by the dropping of one side of the pelvis.

   b. Excessive trunk rotation may be caused by an exaggerated arm swing, or by restriction of the arm swing. Normally the arm swing exactly counterbalances the hip swing.[13]

   c. Straight, sagittal plane action of the leg is assured by keeping the knee and the foot pointing straight forward in all phases of the gait.

   d. The rotation of the pelvis should be only just enough to enable the leg to move straight forward. Too little or too much rotation tends to cause a weaving gait.

   e. Minimal lateral motions occur when the feet are placed in such a way that their inner borders fall approximately along a single straight line.

6. The tendon action of the two-joint muscles of the lower extremity contributes to economy of muscular action in walking (see p. 45).

7. Properly functioning reflexes contribute to a well coordinated gait.

8. The stability of the weight-bearing limb and the balance of the trunk over this limb are important factors in the smoothness of the gait.

Individual Variations in the Gait.   Although the basic anatomic analysis of the gait is valid for all physically normal persons, individual characteristics are present to such a degree that persons are often recognized by their gaits. These variations may be either structural or functional in origin. The structural differences include unusual body proportions, as well as differences in the limbs themselves such as knock-knees and bowlegs. Extreme variations in the angle between the neck and the shaft of the femur and in the obliquity of the femoral shaft are also responsible for characteristic gaits.

Variations in forward-back distribution of weight and in length of stride have already been mentioned. Other variations in movement patterns which are not structural in origin are often related to characteristics of the personality. This was brought home forcefully to the author when she attempted to help college students whose gaits were awkward. Almost invariably the students who had the most awkward gaits were those who were extremely shy or lacking in self-confidence. A study investigating the possible relationship between the two might be rewarding.

RUNNING

Easy running, like walking, is a pendulum type of movement. It is doubtful, however, whether running at top speed can be so classified. The most notable factors differentiating the run from the walk are the period of double support, characteristic of the walk, but not present in the run, and the period of no support (a "sailing-through-the-air period"), characteristic of the run, but not present in the walk. In the run the foot hits the ground, not in front of the body as in the walk, but almost directly under the body's center of gravity. This reduces the restraining part of the supporting phase and gives greater emphasis to the propulsive part. As the speed increases, the restraining part of the supporting phase diminishes, disappearing completely as maximum speed is attained. The use of the term "driving phase" for the supporting phase in running indicates its propulsive nature.

In running, as in walking, the force exerted to produce the movement has two components, horizontal and vertical. In running, however, because of the tremendous increase in horizontal force, the vertical component is negligible.

Whether the run is an easy jog or a full-speed sprint, economy of effort is a highly desirable objective. To achieve this it is essential that the runner, either consciously or unconsciously, observe the principles which apply to efficient running. The most noteworthy of these are listed below.

Mechanical Principles of Running

1. In accordance with the first law of motion, a body at rest remains at rest unless acted upon by a force. In running, the problem of overcoming inertia decreases as the level of speed is reached. It is greatest at the take-off, and least after acceleration has ceased.

a. The crouching start enables the runner to exert maximum horizontal force at the take-off by:

(1) Providing a surface against which the foot can push horizontally;

(2) Putting the legs in a more horizontal position;

(3) Enabling the runner to use maximum hip, knee and ankle extension in both legs.

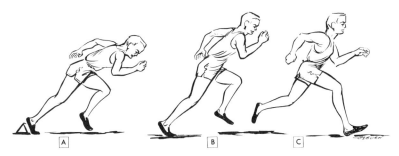

Figure 22–4. Sprinting. *A*, Take-off; *B*, acceleration; *C*, full speed.

b. During acceleration the horizontal component of the leg drive gradually diminishes until a level of speed is maintained, during which period it remains uniform. The period of acceleration is characterized by a gradual decrease in the forward inclination of the trunk, a lengthening of the stride (made possible by the raising of the center of gravity as the trunk becomes more erect), and decrease of the knee thrust, resulting from the gradual straightening of the knee at the moment of contact between the foot and the ground.

2. Also in accordance with the first law of motion, a moving body will move in a straight line unless it is acted upon by a force causing it to change its direction. In order to run in a curved pathway, as when running around a circular or oval track, an additional force is needed to overcome the body's tendency to continue in a straight line. This is achieved by leaning toward the inside as the slant of the body will introduce a lateral component to the pressure of the foot against the ground.[5] The well banked curves of indoor tracks do this for the runner.

3. In accordance with the second law of motion, acceleration is directly proportional to the force producing it. Hence, the greater the power of the leg drive, the greater the acceleration of the runner.

4. In accordance with the third law of motion, every action has an equal and opposite reaction.

5. Since a long lever develops more speed at the end than does a short lever, the length of the leg during the driving phase of running should be as great as possible when speed is a consideration. This is achieved by full extension at the knee joint at the end of the driving phase.

6. The smaller the vertical component of force, the greater the horizontal or driving component.

a. In the most efficient run, vertical movements of the center of gravity are reduced to a minimum.

b. The vertical component of force should be just enough to counteract the downward pull of gravity, but not enough to produce an unnecessary bounce in running.

7. The more completely the horizontal component of force is directed straight backward, the more it will contribute to the forward motion of the body. Lateral movements of the arms, legs and trunk detract unnecessarily from forward propulsion. To assure forward motion of the body:

a. The knees should be lifted directly forward-upward with the entire lower extremity kept in the sagittal plane. (Unathletic girls frequently run with a minimal knee lift and with an inward rotation of the thighs, the feet and lower legs being thrown out to the side.)

b. The arm swing should exactly counterbalance the twist of the pelvis and should not cause additional lateral motion.

8. Efficiency in running, as in any movement, requires the elimination of all unnecessary force.

a. The shorter the lever, the less the force required to move it, and the less the reaction to it. By flexing the leg at the knee and carrying the heel high up under the hip in the recovery phase, the leg is moved more rapidly, as well as more economically.

b. Internal resistance caused by the viscosity of the sarcolemma is reduced by warming-up activities.

c. Internal resistance caused by tight muscles, fasciae and ligaments is reduced by systematic stretching exercises.

d. Unnecessary force in the form of excessively rapid muscular contractions is eliminated by developing as long a stride as can be controlled.

SUPPLEMENTARY MATERIAL

The following five studies are of particular interest because they represent the use of five different techniques.

Electromyographic Study of the Muscles of the Foot in Walking.[16] Sheffield, Gersten and Mastellone investigated the action of the ankle and foot muscles used in walking. The subjects who participated in the study were ten normal adult males, and the walking was performed on the level at a rate of 60 steps per minute, one step consisting of the two phases, support and swing. The results are briefly summarized below.

TIBIALIS ANTERIOR, EXTENSOR DIGITORUM LONGUS AND EXTENSOR HALLUCIS LONGUS. Active throughout both phases with two peaks of intensity, the first during the early part of the swing phase when dorsiflexion was necessary in order to clear the ground, and the second at heel strike, apparently to lower the foot gradually instead of slapping it down.

FLEXOR DIGITORUM LONGUS, FLEXOR HALLUCIS LONGUS, PERONEUS LONGUS AND TIBIALIS POSTERIOR. The maximum activity of these muscles commenced near the beginning of the support phase, when the metatarsal region struck the ground, and continued until this region was off the ground. There was no activity during the swing phase.

GASTROCNEMIUS AND SOLEUS. In eight subjects the gastrocnemius became active at the time the metatarsal region touched the ground; in the other two there was slight activity beginning at the time the heel touched the ground. In all ten subjects these muscles showed a high degree of activity throughout the support phase.

On the whole the findings of these investigators substantiate those of the Advisory Committee on Artificial Limbs of the National Research Council in a similar study.[1] The latter group studied the muscular activity of six subjects as they walked at a normal pace, a rapid pace, up and down stairs and up and down a ramp. The electromyograms made during rapid walking closely resemble the muscular activity described by Sheffield and his co-workers. There are a few minor discrepancies, however. Sheffield's group appeared to find a greater degree of activity of the dorsiflexor muscles during the early part of the swing phase. They also found that the maximum activity of the second group of muscles began later than had been reported by the Research Council group. The apparent discrepancies may be due to this reviewer's interpretation, however, since she compared the electromyographic tracings of one study with the written report of another.

Analysis of the Support Phase of Walking.[2] Barnett introduced the use of a new type of pedograph that gives quantitative results for the functions of the foot in walking. In his study, reported in 1956, he obtained records for 100 normal subjects, aged 17 to 25. These records consisted of radiographs, footprints and profile photographs of the feet and ankles taken at intervals of 1/30 second. The moments of weight-bearing over different regions of the foot were recorded by means of horizontal bands placed at intervals across the sole. On the basis of these records Barnett made the following observations:

1. HEEL PHASE. (First 10–20% of support phase.) The initial contact is made by the posterolateral part of the heel, but the entire heel shares equally in weight bearing almost immediately. It is this initial contact that is responsible for the wearing down of the outer posterior edge of the heel of the shoe.

2. STANDING PHASE. (Next 30–35% of support phase.) The weight is borne by the heel, the outer side of the sole and the heads of the metatarsal bones. It is during this phase that the center of gravity is directly above the foot.

3. METATARSAL PHASE. (10% or less of support phase.) Comparing his findings with Morton's observations regarding a "short first metatarsal"[10] Barnett observes that this occurs in approximately 50% of the population and therefore considers this to be a normal variation. The more the first metatarsal protrudes beyond the second, the greater is its share of weight bearing. In feet having a so-called short first metatarsal the weight bearing is well distributed across the other metatarsals and does not exceed 4 kg. per sq. cm. beneath the second metatarsal "presumably because other factors can compensate for the normal degree of protrusion of this bone." He observes that in ordinary walking the pressure beneath the second metatarsal head can be decreased by turning the toes out and by extending the interphalangeal rather than the metatarsophalangeal joint of the big toe. It might be of interest to check the relative length of the first and second metatarsal bones in persons who habitually walk with the toes turned out.

4. FOREFOOT PHASE. (Next 30% of support phase.) The weight is borne by the metatarsal heads and the toes with the big toe usually predominating. Barnett observes from the pedograph records that the other toes, especially the second, share a considerable part of the weight and suggests that this is due to the fact that the oblique axis of the ankle is almost parallel to the heads of the outer four metatarsals.

5. STEP-OFF PHASE. (Next 3–10% of support phase.) The weight is borne entirely by the toes, especially the big toe, but the total amount borne by this foot is small as this is the period of double

support and the other foot is bearing most of the weight. Barnett comments that the fifth toe plays a greater part in the step-off than one might expect.

In discussing abnormalities, Barnett states that the majority of complaints are related to the standing phase. The most common cause of pain during the metatarsal phase, he considers, is the prolongation of this phase, usually because of a high longitudinal arch and claw foot and consequent delay in using the toes. He suggests that this lack of toe function may be the cause of metatarsalgia in the foot that appears normal in a clinical examination. (Perhaps the implication for the physical educator is that children and youths should be encouraged to use their toe muscles.)

Temporal Components of Motion in Gait. In 1960 Smith, McDermid and Shideman developed a technique for analyzing the temporal components of motion in walking using an electrobasometer.[17] They state that this makes possible a "flexible precise analysis of both shod and unshod gait in all types, conditions, and patterns of locomotion." Based on such analyses, they developed what they termed a psycho-physiological theory of gait as contrasted to a mechanical theory.

Accelerographic Study of Gait. In 1962 Liberson, Holmquest and Halls developed a method of recording simultaneously accelerograms, electromyograms and high speed motion pictures of normal and pathological gaits.[9] In their opinion one advantage of their technique is its application to the swing or recovery phase of the gait as well as to the stance phase. Their interest in developing this technique was in its usefulness in analyzing and correcting pathological gaits.

Electrogoniometric Study of Hip Joint Action in Walking. In 1969 Johnston and Smidt used the relatively new device, an electrogoniometer, to measure the movements of the thighs at the hip joints in walking.[8] This provided objective evidence of the following sequence of movements:

Hip extension: From just prior to heel-strike, gradually increasing, to just prior to toe-off.

Hip flexion: From just prior to toe-off to just prior to heel-strike.

Abduction: During latter part of stance phase to just after toe-off.

Adduction: Just after toe-off to latter part of stance phase.

Outward rotation: In late stance phase through much of swing phase.

Inward rotation: Just prior to heel-strike until late stance phase.

The average motion taking place at the hip joint was 52 degrees in the sagittal plane, 12 degrees in the coronal plane, and 13 degrees in the transverse plane. A major purpose of the study was to test the use of the electrogoniometer as a method of measurement in the study of hip joint disease. The authors were favorably impressed with it as being a practical and valuable instrument for this purpose. They found the method to be "accurate, simple, and relatively inexpensive."

Additional Studies of Walking. Extensive studies on various aspects of walking have been made by Murray and by Basmajian and their respective co-workers. For other electromyographic studies of the muscles used in walking, it is suggested that the reader refer to the current edition of Basmajian's book, *Muscles Alive*.[3]

DEMONSTRATIONS AND LABORATORY EXERCISES

1. Try this as a class exercise, working in pairs. *A* stands with heels against a wall with the feet otherwise in a comfortable, "natural" position in readiness to walk. *B* holds a ruler across the toes of *A*'s feet and draws a line against the ruler. *A* then stands with feet parallel at right angles to the wall, and again *B* draws a line. Measure the distance between the two lines. This measurement is likely to vary from $1/4$ in. to 1 in. in a sizable class. *A* and *B* now change places and repeat.

Assume that you are to engage in a walking race of 1000 yards; also assume that if you toed straight ahead, each step would be 1 yard long. It would therefore take you 1000 steps to cover the distance. But suppose you toed out so that each step was (your measurement)_____ short. How many yards short of the finish line would you be when you had taken 1000 steps? (Ans. If the difference between the two lines had been $3/16$ in. you would be $3/16 \times 1000 = 187.5$ in. or 5.2 yards short.)

Implication. If you are walking against an opponent who walks at the same rate as you, but who toes straight ahead, you would be 5.2 yards behind him when he crosses the finish line. Yet, presumably you took the same number of steps.

2. Observe the gait of people on the street or campus; detect individual characteristics; and analyze them in terms of anatomic and mechanical principles.

3. Get a subject to walk in each of the following ways. Observe and note differences in the movements of the head, shoulders, hips, etc.

    a. Placing one foot directly in front of the other.
    b. Keeping a lateral distance of 10 to 12 inches between the feet.
    c. Pointing the toes out.
    d. Pointing the toes in.
    e. Pointing the toes straight ahead.
    f. Taking a short stride.
    g. Taking a long stride.

4. Select four or five individuals who are not alike in leg length. Get them to practice walking until each one finds the stride and speed that feels most comfortable to him. Compare their strides and measure the distance between footprints for each individual.

5. Observe several individuals as they run. Look for the application of the principles listed.

6. Observe other forms of locomotion and discover for yourself what principles apply to them.

REFERENCES

1. Advisory Committee on Artificial Limbs, National Research Council: The Pattern of Muscular Activity in the Lower Extremity during Walking. Berkeley, Cal., Prosthetic Devices Research Project, Institute of Engineering Research, University of California, 1953.
2. Barnett, C. H.: The phases of human gait. Lancet, 271:617–621, 1956.
3. Basmajian, J. V.: Muscles Alive, 2nd ed. Baltimore, The Williams & Wilkins Company, 1967.
4. Bresnahan, G. T., and Tuttle, W. W.: Track and Field Athletics. St. Louis, C. V. Mosby Company, 1937, Chapter 3.
5. Broer, M. R.: Efficiency of Human Movement, 2nd ed. Philadelphia, W. B. Saunders Company, 1966.
6. Carlin, E. J.: Human gait. Am. J. Phys. Med., 42:181–184, 1963.
7. Hogue, R. E.: Upper-extremity muscular activity at different cadences and inclines during normal gait. J. Am. Phys. Ther. Assn., 49:963–972, 1969.
8. Johnston, R. C., and Smidt, G. L.: Measurement of hip-joint motion during walking. J. Bone & Joint Surg., 51A:1083–1094, 1969.
9. Liberson, W. T., Holmquest, H. J., and Halls, A.: Accelerographic study of gait. Arch. Phys. Med. & Rehab., 43:547–551, 1962.
10. Morton, D. J., and Fuller, D. D.: Human Locomotion and Body Form. Baltimore, The Williams & Wilkins Company, 1952.
11. Murray, M. P., Drought, A. B., and Kory, R. C.: Walking patterns of normal men. J. Bone & Joint Surg., 46A:335–360, 1964.
12. Murray, M. P., Kory, R. C., Clarkson, B. H., and Sepic, S. B.: Comparison of free and fast speed walking patterns of normal men. Am. J. Phys. Med., 45:8–24, 1966.
13. Murrary, M. P., Sepic, S. B., and Barnard, E. J.: Patterns of sagittal rotation of the upper limbs in walking. J. Am. Phys. Ther. Assn., 47:272–284, 1967.
14. Saunders, J. B. deC. M., Inman, V. T., and Eberhart, H. D.: The major determinants in normal and pathological gait. J. Bone & Joint Surg., 35A:543–558, 1953.
15. Schwartz, R. P., Heath, A. L., Morgan, D. W., and Towns, R. C.: A quantitative analysis of recorded variables in the walking pattern of "normal" adults. J. Bone & Joint Surg., 46A:324–334, 1964.
16. Sheffield, F. J., Gersten, J. W., and Mastellone, A. F.: Electromyographic study of the muscles of the foot in normal walking. Am. J. Phys. Med., 35:223–236, 1956.
17. Smith, K. U., McDermid, C. D., and Shideman, F. E.: Analysis of the temporal components of motion in human gait. Am. J. Phys. Med., 39:142–151, 1960.
18. Steindler, A.: Kinesiology of the Human Body. Springfield, Ill., Charles C Thomas, Publisher, 1955, Lectures 37 and 38.
19. Wright, D. G., Desai, S. M., and Henderson, W. H.: Action of the subtalar and ankle-joint complex during the stance phase of walking. J. Bone & Joint Surg. 46A:361–382, 1964.

RECOMMENDED READINGS

Brunnstrom, S.: Clinical Kinesiology. Philadelphia, F. A. Davis Company, 1962, Chap. 11.
Bunn, J. W.: Scientific Principles of Coaching. Englewood Cliffs, N.J., Prentice-Hall, Inc., 1959, pp. 110–112.
Deshon, D. E., and Nelson, R. C.: A cinematographical analysis of sprint running. Res. Quart. Am. Assn. Health, Phys. Ed. & Recrn., 35:451–455, 1964.
Dyson, G. H. G.: The Mechanics of Athletics, 2nd ed. London, University of London Press Ltd., 1963, Chapter 6.
Elftman, H.: Biomechanics of muscle; with particular application to studies of gait. J. Bone & Joint Surg., 48A:363–376, 1966.
Gray, E. G., and Basmajian, J. V.: Electromyography and cinematography of leg and foot ("normal" and flat) during walking. Anat. Rec., 161:1–16, 1968.
Morton, D. J.: The Human Foot. New York, Columbia University Press, 1935, Chaps. 15 and 18.

CHAPTER 23

Kinesiologic Aspects of Selected
Sport and Gymnastic Skills

The teaching and coaching of sports and gymnastics are among the chief concerns of physical education teachers. It is therefore to the interest of teachers-in-training to learn the most effective way of introducing a particular sport or gymnastic stunt to beginners, presenting the motor skills involved, recognizing the problems commonly experienced by learners, analyzing the performance of each individual and detecting his faults and weaknesses, and coaching both mediocre and skilled performers so as to enable them to attain their potentials. A sound foundation in kinesiology can provide the prospective teacher with the necessary tools for accomplishing all of these objectives. Inasmuch as physical education students are both performers and potential teachers, they have a dual motivation for learning the principles, fine points and teaching aids that may contribute to their skill both as performers and as teachers.

Three dissimilar activities have been selected for analysis in this chapter: the forehand drive in tennis, representing a land sport that features giving impetus to an external object; the sprint crawl stroke in swimming, representing the movement of the body through the water; and trampolining, representing movements performed in the air without any support. Some additional applications of kinesiology are presented as examples of the variety of ways the instructor can use his scientific background to make his teaching more effective and more meaningful to his students.

THE FOREHAND DRIVE

Although the reader is no doubt familiar with the forehand drive, a brief description is presented here in order to provide a basis for reference in the discussion that follows.

Description (Fig. 23–1)

STARTING POSITION. The left side is toward the net, the feet about 18 inches apart, the knees slightly flexed and the weight on the balls of the feet. The racket is held with the eastern grip, as though shaking hands with it.

BACKSWING. The weight is transferred to the right foot and the trunk rotated to the right as the racket is swung back at about waist height. The elbow is kept away from the body. (It is assumed that the straight backswing is being used, rather than the circular.) There is a pause at the end of the backswing before the forward swing is begun.

FORWARD SWING AND FOLLOW-THROUGH. The arm and racket swing forward and slightly upward in a continuous sweep. The racket is held with its head slightly above the level of the wrist at all times. The racket face is either flat or facing slightly upward at the moment of impact, and the grip is firm. The weight is transferred from the right to the left foot, and the body is rotated to the left so that, at the finish of the follow-through, the right shoulder is pointing in the direction of the ball's flight. As the weight is shifted from the right to the left foot, the racket is in contact with the ball and is moving forward in a straight line, rising slightly. The racket is above shoulder height for the follow-through and may finish in a slightly closed position, that is, facing somewhat downward.

Mechanical and Anatomic Factors

The movement involved in the forehand drive is classified as "giving impetus to an object," in this instance, striking a ball with a racket. (See page 129 for the principles of giving impetus to an external object and page 134 for specific principles that apply to striking.) The action is ballistic in nature and, as such, is initiated by muscular force, continued by momentum, and finally terminated by the contraction of antagonistic muscles. The chief lever participating in the movement consists of the arm and racket together with the fulcrum located at the shoulder joint, the point of force application at a point on the humerus that represents the combined forces of the muscles producing the movement (mainly the anterior deltoid and the pectoralis major), and the resistance point at the center of gravity of the arm-racket lever. At the moment of impact, however, the resistance point may be considered the point of contact of the ball with the racket face. The additional lever action due to the shift from rear to forward foot and to the rotation of the trunk from right to left should also be recognized (Note first two positions in Fig. 23–1).

In considering the force that is involved in the forehand drive it is important to distinguish between the force that is applied *to the lever* and the force that is applied *by the lever to the ball*. Whereas the force applied to the lever is muscular force, the force applied to the ball is the force of momentum. It is determined by both the mass and the velocity of the implement that makes contact with the ball. These, in turn, are related to the distance of the point of contact from the fulcrum—in other words, the length of the temporary resistance arm of the lever ("temporary" because the distance from the fulcrum to the point of contact with the ball constitutes the resistance arm of the

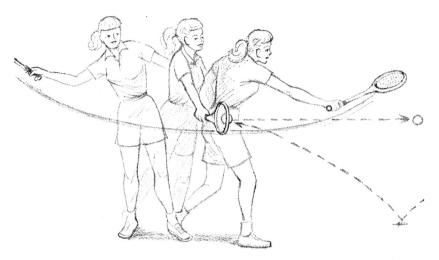

Figure 23–1. The forehand drive. (From Vannier, M., and Poindexter, H. B., Individual and Team Sports for Girls and Women, 2nd ed. Philadelphia, W. B. Saunders Company, 1968.)

lever only for the brief moment of impact). In addition to the angular movement of the arm-racket lever and the rotatory movement of the trunk, the linear motion produced by the forward movement of the body (due to weight shift) adds to the force which meets the ball.

The purpose of the forehand drive is to return the ball so that it will not only land within the opponent's court, but will land in such a place and manner that it will be difficult for him to return it. For the player to achieve this requires both high speed and expert placement of the ball. Hence, imparting maximum speed to the ball and, at the same time, placing it with accuracy, are the two major skills that the player seeks to develop.

The force of impact is determined by the speed of the racket at the moment of contact with the ball and maximum velocity can be obtained only when maximum distance is used for accelerating. The function of the backswing is to provide this distance. There are two types of backswing, the straight and the circular. The straight backswing has the advantage of greater ease in controlling the direction of the racket and in timing the movement, but the disadvantage of necessitating the overcoming of inertia in order to reverse the direction from the back to the forward swing. The circular backswing, on the other hand, permits the arm to move in one continuous motion and it therefore provides twice the distance for building up momentum. For the more skillful player who is able to control both the direction of the racket and the timing of the entire movement, it is the more efficient method.

Whichever backswing is used, two important anatomic factors are the player's range of motion at the shoulder joint and the strength of the muscles responsible for swinging the arm horizontally forward. These are the pectoralis major, anterior deltoid, subscapularis, coraco-brachialis, and biceps brachii. A good forehand drive, however, depends upon more than just the arm movement. The shifting of the weight, the rotation of the trunk, and the coordination of all these movements are a vital part of the total skill. Each movement in turn gets under way before the next one commences. If the timing is correct, the cumulative effect of these movements is to produce maximum velocity. If any of the movements is added to the preceding one either too early or too late the potential velocity will not be realized.

Force. Other important factors that contribute to the force applied to the ball, and therefore to the speed of the ball on its return flight, are presented below.

1. The use of the arm in an almost fully extended position increases the length of the lever, thereby giving greater velocity to the racket head than would be the case if the upper arm were close to the body.

2. The concentration of mass at the level of the shoulders moving forward at the moment of impact assures maximum speed for striking.

3. A skillful player tends to use a relatively heavy racket because, other things being equal, the greater the mass of the striking implement, the greater the striking force, and hence the greater the speed of the struck ball.

4. A new ball and a well strung racket assure a good coefficient of restitution (i.e., elasticity), thereby increasing the speed of the struck ball.

5. A firm grip on the racket and the use of good wrist control assure the transmission of force from the body to the instrument, and hence to the ball.

Placement. Placement of the ball is a matter of direction. It will be recalled that the direction taken by a struck ball is determined by four factors:

1. The direction of the striking implement at the moment of impact.

2. The relation of the striking force to the ball's center of gravity — in other words, the control of spin.

3. Firmness of grip and wrist at the moment of impact.

4. Angle of incidence.

The first of these is obvious. The beginner may be less aware of the importance of the other three factors. For successful placing of the ball, an understanding of the effect of spin and the skill of imparting the desired spin to the ball are essential. Firmness of grip is dependent upon wrist and finger strength and is closely related to the angle at which the racket face makes contact with the ball. Since the angle of rebound equals the angle of incidence (actually slightly less than this in the case of tennis balls because of their compressibility), it will be seen that firmness of grip is therefore an important factor in the direction taken by the struck ball.

THE SPRINT CRAWL

The technique upon which this analysis is based is described by Armbruster, Allen and Billingsley in their book, *Swimming and Diving.** The position of the head and trunk and the movement of the head in breathing are described briefly. The arm and leg strokes are described in somewhat greater detail and their propulsive phases are analyzed anatomically.

Mechanics of the Crawl Stroke

As an introduction to the kinesiologic aspects of any swimming stroke, the principles of moving one's body through the water should be reviewed with care. (See pages 113–116.) Armbruster et al. describe the position of the body for the sprint crawl stroke in considerable detail and, in so doing, demonstrate the importance of seemingly minor details in streamlining the body for minimizing the resistance of the water to forward progression.[1] Counsilman devotes the entire first chapter of his book *The Science of Swimming* to a discussion of the mechanical principles involved in swimming.[4] His illustrations for this chapter are particularly helpful, both to the kinesiology student and to the swimmer, for understanding the forces that must be combated in the water.

THE HEAD AND TRUNK

The head and trunk have three important functions in swimming, particularly in speed swimming. These are minimizing resistance, enabling the swimmer to breathe, and providing a stable anchorage for the arm and leg muscles. The position of the body is the key to reducing resistance. The body is almost horizontal, but not quite, because the feet and buttocks are below the surface of the water, and the head and shoulders are partly above it. The head is held with the chin slightly lifted and the eyes close to the surface of the water, in some cases just below it, and in some cases just above it. The exact position of the body varies with the anatomic build and the buoyancy of the individual, as well as with the speed of the stroke. A common mistake is to lift the head too much. If it is held too high, or tipped back too far, it makes the swimmer overtense and hence reduces his endurance. Armbruster et al. emphasize the importance of keeping the chin and nose in the midplane of the body in order to keep the body on an even keel. By static contraction of the rectus abdominis the spine is held in a position of slight flexion — or at least of incomplete extension — and the pelvis in a position of slightly decreased inclination.

The turning of the head for inhaling must be accomplished with the least possible interference with the rhythm of the arm and leg action and with the progress of the body through the water. It is

*For an analysis of the crawl stroke for teachers of beginning swimmers, see Basic Swimming Analyzed, by Marjorie M. Harris.[6]

essential not to lift the head for breathing, but to rotate it on its longitudinal axis while at the same time tucking the chin in close to the side of the neck. In this position the face appears to be resting on the bow wave, and the mouth is just above the surface of the water. After a quick inhalation the face is again turned forward with the eyes in the horizontal plane and the nose and chin in the midsagittal plane of the body.

In order to provide a firm base of attachment for the muscles of the arms and thighs the trunk must be held steady. By the alternating action of the left and right oblique abdominals and spinal extensors the spine and pelvis are stabilized against the pull of the shoulder and hip muscles. Thus they permit the latter to exert all their force on the limbs for the propulsive movements.

THE ARM STROKE

Entry and Support. Since the arm stroke provides approximately 85% of the total power, it is most important that the entry of the arm into the water should place it in the most advantageous position for exerting force which will be effective in driving the body forward. Its position on entry is with the forearm high and the elbow pointing to the side. The hand passes in front of the shoulder in preparation for the entry, and then, reaching forward with the shoulder held high, it is driven forward into the water directly in front of the shoulder. The brief moment between entry and the beginning of the chief propulsive action is known as the support phase, its purpose being to keep the head and shoulders above the surface. The pressure of the forearm and hand is chiefly downward, passing into backward.

Catch, Pull and Push. The moment at which the chief propulsive action changes from downward to backward constitutes the catch. This usually occurs when the hand is five to ten inches below the surface and involves a quick inward movement of the hand and arm which serves to bring the hand to a position in front of the axis of the body in such a way that the body weight is balanced above the arm. The upper arm is approximately vertical, a position which favors the large muscles (sternal portion of the pectoralis major and latissimus dorsi) for their task of pulling the arm downward and backward. Since the purpose of the stroke is to drive the body forward, it is essential to apply maximum force backward. Armbruster et al. state that this is best done by keeping the arm in a near vertical position during the pull and push with the hand pulling along a line below the long axis of the body. In order to keep the hand in this plane the elbow must gradually flex. They refer to the hand and forearm serving as an anchorage for the shoulder to be pulled forward over them. In order to keep the hand and forearm in the best position for pressing against the water the elbow is flexed slightly and the hand drawn inward and

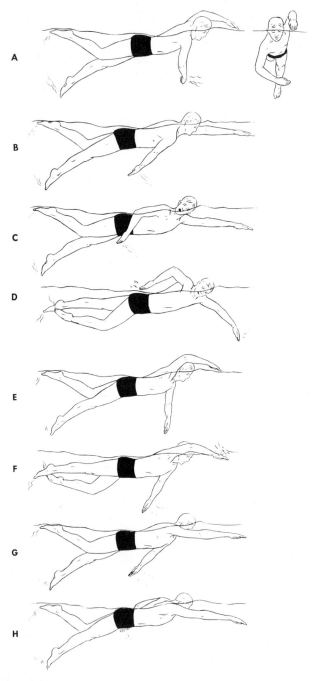

Figure 23–2. The sprint crawl. (From Armbruster, D. A. et al.: Swimming and Diving, 5th ed. St. Louis, C. V. Mosby Co., 1968.)

slightly upward toward the chest. They give the following three reasons for flexing the elbow during the pull:

1. It permits the hand and forearm to assume a position in which they can exert their force more nearly in line with the body's long axis.

2. It shortens the lever arm and thus permits greater speed with less energy expenditure.

3. It favors the transition from pull to push.[1]

The transition from pull to push occurs as the arm passes under the shoulder. The upper arm remains nearly vertical as the forearm gradually extends until it is in front of the hip, at which time the upper arm extends and the hand gives a quick push backward.

Release and Recovery. The elbow is now near the surface with the hand slightly lower and posterior to it and the palm facing mostly upward. The pressure of the forearm and hand now being relaxed, the elbow and shoulder are raised until the hand is out of the water. As this occurs, the palm turns toward the body. The arm is then carried forward through the air with the hand moving from a position near the hip to a position in front of the shoulder, preparatory to a new entry. The movement of the arm from release to the completion of recovery is continuous. It is important that no break occur as this would mean loss of momentum and would necessitate additional force for overcoming inertia, or at least for regaining the lost velocity.

The movement of the arm during the recovery starts with a lift of the entire arm and shoulder from the water by raising the elbow until the hand is clear of the water. This is followed by "an outward and forward circular motion with the shoulder acting as the axis"[1] and the hand being carried forward with the palm downward and the thumb leading.

Armbruster, Allen and Billingsley state that as the elbow is brought forward it remains above the level of the hand throughout the recovery and entry, the forearm being virtually horizontal as the arm moves forward past the shoulder and the hand staying in line with the forearm. Finally, as the hand passes the head, the arm reaches forward in preparation for the entry, the shoulder girdle remains high, the tip of the elbow is above shoulder level pointing to the side, and the forearm then points downward from the elbow with the wrist slightly flexed, the palm facing the water, and the fingers aiming forward into the water.

Armbruster and his co-authors mention that there are various other styles of arm recovery in the crawl stroke, the chief differences being in the position of the elbow. Counsilman also discusses various forms of arm recovery and attributes the variety to variations in shoulder flexibility. He even goes so far as to express the opinion that if all swimmers had equal degrees of flexibility they might all use similar recoveries.[4]

Brief Anatomic Analysis of Propulsive Phase of Arm Stroke (Catch, Pull and Push)

Shoulder joint: Strong extension, slight inward rotation, slight "horizontal" flexion-adduction in oblique plane, followed by con-

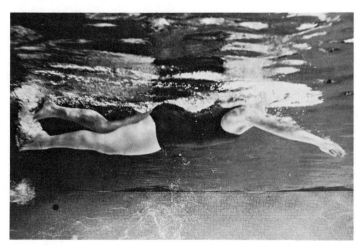

Figure 23-3. The crawl stroke. Taken through underwater window in Wellesley College swimming pool. The right arm is completing the glide and is about to begin the pull. (Photo from files of Department of Physical Education, Wellesley College.)

tinued extension and possibly slight hyperextension. Muscles: Latissimus dorsi, teres major, sternal portion of pectoralis major, posterior deltoid.

Shoulder girdle: Downward rotation, adduction, slight upward tilt. Muscles: Rhomboids and pectoralis minor.

Elbow and radioulnar joints: Flexion, slight pronation; partial extension toward end. Muscles: Brachialis, brachioradialis, probably biceps brachii because of resistance, pronator teres, pronator quadratus; triceps, anconeus.

Wrist: Held in midposition, possibly slight flexion toward end of propulsion. Muscles: Palmaris longus, flexor carpi radialis (longus and brevis), flexor carpi ulnaris.

Fingers: Held in extension and adduction. Muscles: Probably flexors and adductors in static contraction.

THE LEG STROKE

Position and Nature of Movement. The legs are relatively close together in a position of easy extension. They oscillate in an up and down movement with the feet attaining a stride of about 18 to 26 inches. In both the upstroke and downstroke the movement, described as whip-like or lashing, starts at the hip joint and progresses through the knees to the ankles and feet. The action of the latter is said to be similar to that of pedaling a bicycle, but obviously with a much smaller range of motion since the ankle joints remain in varying degrees of plantar flexion throughout the entire leg stroke. Unlike the arms, whose movements alternate between propulsion and recovery, both phases of the leg stroke are propulsive. In the downstroke the water is pushed back along the front of the thigh, then the shin, and finally the front of the ankle and dorsal surface of the foot. In the upstroke the water is pressed back along the posterior surface of the thigh, then the calf of the leg, and finally along the sole of the foot. A quick, forceful plantar flexion at the very end of the upstroke provides a powerful backward and upward push of the sole of the foot against the water, driving the body forward.

Downstroke. As the plantar flexors relax, the hip flexors, followed almost immediately by the knee extensors, start to contract. The thigh flexes only slightly and the knee, which was in a position of slight flexion at the completion of the upstroke, extends completely during the downstroke. The ankle and foot remain in plantar flexion, probably being held in this position by the pressure of the water against the dorsal surface of the foot. It seems likely that the dorsiflexors contract statically to stabilize the foot against this pressure. Throughout the downstroke the foot remains in a slight toeing-in position. Armbruster et al. warn that the heels should not be allowed to drift apart in an attempt to facilitate the in-toeing as this would involve rotation of the thigh and would cut down on the driving power of the limb.

BRIEF ANATOMIC ANALYSIS OF DOWNSTROKE

Hip joint: Partial flexion. Muscles: Iliopsoas, tensor fasciae latae, pectineus, sartorius and gracilis.

Knee joint: Strong extension. Muscles: Quadriceps femoris.

Ankle joint: Incomplete plantar flexion probably caused by pressure of water. Muscles: Tibialis anterior, peroneus tertius, extensor digitorum longus, and extensor hallucis longus may contract statically to stabilize foot against pressure of water.

Tarsal joints: Adduction and inversion. Muscles: Tibialis posterior and anterior, flexor digitorum longus, and flexor hallucis longus.

Upstroke. At the completion of the downstroke the thigh is in a position of slight flexion, the knee is completely extended, the ankle is incompletely plantar flexed, and the tarsal joints are probably neutral in the split second between the downstroke and the upstroke. The upstroke begins with thigh extension, and this is accompanied almost immediately by slight knee flexion. Active plantar flexion, first of the ankle, then of the tarsal joints, occurs with increasing intensity throughout the stroke and reaches a peak at the very end when the sole of the foot exerts a quick, forceful, backward and upward thrust against the water. The movements of the three major segments of the lower extremity are forceful in the upstroke but are under such good control that the foot stops just below the surface of the water. To break through the surface constitutes a major error as it causes an immediate reduction in propulsive force.

BRIEF ANATOMIC ANALYSIS OF UPSTROKE

Hip joint: Strong but incomplete extension. Muscles: Hamstrings and gluteus maximus.

Knee joint: Slight flexion against resistance. Muscles: Hamstrings, sartorius, gracilis, popliteus and gastrocnemius.

Ankle joint: Plantar flexion. Muscles: Gastrocnemius, soleus, peroneus longus and brevis, tibialis posterior, flexor digitorum longus, and flexor hallucis longus.

Tarsal joints: Plantar flexion, especially in final part of stroke. Muscles: Peroneus longus and brevis, tibialis posterior, flexor digitorum longus, and flexor hallucis longus.

ADDITIONAL ASPECTS

Other aspects of the crawl stroke which are important to the swimmer and the coach include the timing and coordination of the arm and leg strokes and of the breathing, the rhythm of the stroke as a whole, the relaxation of the body and the flexibility of the joints, particularly of the shoulders and ankles. Of these, possibly the last named is of greatest interest to the kinesiologist. The serious swimmer will want to know how to increase the range of motion in his shoulder joints and ankles; specifically, how to stretch the pectorals and anterior ligaments of the shoulders, and gain greater plantar flexion of the feet. Armbruster et al. and Counsilman have suggested a few exercises for these purposes.[1, 4] The kinesiology student should be able to originate several others.

TRAMPOLINING

There are two basic and interacting principles that apply to trampolining and to diving alike. These are (1) Newton's law of action and reaction (see page 83) and (2) the principle of the transfer of momentum from the part to the whole.

According to Newton's third law of motion, for every action there is an equal and opposite reaction. A body which is supported is able to move by pushing against the supporting surface because the latter pushes back against it with equal force. If the individual is in the air, however, having just taken off from a diving board or a trampoline, there is absolutely nothing he can do to alter the course of his flight. This was set by the conditions of his take-off and no attempts at stepping or jumping will alter the course of his center of gravity one iota. His body may twist or turn, fold or unfold, but his center of gravity continues on its predetermined course influenced normally only by the force of gravity or possibly by a strong wind.

According to the principle of the transfer of momentum, the momentum of a *supported* body can be transferred to the rest of the body *because of the reaction of the supporting surface.* For instance, a person sitting on the edge of a platform or large table with legs hanging down may rock back onto his back bringing his legs up at the same time. If, from this position, he swings his feet over his head keeping his knees straight, quickly reverses the movement and vigorously flings his legs forward, and then suddenly stops them after

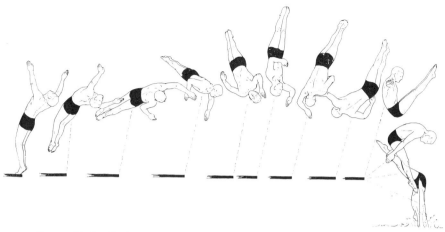

Figure 23-4. Back one and one half somersault, one and one half twist, free. (From Armbruster, D. A. et al.: Swimming and Diving, 5th ed. St. Louis, C. V. Mosby Co., 1968.)

they pass the vertical, his head and trunk will lift and he will rise to a sitting position. The movement of his legs will have been transferred to the rest of his body causing it to follow in the direction of his legs.

Similarly, if one should stand on a carpet or pavement with the right forearm across his chest and then, with vigor, fling the right arm horizontally to the right and as far back as possible, his body would tend to rotate in the same direction, again demonstrating the transfer of momentum from the part to the whole. But if one were to attempt the same thing in the air he would find that his body tended to turn in the opposite direction from his arm. This illustrates the fact that momentum of a part of the body cannot be transferred to the rest of the body if the body is unsupported. The principle that is followed here is that of action and reaction. Having no supporting surface to provide the reaction, another part of the body must provide it. The implication for trampolining activities is as follows. There are two methods of performing twists available to the performer. Either he can start before losing contact with the trampoline by giving a slightly sideward push-off and at the same time start to twist some part of his body—head, shoulders, arms, pelvis or feet—or he can start the twist in the air, usually by flinging first one arm, then the other, in the same direction in a plane at right angles to the long axis of the body.

The movements of the body in trampolining appear to be governed by four factors.

1. The rebound from the trampoline, including both the magnitude and the direction of the force.
2. The force of gravity, the effect of which may be broken down to three phases.
   a. Upward phase: continuous slowing of upward motion until zero point is reached.

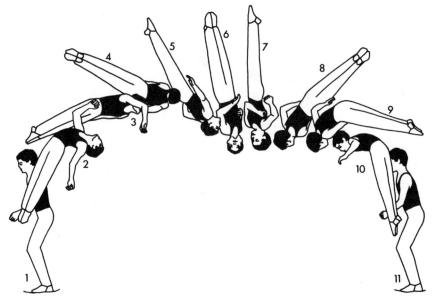

Figure 23–5.   Double twisting back somersault. (From Hennessy, J. T.: Trampolining. Dubuque, Iowa, Wm. C. Brown Co., 1968.)

       b. Zero point: split second between upward and downward motion.

       c. Downward phase: downward acceleration at rate of 32 feet per second per second.

    3. Newton's third law of motion of action and reaction.

       a. Between body and resisting object with which it is in contact. (This is usually thought of as a supporting surface but it could be an obstacle touched by the body in the air.)

       b. Between one part of body and another part when there is no contact with a resisting surface.

    4. Transfer of momentum from one part of the body to the whole when the body is supported.

There is an additional factor of air resistance which may have a slightly retarding effect on the upward or downward momentum of the body.

No attempt is made here to analyze a specific trampoline skill,* but a few simple demonstrations are suggested for illustrative purposes and for giving the observers practice in identifying the underlying principles. Some questions are posed concerning these as a means of sharpening the powers of observation of those about to learn the basic skills of trampolining. Only skillful performers should be selected for participating in these demonstrations.

---

*For specific skills see J. T. Hennessy (*Trampolining*)[7] and B. A. Gowitzke (article in *Kinesiology Review 1968*).[5]

Demonstrations

1. Practice the fundamental bounce a few times and then, upon starting downward, try hard to move forward about six inches.

Questions. *a.* Did the up phase of the final bounce resemble exactly the up phases of the preceding bounces? *b.* What happened in the down phase?

2. At the height of a jump follow the directions of the instructor to turn the head to the left or right.

Questions. *a.* What happened? *b.* How do you explain this?

3. Perform a few preliminary bounces with the arms extended sideward at shoulder level. When at the top of a bounce, in response to the instructor's directions, swing the left or right arm sharply forward from the shoulder.

Questions. *a.* What happened to the rest of the body? *b.* What principle did this illustrate?

4. After a few preliminary bounces perform a half twist to the left. The observers should watch this several times, looking in turn at the head, arms, hips, and feet.

Questions. *a.* Did the four parts of the body show any unusual movement? *b.* What movement initiated the twist? *c.* What principle did the movement illustrate?

5. After a few preliminary bounces, at the height of the jump twist to the left or right in response to the directions of the instructor.[*]

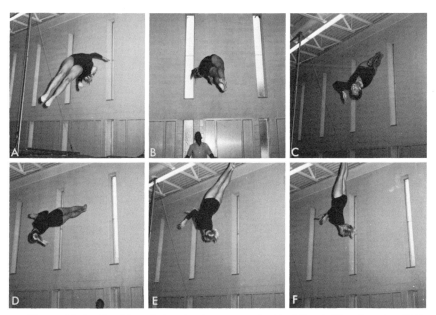

Figure 23–6. Double twisting back somersault. (Judi Ford, Miss America 1969, Junior Women's National A. A. U. Trampolining Champion, 1968. Courtesy of Mrs. Virgil Ford.)

---

[*]Suggested by John W. Bunn in personal correspondence.

Questions. *a.* How was the twist initiated? *b.* What principle did this illustrate?

ANALYSIS OF COMMON FAULTS IN SELECTED SPORT TECHNIQUES

One particularly useful application of kinesiology for the sports instructor is the analysis of common faults. A number of such analyses have been made by Vollmer in an original study at Wellesley College. The material in this section is condensed from portions of her study.[*] It is included in this text as a means of demonstrating to the reader how he can analyze common faults in sport techniques and use these analyses as the basis for his teaching suggestions. Prior to making the analysis of a fault it is essential to note the respects in which the fault differs from the correct form of the technique. The next step is to analyze the fault kinesiologically. This may include both anatomic and mechanical analyses, or it may be limited to either one or the other, depending upon the nature of the fault. The final step is to devise teaching suggestions. These should be the natural and logical outgrowth of the analysis. Practice of this sort should enable the student-teacher to think analytically about his teaching and should sharpen his awareness of cause and effect relationships. Being fore-warned of the nature and cause of the faults, he should be able to teach the techniques in such a way that his pupils will avoid the common faults. If some students do develop them, he will presumably be prepared to make appropriate suggestions for overcoming them.

FAULT IN THE CRAWL STROKE: RIGID FLUTTER KICK

Description. In the rigid flutter kick the movement is one of alternate flexion and extension of the entire lower extremity, with the movement confined to the hip joint instead of being transmitted successively through the thigh to the knee joint and thence through the leg to the ankle and foot. The knee joints are fully extended throughout the kick, and the feet and ankles are held in an unchanging position of plantar flexion, the exact degree of this flexion varying with individuals. The swimmer who commits this fault finds that to cover the same distance he has to kick more times than a swimmer who kicks correctly. This results in a narrower kick. A rigid flutter kick is obviously less efficient than the correct kick. In brief, the rigid flutter kick deviates from the correct form in that there is an absence of knee and ankle flexion, an absence of relaxation at the end of the downkick or beginning of the upkick, and an absence of "fishtail" action of the sole of the foot against the water.

---

[*]Used by permission of Mrs. Lola Vollmer Shepherd.

Anatomic Analysis. In the correct downkick the upward pressure of the water against the lower leg causes flexion at the knee. In the rigid kick, however, this is prevented by the tension of the quadriceps extensors. Normally the slight flexion at the knee is followed by extension during the course of the downstroke, but when the knee is already rigidly extended, this extension cannot take place. Similarly, the reduction of plantar flexion which should take place at the end of the downstroke fails to occur because of the continuous contraction of the plantar flexor muscles (soleus, peroneus longus and brevis, tibialis posterior, flexor digitorum longus and flexor hallucis longus).

In the upstroke the tension of the quadriceps extensors again prevents the slight knee flexion which occurs when the kick is correctly performed. (See Figs. 23–2 and 23–3.) Throughout the stroke the extensors of the lower back and the abdominal muscles contract to stabilize the pelvis against the pull of the hip flexors and extensors. Normally they relax momentarily just before the legs reverse their direction. The tension in the muscles of the lower extremities spreads to these, however, and the excess tension of these muscles causes interference with the action of the diaphragm. This, in turn, results in less efficient breathing and is an additional factor in causing fatigue.

Mechanical Analysis. The propulsive component of force which drives the body forward is that which pushes the water directly backward. In the downstroke this is provided most effectively by the instep of the foot, and in the upstroke, by the sole. The amount of propulsive force developed depends upon the angle at which the instep and the sole of the foot are held with respect to the surface of the water. In the upstroke the best angle for the sole of the foot is possible only when the knee is slightly flexed. In the rigid kick the knee is straight, and the sole of the foot is therefore not in the best position for providing propulsive force.

In the correct form each limb acts as a series of levers—thigh, lower leg and foot—but in the rigid kick each limb acts as one long lever with the force arm extending from the distal attachments of the hip flexors and extensors to the axis of the hip joint. The resistance arm consists of the entire length of the lever from the instep or from the sole of the foot to the hip joint. The force acting on this lever comes solely from the muscles of the hip joints. The muscles of the knee and ankle do not contribute to the motion of this lever but when the limb is used as a series of levers, they provide additional force.

Inertia must be overcome with each reversal of direction in the kick. Since, in the rigid flutter kick, the stroke is shorter and faster than it should be, the muscles of the hip joint, which have the double task of overcoming both the inertia of the limb and the resistance of the water, are overburdened. They must work harder and faster to meet the demands made on them by the frequent changes of direction and the increased resistance of the water due to the speed of movement. Ordinarily the upstroke has an advantage over the downstroke because, when the stroke is performed correctly, the sole of the foot

is in a better position to push back against the water than is the instep
on the downstroke. In the rigid kick this advantage is lost.

Teaching Suggestions. "The rigid crawl flutter kick is associated with undue tension of the quadriceps extensors at the knee joint,
and of the plantar flexors at the ankle joint, during the changes of
direction in both the downkick and the upkick. There may also be
unnecessary tension of the abdominal muscles and the spinal extensors. As the kick is inefficient, it is carried on at a faster rate and
through a narrower arc than would be the correct kick for the individual swimmer. Conversely, a rapid, narrow kick tends to be a rigid
kick. These factors aid in its recognition. In the teaching of the kick,
it would seem the best procedure to insist on a slow, deep kick in the
student's first attempts, and to increase the rhythm gradually to the
desired rate. Motivation should not be directed toward speed in the
performance of the 'kick glide' in the teaching progression. Neither is
it desirable to emphasize that the legs be held straight at the knees.
The emphasis should be put on the increased action at the hips and at
the ankles. Furthermore, land drills to increase ankle flexibility seem
to be advisable."[15]

FAULT IN ARCHERY: CREEPING ON THE RELEASE

Description. The fault known as creeping may be caused by
either arm. It may be due to a forward movement of the right hand
prior to, or at the moment of, the release; or it may be due to the
relaxation of the left arm at both the shoulder and the elbow joints.
If the creeping is due to the right arm, the normal follow-through
is omitted entirely; if it is due to the left arm, the follow-through is
reduced because of the loss of tension between the bow and the string
preceding the release.

Anatomic Analysis. The arms are maintained at shoulder
level by the deltoid and supraspinatus muscles and are drawn back in
horizontal extension chiefly by the posterior deltoid, infraspinatus and
teres minor, assisted by the latissimus dorsi. The scapulae are strongly
adducted by the rhomboids and middle trapezius. Both the horizontal
extension of the arm and the adduction of the scapula are stronger on
the side of the drawing arm than of the bow arm. The muscles of the
drawing arm are in phasic contraction, whereas those of the bow arm
are in static contraction. The elbow extensors and the ulnar flexors
of the wrist are in strong static contraction to resist the pressure of the
bow.

When creeping is the fault of the right arm (i.e., the drawing
arm), it is caused by premature relaxation or by lengthening contraction of the scapular adductors and the horizontal extensors of the
shoulder joint. This results in insufficient resistance to the pull of the
string. When creeping is the fault of the left, or bow, arm, it is caused

by tiring, and consequent relaxation, of the muscles which must resist the pressure of the bow, particularly the triceps muscle.

Mechanical Analysis. "Creeping before or during the release reduces the tension between the string and the bow, and thereby reduces the potential energy which the string has acquired. Thus the amount of force imparted to the arrow by the string is decreased. Furthermore, this fault introduces a variable factor, as the amount of creeping will tend to vary with each shot.

"A study has been made on the effect of creeping when the archer holds his anchor and aims correctly.[8] A reduced draw, or a creep, of one half inch resulted in hits 5.9 inches below the target center at forty yards, and 9.4 inches below the center at fifty yards. A creep of three quarters of an inch resulted in hits 8.8 inches below the center of the target at forty yards and 13.8 inches below at fifty yards."[15]

Teaching Suggestions. The student should be instructed to keep drawing actively with the right arm and to be constantly aware of the pull between his shoulder blades until after the release. Absence of a follow-through is usually an indication of creeping. Since creeping may be caused by using too heavy a bow, the teacher should check to see that the bow is the right weight for the student. He should also make sure that the student has a correct anchor and that he is not holding the draw position too long. If the student has difficulty finding his aim, he should relax his draw and rest a moment before drawing again.

If the student-teacher will select a number of common faults, comparable to those just cited, and will analyze them in a similar manner, he will find this practice to be of value in helping him to become more observant and analytical in his teaching and coaching.

USE OF KINESIOLOGIC EXPLANATIONS IN THE TEACHING OF SPORT SKILLS

Physical education teachers have found that their students learn sport skills more rapidly and practice them more intelligently when they have at least a rudimentary knowledge of the basic principles which underlie successful performance.[9, 12, 13] The student of kinesiology should keep this in mind and, as he reviews the anatomic and mechanical principles of movement, should think of ways of explaining them in simplified terms. This is a practical application of kinesiology which has received all too little attention in the past.

As an illustration of the way simplified kinesiologic explanations and demonstrations may be utilized by the sports instructor in his teaching, a portion of an original study by McAuley is presented below (by permission of Janet McAuley) in somewhat abridged form.[11]

Softball Overhand Throw*

Kinesiologic Explanations   *Demonstrations*

Leverage

The ball is held in the finger tips because the fingers lengthen the throwing lever. The improved leverage serves to increase the speed that can be developed. The longer the lever, the greater the speed that can be developed at its end. Hence the greater the momentum that can be imparted to the ball.

To demonstrate the difference between using a short and a long lever in throwing a softball, have the students throw, first using just the hand and forearm, and then using the entire arm.

Movement of the Body

The weight shifts to the right foot in the preparatory phase so that in the actual throw the momentum caused by the forward shifting weight can be added to the ball as it leaves the hand. The rotation of the trunk to the right in the preparatory phase ensures a larger arc to swing through in the delivery phase.

To demonstrate the value of the weight shift and rotation in throwing a softball, have the students throw, first with a narrow stance and without moving the feet or shifting the weight, and then using the correct form. They should compare the two methods with respect to the distance of the ball's flight.

Angle of Release

If distance is desired, the ball should be released at approximately a 45-degree angle from the horizontal. This assures sufficient vertical force to overcome the force of gravity, yet at the same time provides optimum horizontal force. If the ball is to be thrown a short distance at maximum speed, it should be released in as nearly a horizontal direction as possible.

To demonstrate the effect of the angle of release on the flight of the ball, have the students throw balls, releasing them at various angles and note the results. If they work in pairs, the partner can check on the angle of release.

Volley Ball Underhand Serve

Relation of Body Position to Flight of Ball

To assure a straight forward swing with the right arm moving in the sagittal plane, the feet are pointed forward toward the net. A moderate stride, with the left foot slightly forward, assures stability for the serve.

The teacher should demonstrate the effect of body position on the flight of the ball, and show how a side-arm swing is required if the side is turned to the net. Note that a ball thus hit will be directed to the side of the court. Have the class try standing incorrectly a few times and serve with some side-arm action, and then have them practice correctly, swinging straight through to the opposite court.

*The authority for all the sport skills referred to in this section is *Team Sports for Girls and Women,* by Meyer and Schwartz.[12]

Relation of Stance to Application of Force

A moderate stride with the left foot slightly forward, the left knee slightly flexed, and the weight over the right foot enables the server to shift the weight forward toward the end of the serve. This contributes to greater force in hitting the ball, hence to greater speed of the ball in its flight.

The teacher should demonstrate the way a stiff forward knee acts as a brake to the momentum of the body and necessitates "tipping over" the stiff leg. Point out the way this "tipping" action tends to make the player hit up and to lose momentum. Have the class concentrate for a while on bending the left knee as they practice serving.

Effect of Hitting Ball Off-Center

The direction taken by the ball after it has been struck is determined in part by the angle of contact. For a straight flight, the ball must be hit directly behind its center with the hand moving in the desired direction of flight. In order to hit the ball properly it should be held at the right side of the body.

The teacher should hit the ball first to the left of its center, and then to the right. The students should note the effect on the ball's flight. The effect of hitting off-center can be shown even more clearly by placing the ball on the floor and hitting it gently, first to the left of its center, then to the right, and then in line with its center.

Angle of Application of Force

If the force is applied to the ball at a 45-degree angle from the horizontal, both optimum horizontal distance and height are assured. The ball then has equal forward and upward components of motion. The upward component carries the ball high enough for it to clear the net, and the forward component carries it an adequate distance onto the court. The application of force to the ball at a 45-degree angle depends upon the height at which it is held by the left hand, as well as upon the movement of the right hand. The ball should be hit about midway between center back and bottom. If the ball is contacted from beneath, its flight has too large a vertical component. If it is contacted too high, the horizontal component is too large. These two faults result respectively either in netting the ball, or in causing it to "pop up." If the ball succeeds in crossing the net on a "pop-up," it usually drops so close to the net on the other side that the front line players are able to spike it.

Demonstrate hitting the ball:
1. Midway between center back and bottom;
2. From beneath;
3. Too high.

Have the class note the flight of the ball resulting from each kind of hit. Then have the class work in pairs and take turns practicing serving, attempting to hit the ball at a 45-degree angle. The partner should stand at the side and announce the approximate angle at which each ball is struck. Both partners should note the effect of this angle on the flight of the ball, with reference both to direction and to distance.

Relation of Length of Lever to Speed of Backswing

The right arm is slightly flexed at the elbow to facilitate rapid completion of the backswing. This is based on the principle that "the shorter the lever, the more rapidly it can be moved." If the arm is straight on the

The instructor should provide himself with two laths or similar sticks. One of these should be sawed in half and the two pieces nailed together at right angles to each other. To demonstrate the relation of the length of the backswing, the swing will take longer and the reversal of direction will be more difficult because more momentum is developed. This additional momentum is likely to cause loss of balance.

lever to the speed of the swing, both the straight and the bent levers should be suspended by one end, lifted together through approximately a 90-degree arc, and then allowed to swing free. The class should note the difference in the speed of their swings.

APPLICATIONS OF KINESIOLOGIC PRINCIPLES TO THE TEACHING OF NEW SKILLS

When the physical education instructor presents a new skill to his class, he will find his teaching more effective if he can point out to his students the similarities between the new skill and a skill with which they are already familiar. Broer made a helpful contribution to this problem by identifying three basic arm patterns used in throwing, striking and rolling skills — underarm, overarm and sidearm — and by pointing out the similarity of mechanical principles and anatomic action involved in the skills within each pattern. In the sidearm pattern, for example, the similarities in three such diverse sport skills as a basketball throw, a tennis drive and baseball batting, were striking.[2]

In a later book, Broer and Houtz reported the results of their electromyographic studies of selected sport skills representing the three patterns mentioned. These gave dramatic evidence of the similarity in the muscular activity that took place in the skills within a given pattern.[3] The implications for the physical education instructor should be obvious.

If the physical education instructor is confronted with the problem of teaching a sport with which he has had little or no experience, he will find that by analyzing it kinesiologically and noting the similarity of the skills involved to skills with which he is already familiar that his problem will already be half solved. As has already been suggested, the value of a classification, such as that found on page 14, is that it enables the instructor to see basic similarities. An awareness of these similarities helps him to recognize the kinesiologic principles which apply to the unfamiliar skill.

Let us assume, for instance, that an instructor is given the assignment of teaching soccer, a sport with which he has had no experience. He has, however, had considerable experience both in playing and in teaching football, baseball and basketball. His first step is to study the rule book and any other books he can find on soccer. If he can observe a game or a film, it will be helpful. His next step should be to identify the various skills involved in soccer, such as running, punting, trapping, and so on. He should then analyze these to see to which category of skill each belongs and to discover the principles which apply to each technique. In the skills involving the giving of impetus he should note whether the emphasis is on distance, speed or direction, and should select the appropriate principles. Whatever the technique under consideration, he should discover how the principles can be applied without violating the limitations of the prescribed form. In field hockey, for instance, the principles of giving impetus to an external object need to be modified when they are applied to a drive in order to conform to the ruling concerning "sticks." This kind of preparation for teaching an unfamiliar sport will give the instructor a basis for confidence which he might not otherwise possess, and will greatly add to the effectiveness of his teaching.

This chapter has attempted to give examples of various ways in which kinesiology may be applied by the physical educator to some of the problems related to the teaching of activities. No attempt has been made to present a series of analyses of the different sports because it is believed that the student will gain more by working these out for himself than by looking up a ready-made analysis in a textbook and applying it to his particular needs.

During the past ten or fifteen years a wealth of material has appeared in the literature and in the research reports presented at physical education conventions. Electromyographic studies and mechanical analyses have been made of nearly every familiar sport, track and field event, and gymnastic activity. The major student and the young instructor will find it well worth their time to keep a notebook on each activity they teach, adding appropriate material whenever it appears. In the course of time they will build up a reservoir of kinesiologic material which will be of invaluable help in teaching, coaching, and problem solving.

SUPPLEMENTARY MATERIAL

Effect of Knowledge of Mechanical Principles on Performance
One question of particular interest to the kinesiologically oriented physical education instructor is, "Is an understanding of the pertinent mechanical principles related to improvement in the performance of athletic skills?" This question was investigated by Mohr and Barrett in relation to four swimming strokes taught at the intermediate level to women college students.[13]

An experimental group of 15 young women were taught the essential mechanical principles that apply to the front crawl, back crawl, side, and elementary back strokes. A control group of 16 were given no information regarding these principles. Both groups, previously equated with respect to ability, received the same instruction in the performance of these four strokes. At the end of the 14 week period of testing and instruction it was found that the experimental group had improved significantly in front crawl sprint, side stroke power, and form ratings for the front crawl, back crawl, and side strokes. The investigators concluded that the results of the study supported the hypothesis that exposing students to an understanding and application of mechanical principles would effect greater improvement than instruction without reference to the principles. They wisely recommended that additional studies be conducted, covering a longer period of time and using larger samples. While the results were gratifying, the investigators admitted that more evidence was needed with respect to the general hypothesis that knowledge of mechanical principles would facilitate the learning of motor skills.

Cinematographic and Mechanical Analysis of Hitting a Baseball. Race conducted this study using 17 professional players who were proficient batters. Only those films were used for analysis that showed effective hitting, the portion of the film so used being limited to the phases of batting from the beginning movement toward the ball to the moment of contact with the ball. The mechanical analysis was based on measurements of velocity of the bat and of different portions of the body. The films were taken at a uniform speed and all subjects used a bat of similar weight. Hence variations in velocity were assumed to be due to individual differences in form and speed of bodily movements. The results indicated that the bat's velocity increased sharply as it approached the ball. Measurements showed that in the effective hitting of this group of experts the hips moved forward at a greater velocity than the striding foot, and the hands and wrists at a greater velocity than the hips. It was also indicated that bodily lean (i.e., weight shift toward ball) appeared to be an important factor in the generation of hitting force.[14]

EMG Study of Batting. Kitzman investigated the actions of the clavicular portion of the pectoralis major, the triceps and the left latissimus dorsi in the forward swing of batting, using as subjects two skilled and two unskilled batters. Photographs were also taken of different phases of the swing. The superior mechanics used by the skilled subjects were obvious in the pictures. One of the unskilled subjects failed to stride toward the ball, and the other took such a long stride that the momentum from his body was obtained at the expense of momentum from his hands and wrists. The skilled subjects were more consistent than the unskilled.[10]

The electromyograms showed that in most instances the peak of muscular action came earlier in the skilled batters than in the unskilled. Although the investigator did not imply this, it would seem that this indicated a more ballistic movement than that used by the unskilled batters. The long head of the left triceps muscle recorded the greatest action potentials for all the subjects. From this, the investigator concluded that right-handed baseball batters could increase their batting force by strengthening this muscle.

ASSIGNMENTS AND PROJECTS

1. Select a team sport, e.g., baseball, field hockey, football, or basketball, and list all the types of skills involved. (Refer to the classification of motor skills on page 14.)

2. Make an analysis of the muscular action of a straight back-

swing in the tennis forehand drive. (The description was given earlier in this chapter. See pages 431ff.)

3. Analyze the difference, in terms of joint and muscular action, between a forehand drive with a straight backswing and one with a circular backswing.

4. Make a kinesiologic analysis of the following sport techniques:
a. Chest pass in basketball
b. Side-arm pass in basketball
c. Drive in golf
d. Batting a baseball
e. Pitching a baseball
f. Crouching start in sprinting
g. Standing broad jump
h. Breast stroke in swimming

Note: In an analysis of a sport technique it will be extremely helpful if motion pictures can be used, particularly if they have been taken in slow motion.

5. Observe the following paired activities and contrast them both anatomically and mechanically.
a. Serve in tennis and in badminton
b. Shot put and baseball throw for distance
c. Standing broad jump and Sargent vertical jump
d. Running front dive and jackknife dive
e. Rowing forward and rowing backward

6. Indicate the mechanical similarities and dissimilarities in throwing a baseball, batting a baseball, serving a volley ball, bowling, and a forehand drive in tennis. Note that all involve a ballistic movement of the arms.

7. Select some sport techniques, such as those mentioned in questions 4 and 5, and observe several performers executing them. The subjects should represent a wide range in ability. Detect the differences in their form and draw up a list of suggestions for each of the poorer performers.

8. Observe several individuals as they swim and look for the application of the principles listed.

9. Analyze any of the standard strokes, e.g., breast, side, elementary back, back crawl, etc. Either observe or practice the stroke before analyzing it.

10. Analyze other forms of aquatic locomotion, e.g., paddling and rowing. Either observe or practice each before analyzing it.

11. Analyze the following common faults kinesiologically and suggest coaching points to avoid or to correct each fault: insufficient body pivot in golf drive, too wide a pull with the arms in the breast stroke, hitting the left arm on the release in archery, a short, choppy stroke in paddling, "catching a crab" in crew rowing.

12. Select a single sport technique and write an elementary explanation of the pertinent kinesiologic principles. This should be worded in such a way that it could be used as teaching material for high school boys or girls.

13. Select a sport with which you have had no experience (e.g., men might select field hockey, and women, football). Identify each skill involved in the sport selected; state its classification (see p. 14), and list several principles which apply to each of the skills identified.

REFERENCES

1. Armbruster, D. A., Allen, R. H., and Billingsley, H. S.: Swimming and Diving, 5th ed. St. Louis, C. V. Mosby Co., 1968.
2. Broer, M. R.: Efficiency of Human Movement, 2nd ed. Philadelphia, W. B. Saunders Company, 1966.
3. Broer, M. R., and Houtz, S. J.: Patterns of Muscular Activity in Selected Sport Skills. Springfield, Ill., Charles C Thomas, Publisher, 1967.
4. Counsilman, J. E.: The Science of Swimming. Englewood Cliffs, N. J., Prentice-Hall, Inc., 1968.
5. Gowitzke, B. A.: Kinesiological and neurophysiological principles applied to gymnastics. *In* Kinesiology Review 1968, Washington, D.C., Am. Assn. Health, Phys. Ed. & Recrn., 1968.
6. Harris, M. M.: Basic Swimming Analyzed. Boston, Allyn and Bacon, Inc., 1969.
7. Hennessy, J. T.: Trampolining. Dubuque, Wm. C. Brown Company Publishers, 1968.
8. Hickman, C. N. et al.: Archery, the Technical Side. Milwaukee, North American Press, 1947.
9. Huelster, L. J.: Learning to analyze performance. J. Health & Phys. Ed., *10*:120–121, 1939.
10. Kitzman, E. W.: Baseball: Electromyographic study of batting swing. Res. Quart. Am. Assn. Health, Phys. Ed. & Recrn., 35:166–178, 1964.
11. McAuley, J. E.: Application of Mechanical Principles to Methods of Teaching Selected Sports Techniques. Unpublished Master's 350 study, Wellesley College, 1950.
12. Meyer, M. H., and Schwartz, M. M.: Team Sports for Girls and Women, 4th ed. Philadelphia, W. B. Saunders Company, 1965.
13. Mohr, D. R., and Barrett, M. E.: Effects of knowledge of mechanical principles in learning to perform intermediate swimming skills. Res. Quart. Am. Assn. Health, Phys. Ed. & Recrn., 33:574–580, 1962.
14. Race, D. E.: Cinematographic and mechanical analysis of the external movements involved in hitting a baseball effectively. Res. Quart. Am. Assn. Health, Phys. Ed. & Recrn., 32:394–404, 1961.
15. Vollmer, L. T.: Kinesiological Analysis of Common Faults in Selected Activities. Unpublished master's study. Wellesley College, 1951.

RECOMMENDED READINGS

Bunn, J. W.: Scientific Principles of Coaching. Englewood Cliffs, N.J., Prentice-Hall, Inc., 1959.
Counsilman, J. E.: The Science of Swimming. Englewood Cliffs, N.J., Prentice-Hall, Inc., 1968. Chapter 1.
Dyson, G. H. G.: The Mechanics of Athletics, 3rd ed. London, University of London Press Ltd., 1964.
Groves, W. H.: Mechanical analysis of diving. Res. Quart. Am. Assn. Health, Phys. Ed. & Recrn., *21*:132–144, 1950.
Lanoue, F.: Analysis of the basic factors involved in fancy diving. Res. Quart. Am. Assn. Health, Phys. Ed. & Recrn., *11*:102–109, 1940.

CHAPTER 24

Motor Skills of Daily Living

Kinesiology is not limited to the sports field, corrective gymnasium and treatment room. It has its place in the home, in the garden, on the farm, in the office and in the shop. Wherever man moves, kinesiology and body mechanics are applicable. Man uses his body constantly. Either he observes the principles of good body mechanics or he violates them. To the extent that he observes these principles, his motions contribute to a strong, efficient upright body; to the extent that he violates them, his motions pave the way for postural strains, abnormal tensions and other pathologic conditions of the bones, joints and muscles. The kinesiologist—be he physical education instructor, physical therapist, occupational therapist or athletic coach—has a real responsibility in pointing out and demonstrating the applications of the basic principles of body mechanics to all the daily life skills. Along with learning how to swim an efficient crawl stroke, serve a tennis ball with speed and accuracy, or drive a golf ball with force and precision, the individual needs to master the more modest skills of lifting a heavy package, moving a large piece of furniture, and using a spade, hoe, rake, broom or vacuum cleaner with efficiency and safety. He should learn to perform these skills both from the point of view of the results accomplished and from the point of view of using his body effectively and without strain. Poor body mechanics means not only a task poorly done, but also a poor machine for doing the task. And conversely, good body mechanics means not only a task efficiently done, but also a strong, capable machine for doing it.

If it is desirable to use the body efficiently in sports and exercises, it is infinitely more desirable to use it efficiently in the movements which characterize one's daily occupation.

The majority of the daily life skills may be classified under the following categories:

1. Locomotion, including ascending and descending.
2. Stooping to reach a lower level; taking a seat; rising.
3. Lifting and carrying.
4. Moving heavy objects by pushing and pulling.
5. Working with long-handled implements (such as those used for housecleaning, gardening, wood chopping and snow clearing).

455

6. Working with small implements and materials at a work surface.

On studying this list it is seen that practically every phase of kinesiology is represented. A complete analysis of representative activities from each category would necessitate a repetition of a large portion of the first two parts of this book. Hence, the procedure adopted is a discussion of the major kinesiologic problems involved and the application of the most noteworthy anatomic and mechanical principles to a few sample activities.

Locomotion, Ascending and Descending. (Fig. 24–1).   Principles which apply to locomotion are presented in Chapters 7 and 22. The problems in the more common uses of locomotion have to do with the anatomic aspects, rather than the mechanical. The alignment of the weight-bearing joints is just such a problem. Poor alignment causes strain and fatigue. If locomotion forms a relatively large portion of a person's daily occupation, the good alignment of his feet, knees, hips and spine is of utmost importance.

One specific problem relating to locomotion in the home is the problem of safety when there is insufficient friction between the feet and the supporting surface. Wet linoleum and scatter rugs on polished floors are familiar everyday hazards. An appreciation of the effects of the horizontal component of force in walking and running would make one more aware of the danger and more cautious in one's locomotion about the house.

Housekeeping frequently involves going up and down stairs. The major problem in going up is economy of effort; in coming down the chief problem is safety. Economy of effort in going up can be achieved by keeping the center of gravity forward, thus minimizing the resistance arm of the thigh lever, and by avoiding superfluous joint and muscle action, such as that involved in plantar flexion of the foot. The most economical way of climbing stairs, therefore, is by inclining the body slightly forward (preferably from the feet, not the

A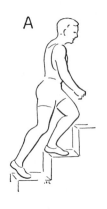

B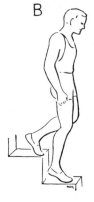

Figure 24–1.   Going up and down stairs.

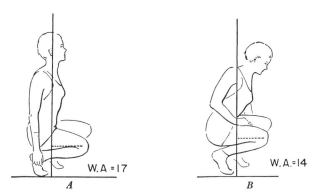

Figure 24–2. Stooping. *A,* Attempting to keep the trunk vertical; *B,* inclining the body slightly forward. (*W.A.* = the weight arm of the thigh lever.)

hips) and by depending upon extension at the knee for lifting the body, rather than extension (plantar flexion) in the ankle joint.

Descending the stairs with safety can be accomplished by keeping the center of gravity approximately over the center of the base of support. Both hurrying and leaning too far forward endanger the equilibrium by causing the line of gravity to come precariously close to the anterior margin of support. Hurrying also increases the danger due to other factors, such as high heels and slippery surfaces.

Stooping, Being Seated and Rising. (Figs. 24–2, 24–3 and 24–4.) The chief problems here are economy of effort, maintaining equilibrium, and avoiding strain. So far as stooping is concerned, these three objectives are interrelated. In taking a seat there may be a more economical way than the one in which equilibrium is preserved, but it is scarcely acceptable from the point of view of aesthetics or social custom.

In stooping to pick up something from the floor or from a low shelf, stability is enhanced if the feet are slightly separated, both laterally and anteroposteriorly. This serves to enlarge the base of support. To perform the movement with maximum efficiency and minimum danger of strain requires that the stooping should be effected by bending at the knees and inclining the trunk slightly forward. The thigh thus becomes the major lever involved. The fulcrum of this lever is the center of motion at the knee joint, the force is furnished by the knee extensors and is applied at their average point of proximal attachment (not the distal, because the thigh is being extended on the lower leg rather than the leg on the thigh) and the resistance is the weight of the body, represented by the line of gravity. Its point of application to the lever depends upon the position of the body. When the trunk is inclined slightly forward, the line of gravity falls through the approximate center of the base of support. This assures a shorter weight arm (i.e., the horizontal distance from the fulcrum to the line of gravity) than is the case when the trunk is held vertically erect. Given a lever in which the force arm and the weight are constant, an increase in the weight arm will necessitate an increase in the force required to balance the lever. Thus stooping with the trunk held in a vertical or near-vertical position actually requires more muscular effort than does stooping with the trunk inclined slightly forward. Figure 24–2 illustrates the two styles of stooping. The position of the line of gravity with reference to the base of support was actually found for the subject in each of these positions and the weight arm of the lever measured. In the original photographs (3⅞ by 2¾ inches) the weight arm in Figure 24–2, A, was 17 mm. and in B, 14 mm. Since the 100-cm. board measured 66 mm. in the photograph, the actual difference in the two weight arms was approximately 4.5 cm. (See p. 16.)

When one bends from the waist to reach the floor, the center of gravity is considerably higher than when one stoops; hence the body is in a less stable position (Fig. 24–3). The close position of the feet also decreases stability. The leverage is not clear-cut. The trunk seems to be the major lever in the motion, but it fails to meet the requirements of a lever in that it is not a rigid bar. It is a flexible bar, turning about the common axis of the two hip joints, and at the same time flexing within itself. The most obvious mechanical disadvantage of this method of reaching the floor is that the horizontal position of the upper trunk permits the force of gravity to act on it with a maximal rotatory component. This requires strong action of the spinal extensors to stabilize the flexible spine, and of the hip joint extensors to control the movement of the trunk as a whole at the hip joints. The strong extensors of the knee, located on the front of the thigh, give no help at all in this movement. All the work is performed by the extensors of the hip and spine. Furthermore, the spinal muscles work in a stretched position. The "approved" method of stooping, by bending the knees and inclining the body slightly forward, has the advantage of giving the major portion of the work to the strong knee and hip extensors, with only a small share taken by the extensors of the spine. This method calls upon the spinal extensors to make a reasonable contribution to the movement, but it does not subject them to strain, nor does it require that they work in a stretched position.

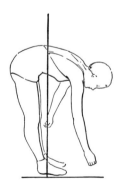

Figure 24–3. Bending from the waist to reach the floor.

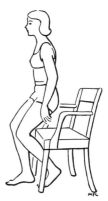

Figure 24–4. In seating oneself gracefully the body is balanced and the movement is controlled.

In seating oneself gracefully, the major problem is to provide a base of support which will remain under the backward-shifting center of gravity. When the style of the chair permits, this can be accomplished by placing one foot well back under the chair, bending at the knees and inclining the body forward just enough to keep the center of gravity over the base of support (Fig. 24–4). The body will be eased into the chair, rather than dropped into it, if the knee extensors are made to control the movement against the pull of gravity. In rising from the chair the problem is to provide immediately a base of support with the feet, so that the transfer of weight can be made gradually instead of suddenly by throwing the body forward or by depending upon the hands for a push-off from the seat of the chair. This is accomplished by placing one foot well back under the chair, inclining the body slightly forward, pushing the feet down against the floor and extending the knees. As the knees are extended the weight is gradually shifted from the rear to the forward foot.

It is more difficult to keep the base of support under the center of gravity when seating oneself on a chair with a low rung or a solid front. With a straight chair having a low rung in front it is possible to put one foot back close to the side of the chair instead of under it and then to lower oneself onto the side of the seat, later shifting to the center. When taking a seat in a deep upholstered chair or davenport which has a solid front, a different technique must be used. With these the only way to keep the base of support under the center of gravity is to stand with the side to the seat, place the near foot forward, bend the knees and lower oneself obliquely onto the front edge of the seat, turning slightly forward at the last moment. One or two additional movements are then needed to complete the forward facing and to get the body well back on the seat. In rising, the reverse procedure is followed. The body is shifted forward and turned sideways; the near foot is placed forward and the other foot backward; the weight is shifted over the feet, the feet pushed down against the floor and the legs and thighs extended.

Lifting and Carrying. (Figs. 24–5, 24–6, 24–7 and 24–8.)   In addition to the problems involved in stooping to reach the object, lifting a heavy object from the floor involves the dual problems of keeping the weight arm of the lever used for lifting as short as possible, and the angle at which the gravitational force applies to the lever as small as possible. This is in the interest both of economy of effort and of reducing the likelihood of strain. When the arm used for lifting is in a horizontal position, whether flexed or extended at the elbow, the gravitational force pulls at right angles to the lever. This means that the force is completely rotatory, and the *true* weight arm of the lever (the perpendicular distance) is coincidental with the *apparent* weight arm. Since $F \times FA = W \times WA$, the longer the weight arm, the more force it takes to balance the lever, other things being equal. If the object were held in the hand with the arm fully extended horizontally, the weight arm of the lever would be extremely long — approximately 30 inches. Great muscular force would be required to balance the lever under these conditions. One instinctively avoids lifting a heavy object in this uneconomical manner, but not everyone recognizes that the most economical manner of lifting is the exact reverse of the above: namely, by keeping the lifting arm vertical, or nearly so, and holding the object as close to the body's line of gravity as possible (Fig. 24–5, A).

In the discussion of stooping, attention was called to the fact that bending over from the waist to reach the floor is not only mechanically disadvantageous, but also requires strong action of the extensors of the spine and hips, and that the spinal muscles are made to work on a stretch. If the body is used in this manner for lifting a heavy object, an additional burden is put upon the muscles of the back, one that they can ill afford to take (Fig. 24–5, B). Strait, Inman and Ralston have made the interesting observation that bending from the waist to touch the floor, without flexing the knees, creates a tensile force of 450 pounds in the erector spinae muscle and a compressional force of nearly 500 pounds on the fifth lumbar vertebra. If a 50-pound weight is held in the hands, the tensile force is increased to 750 pounds and

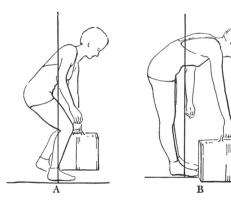

Figure 24–5.   Picking up a suitcase. A, Efficiently; B, inefficiently.

A   B

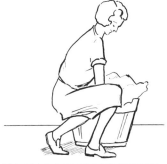

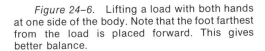

Figure 24–6. Lifting a load with both hands at one side of the body. Note that the foot farthest from the load is placed forward. This gives better balance.

the compressional force to 850 pounds.[1] The spinal extensors are not powerful muscles and are easily strained. It is unintelligent to expose them to the danger of strain when this can be avoided by observing the principles of good mechanics.

In addition to efficient leverage and prevention of backstrain, the stability of the body should be considered. When lifting a suitcase, for instance, one should stand close beside it, the feet in an easy forward-backward stance, with the foot on the far side placed forward. Then if the suitcase proves to be heavier than expected, the near foot can be shifted slightly sideward and balance will quickly be restored. If the near foot is forward, however, it is impossible to do this and the lifter is likely to lose his balance and fall over his own feet.

The same principles of leverage that apply to lifting a heavy object apply also to carrying it. In carrying a weight there is the further problem of assuming a balanced position with the center of gravity centered over the base of support. During the process of lifting, the equilibrium is temporarily disturbed. Once the body is erect, however, it should adjust itself in such a way that it compensates for the load and the new center of gravity (of body and load combined) is above the center of the supporting base. For instance, when one carries a heavy suitcase, it is no longer good body mechanics to keep the body erect with the head and spine carried in the midsagittal plane of the body. In the presence of a heavy unilateral load, good mechanics requires a compensatory movement, e.g., lifting the arm or inclining the trunk to the opposite side. Failure to make this compensation necessitates additional work by the muscles on the opposite side of the trunk (see Figs. 5–6 and 5–7).

In lifting a heavy box down from a high shelf the chief problems are those of avoiding strain and of keeping the movement of the box under control. As the individual tugs on the box to pull it off the shelf he is imparting horizontal momentum to the box. If he pulls quickly or if the box comes free suddenly, as soon as the box is free of the shelf its momentum will be transferred to him. If he is not prepared for this, it may swing his trunk backward and strain his

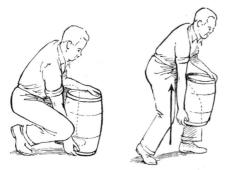

Figure 24–7. A safe and efficient method of lifting a heavy object.

lower back (Fig. 24–8, *A*). To avoid this likelihood he should observe the principles of widening the base of support in the direction of the oncoming force. In other words, he should stand with one foot forward (Fig. 24–8, *B*). This will permit him not only to shift his weight from the forward to the rear foot, but also to take a step backward if necessary. This provides additional space in which the box can lose its horizontal momentum. Whether the box is pulled off the shelf slowly or quickly, there is the problem of maintaining equilibrium when reaching forward for the box and when the weight of the box is first transferred to the hands. For a brief moment, at least, the center of gravity is precariously near the front margin of the base of support.

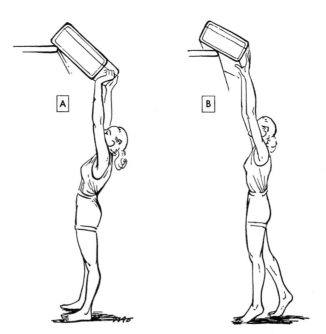

Figure 24–8. Lifting a box down from a high shelf. *A,* Inefficiently; *B,* efficiently.

By placing one foot well forward, the lifter provides an adequate base of support for the anteriorly displaced center of gravity.

Pushing or Pulling Heavy Objects. (Fig. 24–9). The main problem in attempting to move a heavy object either by pushing or by pulling is the efficient application of force. This serves two purposes: first, the successful moving of the object, and, second, the conservation of the mover's energy. There are two factors to be considered in the problem of applying force efficiently. These are the direction of the force, and the point at which it is applied. Whenever feasible, the force should be applied squarely in the direction in which the object is expected to move. When this is not feasible, the undesirable component of force should be as small as possible. For instance, if one desires to push a low trunk across the floor, it would be difficult to stoop low enough to push with the arms in a horizontal position. One should stoop as low as conveniently possible, however, in order to reduce the downward component of force which would tend to increase friction. If it were necessary to move the trunk down a driveway, and no cart or wheelbarrow were available, it would be more efficient to tie a rope to it and to pull it. By using a long rope, the horizontal component of force would be relatively great and the vertical or lifting component relatively small. Some lifting component would actually be desirable because it would serve to reduce friction.

The point at which the pushing or pulling force is applied to the object depends upon which kind of motion is desired, linear or rota-

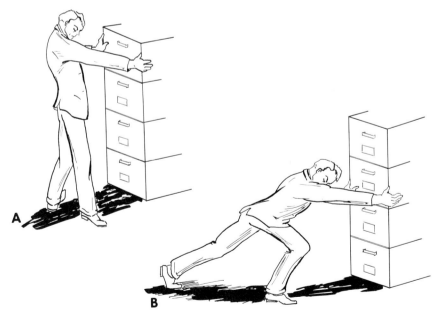

Figure 24–9. Pushing a tall piece of furniture. *A,* Inefficiently; *B,* efficiently. (Notice the low placement of the hands, the horizontal push of the arms, and the use of the rear leg and body weight.)

tory. If one wishes to push a large box or a heavy chair across the floor, he should place his hands in line with the object's center of gravity, provided the amount of friction is inconsequential. This would probably be true of the chair if it had casters. In the case of the box, however, there would probably be considerable friction. In such a situation the force should be applied below the object's center of gravity. The exact spot would have to be determined by experimentation. The criterion would be the object's tendency to tip. There is no tipping in efficient linear motion.

If one wishes to move the box by turning it end over end, he should then place his hands as far above its supporting surface as possible. In this way the box is being used as a lever, with the fulcrum located at its point of contact with the floor. Since the amount of force necessary to turn the box is in inverse proportion to the distance of the hands from the floor (i.e., the force arm of the lever), the higher the hands are placed, the less force is needed. If one wishes to rotate a box horizontally or to move it across the floor by a series of alternating partial rotations, he should place his hands on the top of the box at diagonally opposite corners.

An anatomic principle that applies to pushing and pulling when great force is required is that of using the strong muscles of the body to supplement the weaker ones. This means supplementing the action of the arms with that of the legs. By inclining the body toward the object being pushed, it is possible to add to the force of the push by using the leg extensors. Likewise the force of pulling can be increased by inclining the body away from the object and extending the legs as nearly in a horizontal plane as feasible.

Working with Long-Handled Implements. Working with implements such as a hoe, rake, mop or vacuum cleaner involves a combination of pushing, pulling and, in some instances, lifting. The last is usually only for short distances, but it may occur with considerable frequency. One characteristic of working with implements such as those named is that the body must maintain a more or less fixed posture for relatively long periods of time. This causes tension and fatigue. Hence the chief problem is that of using the body in such a way that tension will be minimized and fatigue postponed as long as possible. If the implement is used back and forth in front of the body, the tendency of the worker is to lean forward. This necessitates static contraction of the extensors of the spine in order to support the trunk against the downward pull of gravity. As implements such as the rake and hoe are lifted at the end of each stroke and carried to position for the next stroke, the force of gravity acts on the implement as well as on the worker's body. Although the implement may not weigh much in itself, its forward position means that the lever has a long weight arm, the effect of which must be balanced by the muscles. This gives an added burden to the back muscles and not infrequently causes a backache. A better method is to stand with the side turned toward the work site and the feet separated in a fairly wide stride, and work the implement from side to side. The reach can then be obtained by bending the knee of the leg on the same side as the implement, and by inclining the body slightly to the same side. Those who are familiar with gymnastics will recognize this as a side lunge position. On the recovery, the knee and the trunk are both straightened. Thus there is an alternating contraction and relaxation of muscles and there is no necessity for any of the trunk muscles to remain in static contraction. Temporary relief can also be obtained by changing sides.

The use of a spade or snow shovel involves primarily the act of lifting. Because the load is taken on the end of a mechanical lever held in a more or less horizontal position, it is inevitable that the weight arm of the lever be relatively long. It can be shortened somewhat, however, by sliding one hand as far down the shaft as possible, using this hand as a fulcrum, and providing the force with the other hand by pushing down on the outer end of the handle. As a variation of this, when getting a particularly heavy load on a shovel, it is possible to bend one knee and brace the shaft against the thigh, thus using the thigh as a fulcrum. This is only for the initial lift, however; the hands must then be shifted to the position previously described in order to carry or throw the load.

Aside from taking and lifting the load on the spade, there is the factor of lowering the body to reach the load and of assuming the erect position for moving it. As in the case of stooping to lift a heavy object from the floor, the chief problems are economy of effort, maintenance of stability and avoidance of strain. These problems are intensified by the additional factor of taking the load on a long-handled implement instead of directly in the hand. As before, separating the feet to widen the base of support, bending at the knees instead of bending from the waist to lower the body and inclining the trunk forward only slightly will respectively increase stability, shorten the anatomic levers involved in the stooping and divide the muscular work among the knee, hip and back extensors intead of making the back muscles assume too large a share of the work. Since the lower back is easily strained by heavy shoveling, it is of great importance to protect it by observing the principles of good body mechanics.

Working with Small Materials and Implements at a Work Surface. The two chief factors to be considered in working with small materials and implements at a work surface are the height of the surface and the position of the materials with reference to the body. So much attention has been given to these in recent years that a detailed discussion would be superfluous. A work surface that is too low makes it necessary for the worker to bend over his work, thus keeping the muscles of his neck and back in static contraction. Hence he becomes fatigued much sooner than he would if he could remain erect. If, on the other hand, the surface is too high, the worker tends to keep his shoulder girdle elevated in order to use his hands effectively. This necessitates contraction of the upper trapezius, levator and rhomboids. If he has to keep his arms elevated for a long time, his deltoid and supraspinatus muscles will be forced to remain in static contraction.

An inefficient arrangement of the materials on the work surface means that the worker has to reach unnecessarily far for some of them and has to make more movements than he would if some thought were given to the advantageous placing of his materials. The time and motion studies by efficiency experts have done much in recent years to show that production can be stepped up considerably by giving attention to small details such as these. Kinesiologically, the problem is a dual one of reducing the length of the reach, thereby reducing the weight arm of the lever (the arms) and of reducing the number of movements, thereby economizing on muscular contractions. These details would not be of great significance for short work periods, but if the motions are repeated hour after hour, attention to these factors makes a great difference in the worker's ability to continue without fatigue.

PROJECTS

1. Experiment to find the best way to shovel snow or dig earth. Describe and analyze the method selected.
2. Experiment to find the best way to pick up and carry a tray of heavy dishes. Describe and analyze the method selected.
3. Experiment to find the best way to pick up and carry a large bag of flour or cement. Describe and analyze the method selected.

REFERENCE

1. Strait, L. A., Inman, V. T., and Ralston, H. J.: Sample illustrations of physical principles selected from physiology and medicine. Am. J. Physics, 15:375–382, 1947.

RECOMMENDED READINGS

Metheny, E. R.: Body Dynamics. New York, McGraw-Hill, Inc., 1952.
Winters, M. C.: Protective Body Mechanics in Daily Life and in Nursing. Philadelphia, W. B. Saunders Company, 1952.

CHAPTER 25

The Prevention of Injury

In all physical activities there is some likelihood of injury. Whether such injury is due to an accident or whether it is due to structural limitations, it can usually be avoided if the proper precautions are taken. Chance plays a relatively small part in injuries resulting from physical activities. "Hindsight" frequently reveals that either a mechanical or a physiological principle was disregarded. Hence familiarity with the principles relating to safety provides the means for preventing such injuries. Acquainting the student with these principles should be as important a part of the physical education program as teaching the activity skills themselves. It is not enough to incorporate the observance of the principles in the technique of the skill; the student should be aware of the principles themselves in order that he may apply them in other situations—in industry, on the street, in the home—wherever and whenever the occasion arises.

The major principles pertaining to the prevention of injury are presented below. They are stated in the form of directions which, if observed, will help to minimize the likelihood of strain and injury.

Principles Relating to the Maintenance of Equilibrium and Prevention of Falls

1. Maintain an adequate base of support.
2. Lower the center of gravity when this is feasible.
3. Keep the center of gravity well centered over the base of support.
4. Increase the size of the base of support in the direction of force or motion.

Principles Relating to the Range of Movement

1. Keep within the normal range of motion for each joint in order to avoid ligamentous and fascial strain. (This requires an understanding of anatomic structures and their limitations.)
2. Strengthen the muscles in order to lessen the likelihood of exceeding the normal range of motion. (For example, strengthen the abdominal muscles in order to help prevent an overthrow in diving.)
3. If attempting to increase the range of motion in a joint or muscle, do it gradually and only after an adequate warm-up.
4. Observe the principles of receiving one's own weight and the impact of external objects in order to avoid joint sprains.

Principles Relating to the Intensity and Quantity of Muscular Exercise

1. Do not exercise past the point of excessive fatigue.

a. Accidents often occur when muscles are fatigued and when the individual is too tired to be alert.

b. Excessive fatigue products in the muscles cause soreness, especially in individuals who are not in good condition.

2. Provide adequate training before permitting participation in strenuous sports. An untrained individual is likely to use his body poorly under the stress of the moment. There should be a careful progression of instruction and practice.

3. Avoid sudden, violent movements whenever possible, and precede all strenuous activity with a warm-up. (Sudden exertion, especially if the muscles are cold, may cause muscle tears.)

4. Observe the principles of receiving, lifting and supporting weights, in order to prevent muscular strain.

Principles Relating to the Transmission of Weight through the Body Segments and Weight-Bearing Joints

1. Provide adequate protection for weak joints.

a. Individuals who have poorly aligned or previously injured joints may have to be excluded from certain activities. (For example, an individual who has knock-knees is likely to have his knees injured in strenuous activities involving running, jumping and bodily contact.)

b. Individuals who have poorly aligned or previously injured joints probably need to wear some form of support or protection.

2. Minimize the rotary components of force. (This requires an awareness of the positions which are likely to put segments under rotatory stress.)

a. If on the hands and knees supporting others, as in a pyramid, the thighs should be perpendicular to the floor.

b. If being supported by another, the weight should be placed in line with the other individual's supporting structures. (For example, a person who is standing on the back of another who is on his hands and knees, should place one foot over the other's shoulders and one over the pelvis.)

3. Only individuals with adequate strength and maturity should support the weight of others.

a. Avoid too great a discrepancy between the strength of the lower man and the weight of the upper man in stunts and pyramids.

b. Avoid using physically immature boys and girls for supporting heavy weights, as in the base of pyramids. (Many of the epiphyses are still not united in teen-aged boys and girls.)

Principles Relating to the Reception of One's Own Weight

1. When landing from a *downward* jump:

a. Insure a gradual loss of kinetic energy by landing on the balls of the feet and immediately letting the ankles, knees and hips bend, controlling the action by means of eccentric contraction of the muscles.

b. Reduce the force of the impact by wearing rubber-soled shoes and by having a soft landing surface.

c. Regain stability by keeping the center of gravity over the center of the base of support on landing. (This may be done by keeping the weight evenly distributed over both feet, or over the hands and feet, and by providing a sufficiently large base of support on landing.)

2. When landing from a *forward* jump and when participating in any activity which involves forward momentum:

a. Insure a gradual loss of the forward kinetic energy by continuing in a roll, run, hop, slide or "frog jump," unless landing in a soft pit, in which case this will not be necessary.

b. Regain stability by providing support in the direction of motion. This is done by landing with the weight forward, using the hands if necessary, in which case the elbows as well as the leg joints should "give."

c. Reduce the force of impact by wearing rubber-soled shoes and by having a soft landing surface.

3. When falling:

a. Insure a gradual loss of the forward kinetic energy by continuing in a roll, slide, or the like, whenever feasible.

b. Absorb the shock of impact (i.e., insure a gradual loss of kinetic energy) by letting the arms "give" as they receive the weight. When falling forward on the knees and catching oneself on the hands, arching the back and turning the face sideward make it possible to rock down on the front of the body without injury. The elbows should bend as soon as the hands touch the floor. This method of self-protection is especially applicable to falling after tripping.

c. Receive the weight on the padded parts of the body, and attempt to land on the various parts in a progressive sequence. For example, after falling on the knee, attempt to fall sideways on the thigh, then onto the side of the arm or the hand which promptly slides out, with the head falling on the extended arm. (This applies particularly to intentional falls in modern dance.)

d. Attempt to land on as large an area of the body as possible in order to minimize the force per square inch.

Principles Relating to Lifting and Carrying External Weights

1. Reduce the rotatory components of weight to a minimum.

a. Get close to the heavy object which is to be lifted from the floor.

b. Carry heavy burdens close to the body.

    (1) A suitcase, with the arm hanging straight down.

    (2) A tray, with elbow bent, forearm vertical, and hand close to shoulder.

    (3) A basket, in the crotch of the elbow with the upper arm vertical.

c. Stoop to reach an object on the floor by bending the knees and inclining the trunk slightly forward.

2. Use the muscles best suited to the task.

For example, when lifting a heavy box from the floor, by stooping as described in *c* above, the strong thigh and buttock muscles will be used, instead of the weaker spine extensors.

3. Insure stability of the body when lifting a heavy suitcase by standing close beside it with the far foot forward. This applies to lifting any heavy object by a handle or cord.

4. Avoid lifting excessive weights.

a. Girls of average strength should not lift weights of more than one quarter or one third of their own body weight, and boys should not lift weights of more than one half of their body weight. These amounts can be increased through training.

b. If an individual wishes to learn to lift heavier weights, he should train gradually.

Principles Relating to Receiving the Impact of External Forces

1. When catching balls and other objects, and when receiving individuals in tumbling and apparatus work:

a. Observe the principles of reducing kinetic energy gradually instead of suddenly.

  (1) "Give" with the arms.
  (2) Shift the weight back from one foot to the other, or take a step backward.
  (3) Move along with the individual when receiving or "spotting" in tumbling and apparatus events.

b. Wear adequate protection, such as a baseball mitt, shin guards, and so on.

c. Put yourself in a favorable position in order to prevent the necessity for overreaching.

d. Point the fingers upward, outward or downward, but not forward.

2. Being hit by a moving body, e.g., a person or a ball:

a. Try to receive the force and ease the shock the same as when catching a ball.

b. Guard against being caught off balance.

c. Wear adequate protection, e.g., shin guards for hockey and padded clothing for football.

d. If possible, avoid lateral blows on the knee, especially when the knee is bearing weight in a flexed position. (This is a common cause of injury to the ligaments and cartilages.)

e. Move along with the striking object. (In boxing this is known as "riding a punch.")

Principles Relating to Circular Motion

1. Since centrifugal force develops in all circular movements, activities such as "snapping the whip," swinging on the flying rings, and so on, should be engaged in only by those who are known to have sufficient strength to keep from being snapped off.

2. Individuals who have a tendency toward chronic dislocation of the shoulder should not be allowed to do strenuous arm circling or swinging movements because of the centrifugal force which develops in such activities.

RECOMMENDED READINGS

Lowman, C. L.: The vulnerable age. J. Health & Phys. Ed., *18*:635–636, 693 (Nov.), 1947.

U. S. Department of Labor, Division of Labor Standards: A Guide to the Prevention of Weight-Lifting Injuries. Special Bulletin No. 11, Washington, D. C., Supt. of Doc., Gov. Printing Office, 1943.

CHAPTER 26

Implications for Teaching

Now that we have this fund of knowledge about human motion, what are we going to do with it? What use are we going to make of it in our teaching careers? There can be no one single answer. Much depends upon the abilities, experience and attitudes of the students we are teaching; much also depends upon the nature of the material to be taught and upon us, ourselves—our experience, our convictions, our philosophy, even our own personalities. The purpose of this concluding chapter is to direct the reader's attention to ways in which the study of kinesiology can contribute meaningfully to effective teaching of physical education.

Looking back on the course that we are now completing, we realize that we have learned something about the mechanism of human movement. We see the body as a living machine functioning in accordance with the universal laws of motion and mechanical principles. We see it as an intricate structure of bones, joints, ligaments and muscles capable of amazing versatility in the movements it can perform. Yet the muscles themselves are only able to pull. Nevertheless, by means of the coordinated action of related segments, each being pulled by the muscles acting upon it, the body as a whole has an almost limitless repertoire of movement patterns. It can not only pull; it can push, lift, strike, throw, kick, walk, run, jump and swim, to name but a few of its amazing capabilities. Note the ways in which these diverse movement patterns can be organized into sports and games, such as tennis, football, or obstacle relay races; gymnastic activities, such as the face vault, the cartwheel, or rope climbing; and the dance, e.g., modern, folk, or tap. These movement patterns are performed with many gradations of skill depending upon the experience and ability of the performer.

The physical education teacher must be prepared to teach a great variety of motor skills. Furthermore, he must teach the ways in which these are modified and combined in order to adapt to the requirements of a particular sport, dance or gymnastic activity. He hopes that his teaching will be such that his students will become proficient both in the individual motor skills and in each total activity of which they form a part. He is vitally concerned, therefore, with knowing the characteristics of skillful performance.

Efficient motion is one of the most important of these. Efficiency refers to the relationship between the amount of work accomplished and the force or energy expended. In mechanics we have seen that efficiency is expressed as the ratio of output to input. In human motion it is the ratio of the external work accomplished to the muscular energy expended. Whereas one of the greatest hindrances to mechanical efficiency is friction, in human motion it is unproductive muscular effort. The poorly coordinated person and the novice tend to make superfluous movements or to tense the muscles unnecessarily. The characteristic of efficient bodily motion is the absence of waste movements, the use of the correct muscles with no more than the needed amount of force, and the relaxation of all muscles which do not contribute either directly or indirectly to the task. It results in smoothness and grace, in what is commonly called well coordinated movement. In relaxation terminology the same quality is known as "differential relaxation." This means simply the ability to relax the unneeded muscles while performing a motor skill. It is an important characteristic of skillful performance, since waste movements and unnecessary tensions not only make for awkward performance, but also hasten the onset of fatigue and increase its intensity. As Steindler has said, ". . . skillful or perfect motion always involves the least expenditure of effort . . ." for the work accomplished.[11] In rapid movements efficiency is characterized by a ballistic type of motion.

Another characteristic of skillful performance is *accuracy.* One may shoot at a basket with a beautifully coordinated and efficient movement, but unless the ball goes into the basket, the player is not considered skillful. Accuracy is based on a combination of factors, namely good judgment of direction, distance and force, proper timing, and good muscular control. It is needed in simple acts such as lifting a forkful of food to the mouth, as well as in more complicated skills such as pole vaulting and pitching a baseball.

Closely related to the characteristics already mentioned are those of *adequate strength, speed* and *power.* Power implies the speed with which force is exerted. It is an important characteristic of skillful performance in such activities as high jumping, broad jumping, throwing, striking and kicking, and in speed events such as sprinting and swimming.

Judgment has already been mentioned as a factor in accuracy. It is more than that, however. In dual and team games and in boxing and wrestling, good judgment is one of the most important characteristics of skillful performance. It implies a sizing up of the situation and choosing wisely between several possible responses. It marks the difference between using one's head and acting blindly, between intelligent and unintelligent participation (see Fig. 26–1).

The general characteristics of skillful performance may therefore be summed up as *efficiency, accuracy, good judgment* and *adequate speed, strength* and *power* for the task. Of course motivation is an

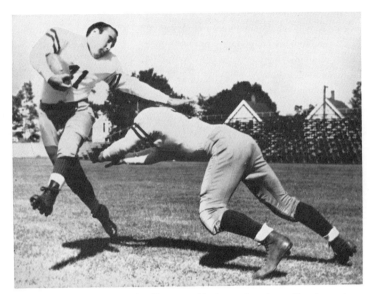

Figure 26–1. An example of split second judgment and reaction to environmental circumstances. (Courtesy of Springfield College.)

all-important factor and there are also the various individual factors of *special aptitudes* which make one person a potential sprinter, and another a potential high jumper. These are related to build, to constitution and to temperament. It is a matter of common observation that greater skillfulness is achieved by individuals who happen to be endowed with greater aptitudes or innate capacities for certain kinds of accomplishments. Great individual differences are seen with respect to the various factors of motor ability such as hand-eye coordination, agility, reaction time and finger dexterity. To be sure, all these can be developed by practice, but not everyone can develop them to the same degree, for there is a wide range in native capacity.

The truly skillful performer is one who habitually obeys the principles of both the anatomic and the mechanical aspects of human motion. His neuromuscular coordination is at peak performance; his muscular function is highly efficient; his kinesthetic sense is well developed; his flexor and extensor reflexes are dependable; the movements of his joints are commensurate with his individual structure; and his techniques of motion are in accord with the laws of his physical environment. In short, he has learned how, and has made it his practice, to observe the principles of skillful motion.

The mechanical principles that apply to specific motor skills have already been emphasized. The anatomic principles are more general in nature. Most of them have been mentioned elsewhere in the text, but it may be helpful to bring them together here.

PRINCIPLES RELATING TO THE STRUCTURE
AND FUNCTION OF JOINTS

Principle I. Since the range of motion may be limited by tight muscles, fasciae or ligaments, it may be increased by the stretching of these tissues.

Principle II. The stretching of tight muscles, fasciae or ligaments should be done gradually and should be preceded by warm-up activities. The danger of rupturing soft tissues is minimized when they have been adequately "warmed-up."

Principle III. Increase gained in the range of motion will be lost unless it is deliberately retained by means of continued exercise.

Principle IV. Flexibility of weight-bearing joints should not exceed the ability of the muscles to maintain the body segments in good alignment.

PRINCIPLES RELATING TO THE MUSCULAR SYSTEM
AND TO NEUROMUSCULAR FUNCTION

Principle I. Muscles contract more forcefully if they are first put on a stretch, provided they are not overstretched. This principle suggests the function of the "wind-up" in pitching and of the preliminary movements in other sport skills.

Principle II. Increase in muscular strength is brought about by increasing the demands made on muscles. This is known as the overload principle. It means that a muscle must be loaded beyond its customary load if strength is to be increased. This principle forms the basis for conditioning exercises and is the principle on which the system of "progressive resistance exercise" is based. *Strength will not be progressively developed by the mere repetition of exercises of the same intensity.*

Principle III. Unnecessary movements and tensions in the performance of a motor skill mean both awkwardness and unnecessary fatigue; hence they should be eliminated. This is achieved by first developing kinesthetic awareness of muscular tension, and then learning how to relax unneeded muscles.

Principle IV. Skillful, efficient performance in a particular technique can be developed only by practice of that technique. Only in this way can the necessary adjustments in the neuromuscular mechanism be made to assure a well coordinated movement.

Principle V. Fatigue from overpractice diminishes skillful performance. It can be avoided by introducing properly spaced rest periods in the practice period.

Principle VI. The most efficient type of movement in throwing and striking skills is ballistic movement. Skills which are primarily ballistic should be practiced ballistically even in the earliest learning stages. This means that from the beginning the emphasis should be placed on form rather than on accuracy. Accuracy will develop with practice. If the emphasis is placed on accuracy in the learning stages, the beginner tends to perform the skill as a "moving fixation" or slow, tense movement. Once this pattern of movement is established, it is extremely difficult to change it later to a ballistic movement.

Principle VII. An important factor in the learning and perfecting of a motor skill is kinesthetic perception. There is no evidence of a general kinesthetic sense, however. Kinesthetic perception appears to be specific for the skill in question.

Principle VIII. Reflex responses of the neuromuscular system should be recognized and should be utilized when such utilization is clearly indicated. (This statement is intentionally general because much more needs to be learned about some of the physiologic reflexes before specific principles can be derived from them.) Of the more familiar reflexes, the extensor reflex is closely related to postural adjustments, and reciprocal innervation is closely related to ballistic motion.

Principle IX. When there is a choice of anatomic leverage, the lever appropriate for the task should be used, i.e., a lever with a long resistance arm for movements requiring range or speed, and a lever with a long force arm for movements requiring strength. For example, kicking is an effective way of imparting force to a football because the leg provides a lever with a long resistance arm, but, for the same reason, it is a poor way of moving a heavy suitcase along the floor.

Dual Purpose of Kinesiology. In the Introduction to the Study of Kinesiology it was stated that such study had a dual purpose for the physical educator, namely, the perfecting of performance in motor skills as well as perfecting the performer himself. (See page 2.) This brings us to a more specific consideration of ways and means. As we look back over the two kinds of basic information that have been represented in the study of kinesiology, we realize that we have received two sets of tools. One set has to do with the mechanical aspects of motor skills, and the other is involved with the anatomic and neurophysiologic aspects. Both sets of tools are related to the human structure and its movements, but their uses differ as widely as do those of woodworking tools and metalworking tools. They serve two totally different purposes. The purpose previously referred to as "perfecting performance" includes presenting the skill and its purpose with such clarity that the students will learn it with a minimum of difficulty. This is what Lawther means when he advocates giving the student a "gross-framework-idea" of the skill.[6] It also includes analyzing the student's performance, diagnosing his difficulties, and making effective suggestions for correcting them.

A student's difficulty may be due to the violation of a mechanical principle, in which case the teacher should make the appropriate suggestion, or it may be due to some physical inadequacy such as lack of strength in a particular group of muscles or limited flexibility in some joint. In these cases it might be desirable to give the student a series of strengthening or flexibility exercises. This would be an example of "perfecting the performer." The entire exercise program—physical fitness, conditioning, and posture correction—belongs in this category. It involves the ability to identify the needs of the individual, to evaluate the exercises from the point of view of their effect on the human structure, and to judge their appropriateness for the age, ability and specific requirements of the individual.

The usefulness of a kinesiology course should now be fully apparent. The more knowledgeable and perceptive the instructor is concerning the role of mechanics in performance, the better equipped he will be to become an effective teacher of motor skills. Likewise, the better his understanding of the proper functioning of muscles and joints and of the effects of specific exercises, the more skillful he will be in prescribing and teaching physical fitness, conditioning, and postural exercises.

There arises another question concerning these two major areas of activity; to what extent does a knowledge of mechanical and anatomic principles *on the part of the student* contribute to the effectiveness of his learning? This embodies two separate questions which should be considered separately.

Knowledge of Mechanical Principles. Whether the learning of motor skills is facilitated by an understanding of the mechanical principles that apply to them is a question of prime interest to physical education teachers and athletic coaches. Of three studies with which the author is familiar, two indicated that a knowledge of mechanical principles was beneficial. Daugherty found that the junior high school boys who were taught certain principles demonstrated greater accuracy and force in selected skills than did the boys who were unfamiliar with the principles.[4] Mohr and Barrett had similar results with college women who were taught the mechanical principles of certain swimming strokes in conjunction with the usual swimming instruction.[9] (See page 451 for a summary of this study.)

The approach of the third investigator, Colville, was somewhat different.[3] She selected three mechanical principles and devised experiments which involved the application of these. The principles investigated and the skills used were as follows:

FIRST PRINCIPLE: The angle of incidence is approximately equal to the angle of reflection.

Skill: Rolling a ball against a surface or surfaces from which it would rebound.

SECOND PRINCIPLE: In stopping a moving object, the force opposing the momentum must be equal to the force of the momentum and if the object is to be caught, this momentum must be dissipated by reducing the resistance of the catching surface.

Skill: Catching a tennis ball in a lacrosse stick and catching a badminton bird on a tennis racket.

THIRD PRINCIPLE: An object set in forward motion through the air by an external force is acted upon by gravitational acceleration.

Skill: Archery.

(For the details of each test the reader should consult the article.)

For all three tests the results gave no indication of a significant difference in performance level between the experimental and control groups. Both methods (instruction with and without using part of the time for learning the principles) resulted in a significant amount of learning which was similar in pattern as well as in amount.

Without having full information about the study one cannot help but have certain questions and comments, for instance: (1) Was instruction given regarding the application of the principles? (2) Might not the first and second tests, because of their artificial nature, have been comparable to nonsense syllables in verbal tests and therefore lacking in motivation for the subjects? (3) It would seem that a better choice of principles might have been made, for instance principles that were more directly related to the quality of performance.

Lawther has reported several additional studies which are listed below.[6]

1. Hendrickson and Schroeder: Transfer of Training in Learning to Hit a Submerged Target. (This has to do with the principle of light refraction as it affects success in hitting underwater targets.)

2. Frey: A Study of Teaching Procedures in Selected Physical Education Activities for College Women of Low Motor Ability. (This investigates the effect of giving detailed reasons for specific forms used in teaching tennis, volleyball, and rhythmic activities.)

3. Cobane: A Comparison of Two Methods of Teaching Selected Motor Skills. (This is somewhat similar to Colville's study but is applied to the teaching of tennis.)

4. Nessler: An Experimental Study of Methods Adapted to Teaching Low Skilled Freshman Women in Physical Education. (There was no report of the methods used, but the implication seemed to be that a knowledge of mechanical principles was one of the factors included.)

5. Broer: Effectiveness of General Basic Skills Curriculum for Junior High School Girls. (This included the factor of instruction in simplified mechanics prior to the teaching of volleyball, basketball, and softball.)

6. Halverson: A Comparison of Three Methods of Teaching Motor Skills. (Knowledge of mechanical principles constituted one factor in this study. The skill was one-handed shooting in basketball.)

Of the nine studies, five reported either negative or negligible results, and four reported positive results. The latter were the studies by Daugherty,[4] Mohr and Barrett,[9] Hendrickson and Schroeder,[6] and Broer.[6] Lawther observed that most of the studies used beginners as subjects. He suggested that a knowledge of the appropriate mechanical principles might be of greater value at the higher skill levels than at the early stages of learning.

The lack of agreement shown by the results of the studies concerning the value to the learner of a knowledge of mechanical principles is also evident in the opinions of physical education instructors. Those who take the negative side may do so for a number of reasons. They may have had poor results in their own teaching experience and assumed that the procedure itself was ineffective without considering the fact that their own presentation may have been at fault. They may have talked too much in their explanation of the mechanical principles (a fault guaranteed to bore the class if not actually cause resentment); they may have failed to make their explanations clear; they may not have been convinced of the value of such explanations in the first place, and consequently they may have lacked enthusiasm in their presentation; they may have been influenced by some of the research studies which reported negative results.

It is significant that instructors who teach kinesiology tend to use this teaching technique in their sports classes and their coaching. McCloy asserted that one of the best ways to be sure that the students would attain the correct objectives was to teach the activities in such a way that the mechanics of each type of skill would be clear to the student. He advocated using simplified vocabulary and explanations so that the students would understand how the skill was to be performed and why the method taught was effective. Furthermore, based on his own experience, he claimed that this technique of teaching could be used successfully with children as young as 10 or 12 years of age.[8]

Broer,[1] Bunn,[2] Dyson,[5] and Rasch and Burke[10] are also among those who advocate giving instruction in mechanical principles when teaching or coaching athletic skills.

Knowledge of Anatomy and Anatomic Principles. The author knows of no research in this area and therefore offers her own opinion which is based upon her teaching experience in the field of corrective physical education. This has included all grades from first grade through college. As a result of this experience, she is convinced of the value of giving brief, simple anatomic explanations accompanied by the use of such visual aids as muscle charts, a human skeleton, various anatomic models, and drawings on the chalkboard. These explanations and demonstrations have been found to arouse the intelligent interest of pupils from about the fourth or fifth grade on. Obviously they must be geared to the age. Whether the students actually perform the exercises with greater energy and zest may be open to question, but there is no question that they tend to perform them with a greater degree of accuracy and precision.

Teaching for Understanding. Any teacher of physical education who has a good knowledge of motor skills can probably teach them to his students. If, in addition, he has a good understanding of kinesiology he will be in a better position to select effective techniques and methods and to diagnose and remedy individual difficulties. He will thus be improving his method of teaching his students how to learn new skills and how to improve their performance. This is desirable but it does not go far enough. Some students may be satisfied with it but the more intelligent student wants to know the *why* of the directions given by the instructor or coach. He wants to understand the reasons for what he does and why one approach is more effective than another.

For the majority of students, greater understanding leads to greater interest, and greater interest leads not only to greater effort but to more productive effort. This constitutes genuine motivation, and finding effective motivation for his students has always been one of the major challenges faced by the instructor.

It is the conviction of this text that the solution to the quest for motivation is to *teach for understanding*, and that an effective way of doing this is to instruct the students in regard to mechanical and anatomic principles and to supplement this with simple demonstrations. If the explanations and the demonstrations are to be meaningful to the student they must be geared to his intellectual and educational level. They should drive home essential points vividly and succinctly if they are to make a lasting impression. An example of a simple and meaningful demonstration may be found in Exercise 1 on page 428. Often such a demonstration will be more effective than a meticulously accurate scientific explanation.

As an aid to the beginning teacher who is interested in explaining the appropriate mechanical and anatomic principles, the following guidelines are suggested.

1. Only those instructors who are convinced of the value of this technique, or who are at least open-minded about it, should use it.

2. The explanations should be kept brief. Preferably, they should not take over five minutes, or occasionally ten at the most, out of a 45- to 50-minute period. It is well to remember Lockhart's warning about keeping oral instructions at a minimum.[7] As she says, most physical education teachers talk too much. This has the unfortunate effect of defeating their purpose. Making oneself understood is desirable, but overexplaining to the point of boring or antagonizing one's listeners may be disastrous.

3. Whenever feasible, visual aids and demonstrations should be used in conjunction with explanations.

4. The explanatory talks on mechanical principles and anatomy should be given only occasionally, not as a part of every lesson.

5. Explain only those aspects of a subject that you consider of vital importance to learning the skill in question and which you believe cannot be taught effectively during the activity practice.

6. Avoid any but the simplest mechanical principles unless you know that your students are familiar with physics.

7. In general, save the finer points of instruction in mechanical principles for intermediate and advanced classes.

8. Do not be surprised to discover that adequate preparation for a brief, effective explanation may take as long as preparation for an hour's lecture. It takes time to select, condense, and simplify.

Finally, the whole purpose of kinesiology can be summed up in three phrases. It is (1) to provide the physical education instructor with the tools he needs in order to teach for understanding, (2) to guide his students in acquiring proficiency in motor skills, and (3) to aid his students in improving their own physiques when such a need is indicated.

REFERENCES

1. Broer, M. R.: Efficiency of Human Movement, 2nd ed. Philadelphia, W. B. Saunders Company, 1966.
2. Bunn, J. W.: Scientific Principles of Coaching. Englewood Cliffs, New Jersey, Prentice-Hall, Inc., 1959.
3. Colville, F. M.: The learning of motor skills as influenced by knowledge of mechanical principles. J. Ed. Psych. 48:321–327, 1957.
4. Daugherty, G.: The effects of kinesiological teaching on the performance of junior high school boys. Res. Quart. Am. Assn. Health, Phys. Ed. & Recrn., 16:26–33, 1945.
5. Dyson, G. H. G.: The Mechanics of Athletics, 3rd ed. London, University of London Press Ltd., 1964.
6. Lawther, J. D.: The Learning of Physical Skills. Englewood Cliffs, New Jersey, Prentice-Hall, Inc., 1968.
7. Lockhart, A.: Communicating with the learner. Quest. VI:57–67, 1966.
8. McCloy, C. H.: The mechanical analysis of motor skills. *In* Johnson, W. R. (ed.): Science and Medicine of Exercise and Sports. New York, Harper & Row, 1960, Chapter 4.
9. Mohr, D. R., and Barrett, M. E.: Effect of knowledge of mechanical principles in learning to perform intermediate swimming skills. Res. Quart. Am. Assn. Health, Phys. Ed. & Recrn., 33:574–580, 1962.
10. Rasch, P. J., and Burke, R. K.: Kinesiology and Applied Anatomy, 3rd ed. Philadelphia, Lea & Febiger, 1967.
11. Steindler, A.: Mechanics of Normal and Pathological Locomotion in Man. Springfield, Ill., Charles C Thomas, Publisher, 1935, p. 13.

RECOMMENDED READINGS

Lawther, J. D.: The Learning of Physical Skills. Englewood Cliffs, New Jersey, Prentice-Hall, Inc., 1968.
Lockhart, A.: Communicating with the learner. Quest, VI:57–67, 1966.
McCloy, C. H.: The mechanical analysis of motor skills. *In* Johnson, W. R. (ed.): Science and Medicine of Exercise and Sports. New York, Harper and Row, 1960, Chapter 4.
Quest, Monograph VI, A Symposium on Motor Learning. A publication of the National Association for Physical Education of College Women and the National College Physical Education Association for Men, 1966. The entire issue.

APPENDIX A

Table of Sines and Cosines

Degrees	Sines	Cosines	Degrees	Sines	Cosines
0	.0000	1.0000	46	.7193	.6947
1	.0175	.9998	47	.7314	.6820
2	.0349	.9994	48	.7431	.6691
3	.0523	.9986	49	.7547	.6561
4	.0698	.9976	50	.7660	.6428
5	.0872	.9962	51	.7771	.6293
6	.1045	.9945	52	.7880	.6157
7	.1219	.9925	53	.7986	.6018
8	.1392	.9903	54	.8090	.5878
9	.1564	.9877	55	.8192	.5736
10	.1736	.9848	56	.8290	.5592
11	.1908	.9816	57	.8387	.5446
12	.2079	.9781	58	.8480	.5299
13	.2250	.9744	59	.8572	.5150
14	.2419	.9703	60	.8660	.5000
15	.2588	.9659	61	.8746	.4848
16	.2756	.9613	62	.8829	.4695
17	.2924	.9563	63	.8910	.4540
18	.3090	.9511	64	.8988	.4384
19	.3256	.9455	65	.9063	.4226
20	.3420	.9397	66	.9135	.4067
21	.3584	.9336	67	.9205	.3907
22	.3746	.9272	68	.9272	.3746
23	.3907	.9205	69	.9336	.3584
24	.4067	.9135	70	.9397	.3420
25	.4226	.9063	71	.9455	.3256
26	.4384	.8988	72	.9511	.3090
27	.4540	.8910	73	.9563	.2924
28	.4695	.8829	74	.9613	.2756
29	.4848	.8746	75	.9659	.2588
30	.5000	.8660	76	.9703	.2419
31	.5150	.8572	77	.9744	.2250
32	.5299	.8480	78	.9781	.2079
33	.5446	.8387	79	.9816	.1908
34	.5592	.8290	80	.9848	.1736
35	.5736	.8192	81	.9877	.1564
36	.5878	.8090	82	.9903	.1392
37	.6018	.7986	83	.9925	.1219
38	.6157	.7880	84	.9945	.1045
39	.6293	.7771	85	.9962	.0872
40	.6428	.7660	86	.9976	.0698
41	.6561	.7547	87	.9986	.0523
42	.6691	.7431	88	.9994	.0349
43	.6820	.7314	89	.9998	.0175
44	.6947	.7193	90	1.0000	.0000
45	.7071	.7071			

APPENDIX B*

OUTLINE FOR STUDYING THE JOINTS AND THEIR MOVEMENTS

Name of joint_____ Bones involved_____

Type of Joint, Movement, and Number of Axes of Motion (Check below.)

____Diarthrodial

    ____Irregular
    ____Hinge
    ____Pivot
    ____Condyloid (ovoid)
    ____Saddle
    ____Ball-and-socket

____Synarthrodial

    ____Cartilaginous
    ____Ligamentous
    ____Fibrous

Type of Movement

    ____Gliding
    ____Axial or rotatory

Axis of Motion

    ____Nonaxial
    ____Uniaxial
    ____Biaxial
    ____Triaxial

Name or describe briefly:

Articulating processes and surfaces_____

_____

Ligaments and cartilages_____

_____

_____

_____

Movements (check)   Comments
____Flexion and extension   _____

____Hyperextension   _____

____Abduction and ad-
    duction or lateral
    flexion   _____

____Rotation   _____

    ____Outward (lat.) and
        inward (med.)   _____

*The check lists in Appendices B and F may be reproduced for class use without specific permission.

Movements (check)   Comments

____Upward and downward   _____

____Right and left   _____

____Supination and
       pronation   _____

Other: _____

_____   _____

_____   _____

APPENDIX C

CLASSIFICATION OF JOINTS AND THEIR MOVEMENTS

Type	Articulation	Movement
	Diarthrodial: Nonaxial	
	Shoulder Girdle	
	Sternoclavicular	Limited motion of outer end of clavicle in all three planes
		Elevation – Depression
		Forward – Backward
		Rotation: Forward-downward – Backward-upward
	Acromioclavicular	Movements of scapula (including motion in both joints)
Irregular;		Elevation – Depression
Arthrodial;		Rotation: Upward – Downward
Plane		Abduction – Adduction
		Upward Tilt – Reduction of same
	Intercarpal	Slight gliding movements in cooperation with movements of wrist and metacarpals
	Intertarsal	Slight gliding movements in cooperation with movements of talonavicular and ankle joints
	Diarthrodial: Uniaxial	
	Elbow	
	Humero-ulnar	Flexion – Extension – Hyperextension (slight)
	Knee	
	Tibiofemoral	Flexion – Extension – Hyperextension (slight)
Hinge;	Ankle	
Ginglymus	Talotibial and talofibular	Dorsiflexion – Plantar flexion (Extension)
	Fingers and thumb	Flexion – Extension
	Interphalangeal	
	Toes	
	Interphalangeal	Flexion – Extension
	Forearm	
Pivot;	Proximal and distal radioulnar	Supination – Pronation
Screw;	Neck	
Trochoid	Atlantoaxial (1st and 2nd cervical)	Rotation: Right – Left

Diarthrodial: Biaxial

	Wrist	
	Radiocarpal	Flexion — Extension — Hyperextension
		Abduction — Adduction
	Fingers	
Condyloid;	Metacarpophalangeal	Flexion — Extension
Ovoid;		Abduction — Adduction
Ellipsoidal	Toes	
	Metatarsophalangeal	Flexion — Extension — Hyperextension
	Head	
	Occipito-atlantal	Flexion — Extension — Hyperextension
		Lateral flexion: Right — Left

Diarthrodial: Triaxial

	Shoulder	
	Glenohumeral	Flexion — Extension — Hyperextension
Ball-and-socket;		Abduction — Adduction
Enarthrodial		Rotation: Outward — Inward
		Horizontal flexion (from abduction)
		Horizontal extension (from flexion)
	Hip	
	Femoro-acetabular	Flexion — Extension — Hyperextension
		Abduction — Adduction
		Rotation: Outward — Inward
		Horizontal flexion (from abduction)
		Horizontal extension (from flexion)
Shallow ball-	Foot	
and-socket	Talonavicular	Dorsiflexion — Plantar flexion (very slight)
		Abduction — Adduction (slight)
		Inversion — Eversion (very slight)
Saddle;		
Seller;	Thumb	
Reciprocal	Carpometacarpal	Flexion — Extension — Hyperextension
reception		Abduction — Adduction
		Opposition (combination of abduction, hyperflexion, and possibly slight inward rotation)

Combination Diarthrodial Nonaxial and Fibrocartilaginous Synarthrodial

Triaxial sim-	Vertebral bodies	
ulated ball-and-	Intervertebral cartilages	⎡ Flexion
socket		⎢ Extension
		⎨ Hyperextension
Nonaxial	Vertebral arches	⎢ Lateral flexion: Right — Left
irregular		⎣ Rotation: Right — Left

APPENDIX D

MUSCULAR ANALYSIS OF THE FUNDAMENTAL
MOVEMENTS OF THE ARM AT THE SHOULDER JOINT*

Abduction (elevation of humerus in plane parallel with scapula)

Movers
- Principal
  - Middle deltoid
  - Supraspinatus
- Assistant
  - Long head of biceps, especially if the forearm is supinated
  - Anterior deltoid, after the arm passes above the horizontal
  - Clavicular portion of pectoralis major, after the arm passes well above the horizontal

*The designation of the precise roles of muscles as principal movers, assistant movers, neutralizers, stabilizers or supporters is entirely arbitrary. It is based on the best available evidence and on an analysis of the circumstances.

Neutralizers...The infraspinatus and teres minor neutralize the flexion tendencies of the anterior deltoid and upper pectoralis major after the arm passes above the horizontal

Stabilizers..{ Trapezius
                                                     Subclavius

Note: 1. Extreme abduction of the humerus is usually accompanied by outward rotation, since a greater range of abduction is possible in this position.

2. In a sense, all the muscles which attach the scapulae to the trunk may be looked upon as stabilizing or supporting muscles in all movements of the upper extremity. These include the subclavius, pectoralis minor, serratus anterior, levator scapulae, rhomboids and trapezius.

Adduction (return from abduction) (Fig. D–1.)

Note: If performed when the body is erect, the movement could be produced by gravitational force alone, without muscular action. If performed more slowly than this, the abductors work in lengthening contraction in order to control the movement, and the adductors are relaxed. If performed more quickly than by the force of gravity, or if performed against resistance, the muscular action is as given below.

Movers
- Principal
  - Latissimus dorsi
  - Teres major
  - Pectoralis major, sternal portion
- Assistant
  - Posterior deltoid (lowest fibers)
  - Coracobrachialis, when the arm is above the horizontal
  - Subscapularis, when the arm is above the horizontal
  - Biceps, when the arm is above the horizontal
  - Long head of triceps

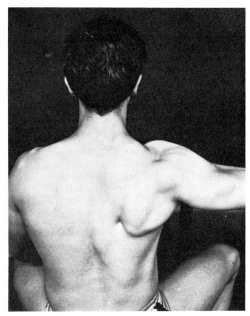

Figure D-1. Sideward depression of the arm against resistance. The latissimus dorsi, teres major and rhomboids are in strong contraction.

Neutralizers..The anterior and posterior muscles neutralize one another's flexion and hyperextension tendencies

Stabilizers..The coracobrachialis, the short head of the biceps and the long head of the triceps are all shoulder stabilizers as well as movers. Each has a relatively large non-rotatory or stabilizing component of force pulling lengthwise through the humerus toward the glenoid fossa. The rhomboids stabilize the scapula. The abdominal muscles and spinal extensors stabilize the trunk if the adduction is forceful

Flexion (forward elevation of humerus in plane perpendicular to scapula) (Fig. D-2.)

Movers ....
- Principal .... {Anterior deltoid / Pectoralis major, clavicular portion}
- Assistant .... {Coracobrachialis / Biceps, especially if elbow is in extended position}

Neutralizers..The infraspinatus and teres minor neutralize the inward rotatory components of the anterior deltoid and pectoralis major

Stabilizers.. {Trapezius / Subclavius}

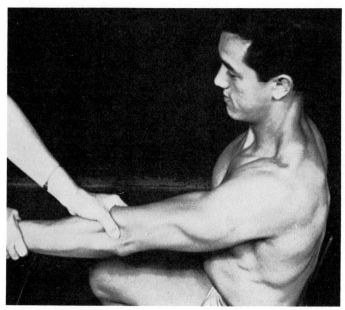

Figure D–2. Forward elevation of the arm against resistance. The anterior and middle deltoid, upper trapezius and serratus anterior are in strong contraction.

Extension (return from flexion) (Fig. D–3.)

  Note: See note under Adduction, regarding the effect of the force of gravity.

Movers	Principal	Latissimus dorsi, especially during the lower 60 degrees of motion Pectoralis major, sternal portion, diminishing as the movement progresses Teres major
	Assistant	Posterior deltoid Long head of triceps, especially if elbow is in flexed position

Neutralizers.....................................The posterior deltoid neutralizes the inward rotatory tendency of the pectoralis major and latissimus dorsi. If the movement is performed with force, the infraspinatus and teres minor also contract to prevent inward rotation

Stabilizers.......................................The long head of triceps and the coracobrachialis stabilize the shoulder joint; the rhomboids stabilize the scapula; the abdominal muscles and internal intercostals stabilize the ribs; and the erector spinae stabilizes the spine. The degree to which these muscles contract depends upon the forcefulness of the act

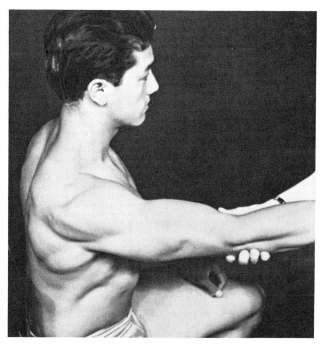

Figure D-3. Forward depression of the arm against resistance. The latissimus dorsi and teres major are in strong contraction.

Hyperextension (backward elevation of humerus in a plane perpendicular to scapula)

Movers ....{ Posterior deltoid
Latissimus dorsi
Teres major

Neutralizers..The posterior deltoid, on the one hand, and the latissimus dorsi and teres major, on the other, are mutual neutralizers with respect to outward and inward rotation

Stabilizers...The levator, trapezius and rhomboids stabilize the scapulae. The erector spinae stabilizes the spine

Outward Rotation (a lateral rotation of humerus around its longitudinal axis) (Fig. D-4.)

Movers ....{ Principal..............Infraspinatus and teres minor

Assistant ....{ Posterior deltoid, when the humerus is adducted and extended

Neutralizers..None in the movement of the humerus. Trapezius IV neutralizes the tendency of the rhomboids to elevate the scapula

Stabilizers...The middle trapezius and rhomboids stabilize the scapulae

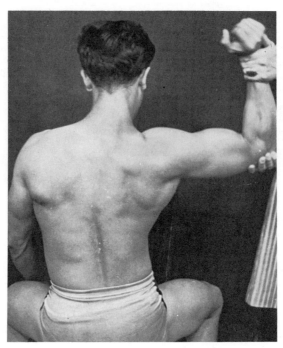

Figure D-4. Outward rotation of the arm against resistance. The posterior deltoid, infraspinatus and teres minor are in strong contraction. (The hyperextension and lateral flexion of the trunk are due to the extreme effort. The latissimus is contracting because he is pushing his elbow down.)

Inward Rotation (medial rotation of humerus around its longitudinal axis)

Movers
- Principal
  - Subscapularis
  - Teres major
- Assistant
  - Latissimus dorsi
  - Anterior deltoid
  - Pectoralis major
  - Coracobrachialis (helps to reduce outward rotation)
  - Short head of biceps (helps to reduce outward rotation)

Neutralizers....................................The anterior deltoid, coracobrachialis and clavicular portion of pectoralis major neutralize the extension function of the latissimus dorsi and teres major

Stabilizers.......................................The pectoralis minor and serratus anterior stabilize the scapulae

Horizontal Flexion (a forward movement of the humerus in the horizontal plane)

Movers
- Principal
  - Subscapularis
  - Pectoralis major
  - Anterior deltoid
  - Coracobrachialis
- Assistant .... Biceps when forearm is extended

Neutralizers.......................................None

Supporters and Stabilizers ....The middle deltoid and supraspinatus support the humerus against the downward
pull of gravity. The pectoralis major on
the opposite side stabilizes the sternum;
the first part of trapezius and possibly the
subclavius stabilize the clavicle; and the
serratus anterior and second part of trapezius stabilize the scapula

Horizontal Extension (a sideward-backward movement of the humerus in the horizontal
plane)

Movers ....
{
  Principal .... {
    Posterior deltoid and posterior portion of middle deltoid
    Infraspinatus and teres minor, especially if the movement is combined with outward rotation
}

  Assistant .... {
    Latissimus dorsi
    Teres major, especially if the movement is combined with inward rotation
}

Neutralizers......................................The middle deltoid and supraspinatus
neutralize the tendency of the latissimus
dorsi and teres major to adduct the humerus. The infraspinatus and teres minor,
on the one hand, and the latissimus dorsi
and teres major, on the other hand, are
mutual neutralizers with respect to outward and inward rotation

Supporters and Stabilizers ....The middle deltoid and supraspinatus support the humerus against the downward
pull of gravity. The lower three parts of
the trapezius and the rhomboids stabilize
the scapula, and the abdominal muscles
stabilize the trunk

MUSCULAR ANALYSIS OF THE FUNDAMENTAL MOVEMENTS OF THE SHOULDER GIRDLE

Elevation

Movers ....
{
  Principal .... {
    Levator scapulae
    Trapezius, parts I and II
    Rhomboids
}

  Assistant .... {
    Sternocleidomastoid, clavicular portion, if the movement is performed against resistance
}

Neutralizers......................................The trapezius and rhomboids are mutually neutralizing with respect to upward
and downward rotation. The serratus
anterior neutralizes the adduction motions of the rhomboids and trapezius

Stabilizers ....If the movement is performed on one side
only, the lateral cervical flexors on the
opposite side stabilize the cervical spine

Depression (return from elevation)

   Note: No muscular action is required in the erect position if the shoulders are
simply allowed to drop from the elevated position. If lowered slowly, the movement is

controlled by means of lengthening contraction of the elevators. If performed against resistance, or in a position other than the vertical, the muscular action is as given below.

Movers ....\{ Trapezius, part IV
Pectoralis minor
Subclavius

Neutralizers.....................................The lower trapezius and pectoralis minor are mutually neutralizing with respect to adduction and abduction; also with respect to upward and downward rotation

Stabilizers.......................................The erector spinae and abdominal muscles stabilize the spine, and the internal intercostals and abdominal muscles stabilize the ribs when the movement is performed against resistance

Abduction and Lateral Tilt (protraction of scapulae)

Movers ....\{ Serratus anterior
Pectoralis minor

Neutralizers.....................................The serratus anterior and pectoralis minor mutually neutralize one another's tendency to rotate the scapula

Stabilizers ....The abdominal muscles, and possibly the internal intercostals, stabilize the ribs if the movement is forceful. The levator scapulae helps to support the scapula

Adduction and Reduction of Lateral Tilt (retraction of scapulae)

Movers ....\{ Principal ....\{ Rhomboids
Middle trapezius, part III

Assistant..............Trapezius II and IV

Neutralizers.....................................The rhomboids and lower trapezius are mutually neutralizing with respect to elevation and depression of the scapula, also with respect to downward and upward rotation

Stabilizers.......................................The abdominal muscles and the erector spinae stabilize the spine. This is particularly true if the movement is performed unilaterally because of the tendency of the spine to rotate

Upward Tilt (a backward projection of the inferior angle of the scapula)

Mover ....Pectoralis minor

Neutralizers.....................................It is doubtful whether there is any neutralizing action in this movement

Stabilizers.......................................Possibly the internal intercostals contract to stabilize the ribs

Note: This is an uncommon movement which occurs only in conjunction with extreme hyperextension of the humerus.

Reduction of Upward Tilt

    Note: Ordinarily no muscular action is needed.

Movers ....Trapezius IV and the lower serratus anterior are in a position to reduce an upward
tilt of the scapula, but they do not need
to contract unless the movement of the
arm is resisted

Neutralizers and Stabilizers..................Impossible to tell by palpation

Upward Rotation (occurs only in conjunction with abduction and flexion of the
humerus)

Movers ....{Trapezius II and IV
                                                   {Serratus anterior

Neutralizers......................................Trapezius II and IV are mutually neutralizing with respect to elevation and
depression

Stabilizers...The abdominal muscles, and possibly the
internal intercostals, help to stabilize the
ribs if the movement is forceful

Downward Rotation (occurs only in conjunction with adduction, inward rotation and
hyperextension of the humerus)

    Note: No muscular action is necessary if the arm is allowed to drop to the side. If
the arm is lowered slowly, the movement is controlled by means of lengthening contraction of the upward rotators. When the arm movement is performed forcefully,
quickly, or against gravity (i.e., when the body is inverted), the muscular analysis of
the shoulder girdle movement is given below.

                                ┌ Principal ....{Rhomboids
                                │   {Pectoralis minor
Movers ....{
                                │   {Levator scapulae (it tends to pull the
                                └ Assistant ....{   scapula upward and inward, but the
                                                        weight of the arm causes the scapula to
                                                        rotate downward)

Neutralizers......................................The rhomboids and pectoralis minor are
mutually neutralizing with respect to
elevation and depression, also with
respect to adduction and abduction.
Trapezius IV helps to prevent elevation of scapula when movement of arm
is resisted

Stabilizers...The abdominal muscles, and possibly the
internal intercostals, help to stabilize the
ribs if the movement is forceful

MUSCULAR ANALYSIS OF THE FUNDAMENTAL
MOVEMENTS OF THE FOREARM AT THE ELBOW AND
RADIOULNAR JOINTS

Flexion

                              ┌ Principal ....{Biceps
                              │   {Brachialis
Movers ....{   {Brachioradialis
                              │
                              │   {Pronator teres (against resistance)
                              └ Assistant ....{Flexors of the hand and fingers (probably
                                                     unimportant as forearm flexors)

Neutralizers......................................The pronator teres and the biceps are mutually neutralizing with respect to pronation and supination of the forearm. The pronator quadratus helps to counteract the supinatory function of the biceps when flexion is resisted or when flexion is performed with the forearm in a pronated position

Stabilizers.......................................If not prevented from so doing, flexion of the forearm will cause slight hyperextension of the arm at the shoulder joint, especially if a weight is held in the hand. If this is not desired, the pectoralis major, anterior deltoid and coracobrachialis will contract to stabilize the humerus. In many instances, as in pulling, the cooperative action of the forearm flexors and upper arm extensors is necessary. In such cases the humerus will not need to be stabilized, but it will require the stabilization of the scapula or of the trunk itself

Extension

Movers ....{ Principal..............Triceps, especially the medial head
.................{ Assistant..............Anconeus

Neutralizers.....................................None

Stabilizers (when forearm is
  extended forcefully).......................{ Pectoralis major, sternal portion
.......................{ Latissimus dorsi
.......................{ Teres major

Pronation

Movers ....{ Principal ....{ Pronator quadratus
.................{ ....{ Pronator teres
.................{ Assistant ....{ Brachioradialis (reduction of supination to neutral position)

Neutralizers.....................................The triceps and anconeus counteract the flexion tendency of the pronator teres

Stabilizers.......................................The contraction of the triceps, anconeus and pronator teres serves to stabilize the elbow joint

Supination

Movers ....{ Principal ....{ Supinator
.................{ ....{ Biceps, when elbow is flexed
.................{ Assistant..............Brachioradialis (reduction of pronation to neutral position)

Neutralizers.....................................If flexion is not desired, the triceps and anconeus counteract the flexion tendency of the biceps

Stabilizers.......................................The contraction of the triceps, anconeus and biceps serves to stabilize the elbow joint

MUSCULAR ANALYSIS OF THE FUNDAMENTAL
MOVEMENTS OF THE WRIST, FINGERS AND THUMB

Wrist

Flexion

Movers ....
- Principal .... { Flexor carpi ulnaris / Flexor carpi radialis / Palmaris longus

- Assistant .... { Flexor digitorum profundus (when prevented from flexing fingers) / Flexor digitorum superficialis (when prevented from flexing fingers) / Flexor pollicis longus / Abductor pollicis longus

Neutralizers.................................. { When strong wrist flexion requires the aid of the finger flexors, the finger extensors contract to counteract the effect of the finger flexors on the fingers, thus permitting them to affect only the wrist joint / Flexor carpi ulnaris is mutually neutralizing with flexor carpi radialis and abductor pollicis longus with respect to ulnar and radial flexion

Stabilizers ....When strong wrist flexion is desired, the triceps provides a firm support for the origins of the wrist flexors by preventing flexion at the elbow

Extension

Movers ....
- Principal .... { Extensor carpi radialis longus / Extensor carpi radialis brevis / Extensor carpi ulnaris

- Assistant .... { Extensor digitorum / Extensor pollicis longus

Neutralizers.................................. { When strong wrist extension requires the aid of the finger extensors, the finger flexors contract to prevent extension of the fingers / Extensor carpi radialis longus and brevis and extensor carpi ulnaris are mutually neutralizing with respect to radial and ulnar flexion

Stabilizers ....When strong wrist extension is desired, the triceps provides a firm support for the origins of the wrist extensors by preventing flexion at the elbow

Ulnar Flexion

Movers .... { Extensor carpi ulnaris / Flexor carpi ulnaris

Neutralizers ....Extensor carpi ulnaris and flexor carpi ulnaris are mutually neutralizing with respect to extension and flexion

Stabilizers .... ⎰ Triceps provides a firm base of support for the ulnar flexors by preventing flexion at the elbow
Palmar interossei prevent abduction of little finger by ulnar flexors

Radial Flexion

Movers .... ⎰ Principal .... ⎰ Extensor carpi radialis longus
Extensor carpi radialis brevis

Assistant .... ⎰ Abductor pollicis longus
Extensor pollicis longus
Extensor pollicis brevis
Flexor carpi radialis

Neutralizers ....Extensor carpi radialis longus and brevis and flexor carpi radialis are mutually neutralizing with respect to one another's extension and flexion tendencies

Stabilizers ....Biceps steadies the elbow joint. Abductor pollicis longus is prevented from abducting and extending the thumb by the stabilizing action of the thumb flexors and adductors

Fingers

Flexion

Movers ....

Principal .... ⎰ Flexor digitorum superficialis (middle phalanges)
Flexor digitorum profundus (distal phalanges)
Flexor digiti minimi brevis (proximal phalanx of fifth finger)

Assistant .... ⎰ Lumbricales (proximal phalanges when other phalanges are extended)
Palmar interossei (proximal phalanges of second, fourth and fifth fingers)
Dorsal interossei (proximal phalanges of second, fourth and fifth fingers)
Opponens digiti minimi (fifth metacarpal)
Abductor digiti minimi (proximal phalanx of fifth finger)

Neutralizers and stabilizers................. ⎰ (These are grouped together because the muscles overlap in the functions of neutralizing and stabilizing)
Extensor carpi radialis longus and brevis and extensor carpi ulnaris stabilize the wrist during flexion of the fingers, thus neutralizing the wrist-flexing tendency of the long finger flexors

If the middle and distal phalanges of the fingers are flexed, but not the proximal phalanges, the extensor digitorum stabilizes the proximal phalanx, and the flexor carpi ulnaris and radialis and palmaris longus stabilize the wrist against the pull of the extensor digitorum

$\begin{cases} \text{If the proximal phalanges of the fingers} \\ \text{are flexed, but not the middle or distal} \\ \text{phalanges, the extensor digitorum} \\ \text{stabilizes the latter two phalanges, and} \\ \text{the flexor carpi ulnaris, flexor carpi} \\ \text{radialis and palmaris longus stabilize the} \\ \text{wrist against the pull of the extensor} \\ \text{digitorum} \end{cases}$

Neutralizers and Stabilizers ....

Extension

Movers ....

Principal ....
$\begin{cases} \text{Extensor digitorum (proximal phalanges)} \\ \text{Extensor indicis (proximal phalanx of index} \\ \text{finger)} \\ \text{Extensor digiti minimi (proximal phalanx} \\ \text{of fifth finger)} \end{cases}$

Assistant ....
$\begin{cases} \text{Lumbricales (middle and distal phalanges)} \\ \text{Palmar interossei (middle and distal pha-} \\ \text{langes of second, fourth and fifth fingers)} \\ \text{Dorsal interossei (middle and distal pha-} \\ \text{langes of second, fourth and fifth fingers)} \\ \text{Abductor digiti minimi (middle and distal} \\ \text{phalanges of fifth finger)} \end{cases}$

Neutralizers and stabilizers ....Flexor carpi ulnaris, flexor carpi radialis
and palmaris longus stabilize the wrist
during extension of the fingers, thus
neutralizing the wrist-extending tendency of the long finger extensors

Abduction

Movers ....
$\begin{cases} \text{Dorsal interossei (second and fourth} \\ \text{fingers)} \\ \text{Abductor digiti minimi (fifth finger)} \end{cases}$

Neutralizers and stabilizers ....Various muscles of the wrist and hand
serve in these capacities, depending
upon the position of the hand, upon
which fingers are being abducted, and
upon the force of the movement

Adduction

Movers ....
$\begin{cases} \text{Palmar interossei (second, fourth and} \\ \text{fifth fingers)} \\ \text{Opponens digiti minimi (fifth metacarpal)} \end{cases}$

Neutralizers and stabilizers ....Various muscles of the wrist and hand
serve in these capacities, depending
upon the position of the hand, upon
which fingers are being adducted, and
upon the force of the movement

Radial and Ulnar Flexion of the Middle Finger

Movers ....Dorsal interossei (both radial and ulnar
flexion of middle finger)

Neutralizers and stabilizers ....Various muscles of the other fingers and
of the wrist serve in these capacities,
depending upon the position of the hand
and the force of the movement

Thumb

Flexion

Movers .... { Principal .... { Flexor pollicis longus (both phalanges)
Flexor pollicis brevis (metacarpal and proximal phalanx)
Opponens pollicis (metacarpal)

Assistant .... Adductor pollicis (metacarpal and proximal phalanx)

Neutralizers and stabilizers .... The extensors of the wrist and other muscles of the wrist and hand, depending upon the position of the hand and the force of the movement

Extension

Movers .... { Principal .... { Abductor pollicis longus (metacarpal)
Extensor pollicis longus (both phalanges)
Extensor pollicis brevis (proximal phalanx)

Assistant .... Extensors pollicis longus and brevis (metacarpal)

Neutralizers and stabilizers .... The flexors of the wrist and other muscles of the wrist and hand, depending upon the position of the hand and the force of the movement

Abduction

Movers .... { Principal .... { Abductor pollicis longus (metacarpal)
Abductor pollicis brevis (metacarpal)
Opponens pollicis

Assistant .... { Extensor pollicis brevis (metacarpal)
Flexor pollicis brevis (metacarpal)

Neutralizers and stabilizers .... The ulnar flexors of the wrist and other muscles of the wrist and hand, depending upon the position of the hand and the force of the movement

Adduction

Movers .... { Principal .... Adductor pollicis (metacarpal)

Assistant .... { Flexor pollicis longus (metacarpal)
Extensor pollicis longus (metacarpal)
Flexor pollicis brevis (metacarpal)

Neutralizers and stabilizers .... None unless the movement is forceful, in which case all the muscles of the wrist and fingers seem to be in static contraction

Opposition

Movers .... { Principal .... Opponens pollicis (metacarpal)

Assistants in different phases of opposition { Flexor pollicis longus (metacarpal and both phalanges)
Flexor pollicis brevis (metacarpal and proximal phalanx)
Adductor pollicis (metacarpal and proximal phalanx)

Neutralizers...In the second part of the movement the tendency of the flexor pollicis longus to flex and radially flex the wrist is neutralized by the extensor carpi ulnaris, extensor carpi radialis longus and extensor carpi radialis brevis. The tendency of the flexor pollicis brevis to flex the metacarpal bone at the same time that it is flexing the first phalanx is neutralized by the extensor pollicis longus and brevis

Stabilizers ....All the muscles of the wrist contract to stabilize it, particularly when the thumb is pressing forcefully against the fingers

MUSCULAR ANALYSIS OF THE FUNDAMENTAL MOVEMENTS OF THE THIGH

Flexion

Movers ....
- Principal ....
  - Tensor fasciae latae, especially during first half of movement
  - Sartorius, continues throughout movement
  - Pectineus, especially during first half of movement
  - Iliopsoas
- Assistant ....
  - Rectus femoris
  - Adductor longus
  - Adductor brevis
  - Gracilis

Neutralizers...The tensor fasciae latae and the pectineus are mutually neutralizing with respect to abduction and adduction

Stabilizers ....Abdominal muscles and lumbar spine extensors stabilize the pelvis

Extension

Movers ....
- Gluteus maximus, especially against resistance and when thigh is flexed beyond a 45 degree angle
- Hamstrings
- Adductor magnus, when thigh is flexed beyond a 45 degree angle

Neutralizers...Gluteus medius netralizes the adductor tendency of adductor magnus

Stabilizers ....Abdominal muscles and lumbar spine extensors stabilize the pelvis

Abduction

Movers
- Principal ....
  - Gluteus medius
  - Gluteus minimus, less effective than medius
- Assistant ....
  - Tensor fasciae latae, when thigh is extended
  - Gluteus maximus, uppermost fibers, only during early part of movement

Neutralizers......................................Gluteus maximus and gluteus medius and minimus are mutually neutralizing with respect to outward and inward rotation

Stabilizers ....These depend upon the position of the body and whether one or both thighs are being abducted. If one thigh is abducted against resistance, the abdominal muscles, spinal extensors and quadratus lumborum help to stabilize the pelvis

Adduction

Movers
- Principal ....
  - Adductor magnus
  - Adductor longus
  - Adductor brevis
  - Gracilis
- Assistant ....
  - Pectineus, when thigh is flexed
  - Gluteus maximus, lower fibers

Neutralizers......................................The adductors magnus and longus are mutually neutralizing with respect to extension and flexion; likewise the pectineus and gluteus maximus

Stabilizers ....The abdominal muscles, spinal extensors and quadratus lumborum help to stabilize the pelvis when one thigh is adducted against resistance

Outward Rotation

Movers ....
- Six deep rotators
- Gluteus maximus

Neutralizers......................................The secondary actions of the six deep rotators neutralize one another

Stabilizers ....When the weight is not on the foot, the abdominal muscles, spinal extensors and quadratus lumborum stabilize the pelvis

Inward Rotation

Movers
- Principal ....
  - Gluteus minimus
  - Gluteus medius, anterior fibers
- Assistant ....
  - Tensor fasciae latae
  - Adductor magnus, lower fibers, when thigh is extended

Neutralizers......................................Adductor magnus neutralizes the abductory tendency of the other movers

Stabilizers ....When the weight is not on the foot, the abdominal muscles, spinal extensors and quadratus lumborum stabilize the pelvis

MUSCULAR ANALYSIS OF THE FUNDAMENTAL MOVEMENTS OF THE LEG AT THE KNEE

Flexion

Movers
- Principal
  - Hamstrings (biceps femoris, semitendinosus, semimembranosus)
  - Sartorius
  - Gracilis
- Assistant
  - Popliteus
  - Gastrocnemius

Neutralizers ....The biceps femoris on the one hand, and the semimembranosus, semitendinosus and popliteus on the other, neutralize one another's rotatory tendencies

Stabilizers ....The hip flexors help to stabilize the thigh against the pull of the hamstrings

Extension

Movers ....Quadriceps femoris

Neutralizers and stabilizers ....The vastus lateralis and vastus medialis neutralize one another's lateral and medial components of force, thus steadying the knee. The hip extensors help to stabilize the thigh against the pull of the rectus femoris

Outward Rotation of Flexed Leg at Knee

Mover ....Biceps femoris

Neutralizers ....The quadriceps femoris checks further flexion if it is not desired

Stabilizers ....Hip adductors

Inward Rotation of Flexed Leg at Knee

Movers
- Principal
  - Semitendinosus
  - Semimembranosus
  - Popliteus
- Assistant
  - Gracilis
  - Sartorius

Neutralizers ....The quadriceps femoris checks further flexion if it is not desired

Stabilizers ....Hip abductors

MUSCULAR ANALYSIS OF THE FUNDAMENTAL MOVEMENTS OF THE ANKLE, FOOT AND TOES

Ankle

Dorsal Flexion

Movers
- Principal
  - Tibialis anterior
  - Peroneus tertius
  - Extensor digitorum longus
- Assistant ....Extensor hallucis longus

Neutralizers.....................................Tibialis anterior and peroneus tertius mutually neutralize one another's tendency to invert and evert the foot

Stabilizers ....None

Plantar Flexion

Movers ....
{
　Principal ....
{
Gastrocnemius
Soleus
Peroneus longus
}
　Assistant ....
{
Tibialis posterior
Peroneus brevis
Flexor digitorum longus
Flexor hallucis longus
}
}

Neutralizers..................................... Peroneus longus and brevis on the one hand, and tibialis posterior on the other, mutually neutralize one another's tendency to evert and invert the foot

Stabilizers .... None

Foot

Dorsal Flexion

　　　The muscular action is the same as for dorsal flexion at the ankle

Plantar Flexion

　　　With the exception of the gastrocnemius and soleus, which do not cross the tarsal joints, the muscular action is the same as for plantar flexion at the ankle

Supination (inversion and adduction) (Fig. D–5, B.)

Movers ....
{
　Principal ....
{
Tibialis posterior
Flexor digitorum longus
}
　Assistant ....
{
Tibialis anterior
Flexor hallucis longus
}
}

Note: The axis of the ankle joint is such that the foot appears to be slightly inverted when it is plantar-flexed. For this reason the gastrocnemius and soleus are sometimes included as inverters of the foot. When one considers the attachment of the tendocalcaneus, however, it is obvious that these muscles can have no direct action on the tarsal joints

Neutralizers.....................................Tibialis anterior and posterior mutually neutralize one another's tendency to dorsiflex and plantar-flex the foot and ankle

Stabilizers ....None

Pronation (eversion and abduction) (Fig. D–5, A.)

Movers ....
{
　Principal ....
{
Peroneus longus
Peroneus brevis
}
　Assistant ....
{
Peroneus tertius
Extensor digitorum longus
}
}

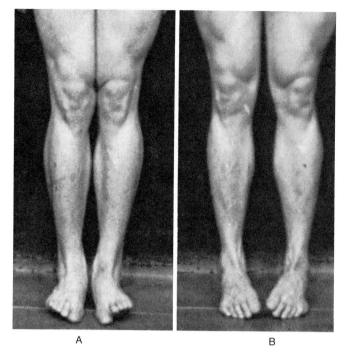

A   B

Figure D–5. The feet and legs in weight-bearing position. *A,* In eversion; *B,* in inversion.

Neutralizers......................................The two principal muscles are mutually neutralizing with the two assistant muscles with respect to plantar and dorsal flexion

Stabilizers .... None

Toes

Note: Only the movers are listed

Flexion

        Flexor digitorum longus
        Flexor hallucis longus
        Short flexors located on the foot

Extension

        Extensor digitorum longus
        Extensor hallucis longus
        Short extensors located on the foot

Abduction

        Short muscles located on the foot

Adduction

        Short muscles located on the foot

MUSCULAR ANALYSIS OF THE FUNDAMENTAL MOVEMENTS OF THE HEAD AND TRUNK

Cervical Spine and Atlanto-occipital Joint

Flexion

Movers
- Principal .... { Sternocleidomastoid / Prevertebral muscles
- Assistant .... { Three scaleni / Hyoid muscles

Neutralizers .... The muscles on the two sides neutralize one another's lateral motions

Stabilizers .... { Clavicular portion of pectoralis major / Subclavius (stabilizes the clavicle for the sternocleidomastoid) / Lower cervical and upper thoracic extensors (stabilize the spine for the prevertebral muscles and the three scaleni) / Rectus abdominis (stabilizes the sternum for the sternocleidomastoid)

Extension and Hypertension

Movers
- Principal .... { Splenius cervicis and capitis / Erector spinae, cervicis and capitis portions / Semispinalis, cervicis and capitis portions / The suboccipitals / The deep posterior spinal muscles, cervicis and capitis portions
- Assistant .... Trapezius I

Neutralizers .... The muscles on the two sides neutralize one another's lateral motions

Stabilizers .... { Extensors of the thoracic and lumbar spine / Rhomboid and trapezius IV (stabilize the scapula for trapezius I)

Lateral Flexion

Movers
- Principal .... { Three scaleni / Splenius, capitis and cervicis / Prevertebral muscles, lateral portions / Sternocleidomastoid / Erector spinae, capitis and cervicis portions / Semispinalis, capitis and cervicis portions
- Assistant .... { Suboccipitals / Deep posterior spinal muscles, cervicis portion / Levator scapulae

Neutralizers .... The anterior and posterior muscles neutralize one another's flexion and extension actions

Stabilizers .... { Flexors and extensors of thoracic and lumbar spine
Subclavius (stabilizes the clavicle for the sternocleidomastoid)
Lower trapezius (stabilizes the scapula for the levator scapulae)

Rotation (Fig. D–6.)

Movers ....

Rotators to the opposite side { Sternocleidomastoid
Deep posterior spinal muscles, cervicis portions

Rotators to the same side { Splenius, capitis and cervicis
Erector spinae, capitis and cervicis portions
Suboccipitals

Neutralizers .... The anterior and posterior muscles neutralize one another's flexion and extension tendencies

Stabilizers .... { Flexors and extensors of thoracic and lumbar spine
Subclavius (stabilizes the clavicle for the sternocleidomastoid)

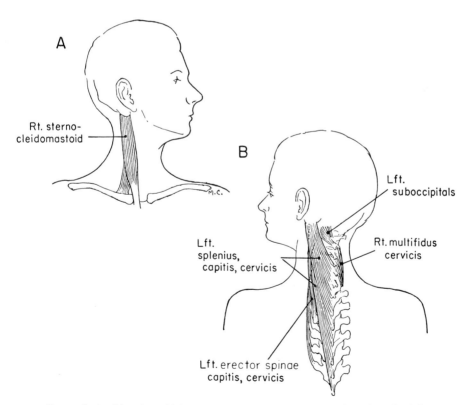

A

Rt. sterno-cleidomastoid

B

Lft. suboccipitals

Lft. splenius, capitis, cervicis

Rt. multifidus cervicis

Lft. erector spinae capitis, cervicis

Figure D–6. Muscles which contract to rotate the head and neck to the left.

Thoracic and Lumbar Spine

Flexion

Movers .... {
Rectus abdominis
External oblique
Internal oblique
}

Neutralizers.................................... The muscles of the left and right sides neutralize one another's lateral flexion and rotational tendencies

Stabilizers .... Hip flexors, particularly when the movement is performed in the supine position

Extension

Movers .... {
Principal .... {
Erector spinae, thoracic and lumbar portions (especially hyperextension from prone position)
Semispinalis thoracis
}

Assistant.............. Deep posterior spinal muscles
}

Neutralizers.................................... The muscles of the left and right sides neutralize one another's lateral motions

Stabilizers .... Hip extensors, particularly when the movement is performed in the prone position

Lateral Flexion

Movers .... {
Principal .... {
Erector spinae, thoracic and lumbar portions
External oblique
Internal oblique
Quadratus lumborum
}

Assistant .... {
Semispinalis thoracis
Rectus abdominis
Psoas
Deep posterior spinal muscles
Latissimus dorsi
}
}

Neutralizers.................................... The anterior and posterior muscles neutralize one another's flexion and extension tendencies

Stabilizers .... Hip abductors on the same side and adductors on the opposite side, particularly when the movement is performed in the side-lying position

Rotation (Fig. D–7.)

Movers .... {
Rotators to the opposite side {
External oblique
Semispinalis thoracis
Deep posterior spinal muscles
}

Rotators to the same side {
Erector spinae, thoracic and lumbar portions, particularly the iliocostalis thoracis
Internal oblique
}
}

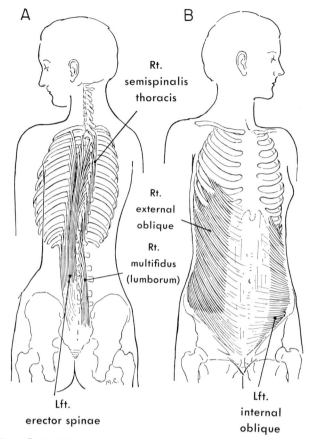

A

B

Rt.
semispinalis
thoracis

Rt.
external
oblique

Rt.
multifidus
(lumborum)

Lft.
erector spinae

Lft.
internal
oblique

Figure D–7.   Muscles which contract to rotate the trunk to the left.

Neutralizers...The anterior and posterior muscles neutralize one another's flexion and exten-
sion tendencies. The muscles on opposite
sides neutralize one another's lateral
flexion tendencies

Stabilizers ....The oblique abdominal muscles serve to
stabilize the pelvis for the erector spinae
and vice versa. The internal intercostals
stabilize the ribs for the levatores
costarum.

APPENDIX E

SUMMARY OF MUSCULAR ACTIONS IN TABULAR FORM

The movements of the majority of skeletal muscles are briefly summarized in tabular form in this section. They are classified according to the segments of the body which they cause to move and to the joints at which the movements occur. This section serves for quick reference to the roles of the muscle as principal and assistant movers in the basic movements of these body segments and should be of use to the student who is learning to identify muscles by the palpation method. Differentiating between principal and assistant movers should not be given too much emphasis, however, because this is often arbitrary and can be misleading.

Obviously tables such as these cannot include information on all of the special factors and circumstances that influence muscle actions. Ideally these should be studied in unabridged anatomy texts and in reports of electromyographic research. The discussions of muscular actions in Part II of this text should be of some help.

PRINCIPAL MUSCLES FOR STUDY

The muscles are classified in Tables 1 to 3 in two ways: (1) according to their action, and (2) according to their position in relation to the joint or, in some cases, location on parts of the skeleton such as forearm, lower leg or in the hand.

KEY TO MUSCLE ACTION

X   Definitely active in the movement
x   An assistant or emergency muscle; acts only under certain conditions, or it acts primarily on another joint and therefore only secondarily on this joint.
?   Action uncertain in the movement; authorities disagree.

TABLE E-1.   Muscles Acting on the Upper Extremity
A. At the shoulder joint
B. On the shoulder girdle
C. At the elbow and radioulnar joints
D. At the wrist joints
E. At the finger joints
F. At the thumb joints

TABLE A. Muscles Acting at the Shoulder Joint

Muscles and Location	Upper Arm									Where to Palpate
	Flexion	Extension	Hyperextension	Abduction	Adduction	Rotation Outward	Rotation Inward	Horizontal Flexion	Horizontal Extension	
Superior										
Middle deltoid				X					X	Lateral surface of upper third of upper arm
Supraspinatus				X		?				Above spine of scapula when scapula is supported, armpit rests over back of chair
Inferior										
Latissimus dorsi		X	X		X		X		X	Posterior border of axilla just below the teres major
Teres major		X	X		X		X		X	Posterior border of axilla just above latissimus dorsi
Anterior										
Anterior deltoid										
Upper	X			?			X	X		In front of the head of the humerus and for a space of 2 or 3 inches below this
Lower					x					
Pectoralis major										
Upper or clavicular	X									Just below the medial two thirds of the clavicle
Lower or sternal		X			X		X	X		Lateral to the sternum, below clavicular portion
Coracobrachialis	x				x		x	X		Anterior surface of upper arm medial to short head of biceps; difficult to palpate
Subscapularis							X	X		Cannot be palpated

A. Muscles Acting at the Shoulder Joint (Continued)

Upper Arm

Muscles and Location	Flexion	Extension	Hyperextension	Abduction	Adduction	Rotation Outward	Rotation Inward	Horizontal Flexion	Horizontal Extension	Where to Palpate
Posterior										
Posterior deltoid		X			x Lower fibers	X			X	Upper and lateral portion of posterior surface of scapula below scapular spine
Infraspinatus						X			X	Posterior surfaces of scapula medial and inferior to posterior deltoid muscle
Teres minor						X			X	
Primary actions at other joints										
Biceps brachii	x							x		See C. Muscles Acting at Elbow and Radioulnar Joints
Triceps brachii Long head		x	x		x	x		x		See C. Muscles Acting at Elbow and Radioulnar Joints

B. Muscles Acting on the Shoulder Girdle

Muscles and Location	Scapula								Where to Palpate
	Eleva-tion	Depres-sion	Abduc-tion	Adduc-tion	Upward Tilt	Reduc-tion of Upward Tilt	Rotation Upward	Rotation Down-ward	
Anterior									
Subclavis		Clavicle X							Cannot be palpated
Pectoralis minor			X		X			X	May be palpated halfway between clavicle and nipple when the arm is elevated backward as far as possible against resistance
Serratus anterior									Anterior lateral surface of upper thorax
Upper			X				x		
Lower			x				X		
Posterior									
Levator scapulae	X							X	Cannot be palpated
Trapezius									Kite-shaped area in upper back and neck
Part I	X								
Part II	X			x					
Part III		X		X			X		
Part IV	X			x			X		
Rhomboids									Cannot be palpated
Major and minor	X			X				X	

C. Muscles Acting at the Elbow and Radioulnar Joints

Muscles and Location	Forearm				Where to Palpate
	Flexion	Exten-sion	Prona-tion	Supina-tion	
Anterior					
Biceps brachii	X			x	Anterior surface of lower two thirds of upper arm
Brachialis	X				Just lateral to biceps if contraction is strong and especially if the forearm is flexed in the pronated position
Brachioradialis	X				On anterior radial aspect of upper half of forearm
Pronator teres	x		X		Cannot be palpated
Pronator quadratus			X		Cannot be palpated
Posterior					
Triceps brachii		X			Posterior surface of upper arm.
Anconeus		X			Lateral margin of olecranon process of back of elbow.
Supinator				X	Cannot be palpated
Primary actions at other joints					
Extensor carpi radialis brevis	x				See D. Muscles Acting at the Wrist Joint
Extensor carpi ulnaris	x				See D. Muscles Acting at the Wrist Joint
Extensor carpi radialis longus	x				See D. Muscles Acting at the Wrist Joint

D. Muscles Acting at the Wrist Joint

Muscles and Location	Hand					Where to Palpate
	Flexion	Exten-sion	Hyper-extension	Radial Flexion or Abduction	Ulnar Flexion or Adduction	
Anterior						
Flexor carpi radialis	X			x		Anterior surface of wrist, just lateral to the tendon of palmaris longus
Palmaris longus	X					Anterior surface of wrist in exact center
Flexor carpi ulnaris	X				X	Anterior surface of ulnar side of forearm
Posterior						
Extensor carpi radialis longus		X		X		Center of dorsal surface of forearm, 2 in. below elbow when forearm is in a pronated position
Extensor carpi radialis brevis		X		X		Dorsal surface of forearm, slightly below the extensor carpi radialis longus
Extensor carpi ulnaris		X			X	Ulnar margin of posterior surface of forearm, halfway between elbow and wrist
Primary actions at other joints						
Flexor digitorum superficialis	x					See E. Muscles Acting at the Finger Joints
Flexor digitorum profundus	x					See E. Muscles Acting at the Finger Joints
Extensor digitorum		x				See E. Muscles Acting at the Finger Joints
Extensor indicis		x				See E. Muscles Acting at the Finger Joints
Extensor digiti minimi		x				See E. Muscles Acting at the Finger Joints
Flexor pollicis longus	X					See F. Muscles Acting at the Thumb Joints
Extensor pollicis longus		x		x		See F. Muscles Acting at the Thumb Joints
Extensor pollicis brevis				x		See F. Muscles Acting at the Thumb Joints
Abductor pollicis longus	x			X		See F. Muscles Acting at the Thumb Joints

E. Muscles Acting at Finger Joints

Muscles and Location	Metacarpophalangeal Joints — Phalanges: Proximal				Interphalangeal Joints — Middle		Interphalangeal Joints — Distal		Where to Palpate
	Flexion	Extension	Abduction	Adduction	Flexion	Extension	Flexion	Extension	
On Forearm									
Flexor digitorum superficialis	x				X				Palm
Flexor digitorum profundus	x				x		X		Cannot be palpated
Extensor digitorum		X				x		x	Dorsal surface, hand and arm
Extensor indicis		X2°							Cannot be palpated
Extensor digiti minimi		X5							Cannot be palpated
In Hand									
Lumbricales	x					X		X	Cannot be palpated
Palmar interossei	x 2, 4, 5			X 2, 4, 5					Cannot be palpated
Dorsal interossei	x		X 2, 3†, 4, X5			x		x	Cannot be palpated
Abductor digiti minimi	x5					x5		x5	Ulnar border of hand
Flexor digiti minimi brevis manus	X5								Palm, just lateral to abductor digiti minimi
Fifth Metacarpal Bone (Articulation with hamate)									
Opponens digiti minimi	X			X					Cannot be palpated

°Numbers refer to fingers: 2 (index), 3 (middle), 4 (ring), 5 (little).
†Actually radial and ulnar flexion of middle finger.

F. Muscles Acting at Thumb Joints

Muscles and Location	Metacarpal					Proximal phalanx		Distal phalanx		Where to Palpate
	Flexion and Hyper-flexion	Exten-sion and Hyper-exten-sion	Abduc-tion	Adduc-tion and Hyper-adduc-tion	Oppo-sition	Flexion	Exten-sion	Flexion	Exten-sion	
On Forearm										
Flexor pollicis longus				x	x	x		X		Cannot be palpated
Extensor pollicis longus		x		x			X		X	With palm on table raise thumb as high as possible and tendon is clearly seen on dorsal surface of thumb, radial side of hand
Extensor pollicis brevis		x	x				X			By extending first phalanx against resistance, tendon stands out between wrist and first metacarpophalangeal joints
Abductor pollicis longus		X	X		x					Just anterior to tendon of extensor pollicis brevis at base of metacarpal
In Hand (Intrinsic)										
Flexor pollicis brevis	x			x	x	X				Along the ulnar margin of the anterior surface of the thenar eminence
Abductor pollicis brevis			X		x	X			x	Anterior surface of thenar eminence
Opponens pollicis	X				X					Along the lateral margin of the thenar eminence, close to metacarpal bone when thumb is pressed hard against the middle finger
Adductor pollicis	X			X	x	x				Inner anterior surface of the metacarpophalangeal joint of the thumb with thumb pressed against one of the fingers

TABLE E-2 Muscles Acting on the Lower Extremity
A. At the Hip Joint
B. At the Knee Joint
C. At the Ankle, Foot, and Toe Joints

A. Muscles Acting at the Hip Joint

Muscles and Location	Flexion	Exten- sion	Abduc- tion	Adduc- tion	Rotation Outward	Rotation Inward	Where to Palpate
Anterior							
Psoas major	X						In the groin on thin subjects when abdominal muscles are relaxed. See text page 255.
Iliacus	X						See psoas
Sartorius	X						At the anterior superior iliac spine
Pectineus	X			x	?		At the front of the pubis, just lateral to the adductor longus
Tensor fasciae latae	X		x			?	About two inches anterior to the greater trochanter
Rectus femoris	X						See B. Muscles Acting at the Knee Joint
Posterior							
Gluteus maximus		X	x upper fibers	x lower fibers	x		Posterior surface of buttocks
Biceps femoris		X					See B. Muscles Acting at the Knee Joint
Semitendinosus		X					See B. Muscles Acting at the Knee Joint
Semimembranosus		X					See B. Muscles Acting at the Knee Joint
Six deep outward rotators					X		Cannot be palpated

A. Muscles Acting at the Hip Joint (Continued)

Muscles and Location	Thigh						Where to Palpate
	Flexion	Extension	Abduction	Adduction	Rotation Outward	Rotation Inward	
Lateral							
Gluteus medius			X			X anterior fibers	About 2 or 3 inches above the greater trochanter
Gluteus minimus			X			X	Cannot be palpated
Medial							
Gracilis	x			X			Medial aspect of posterior surface of knee anterior to the semitendinosus
Adductor longus	x			X			Just below origin at the medial aspects of the groin
Adductor brevis				X			Cannot be palpated
Adductor magnus	x	X		X		x condyloid portion	Medial surface of middle half of thigh

B. Muscles Acting at the Knee Joint

Muscles and Location	Lower Leg				Where to Palpate
	Flexion	Extension	Rotation Outward	Rotation Inward	
Anterior					
Rectus femoris		X			Anterior surface of thigh
Vastus intermedius		X			Cannot be palpated
Vastus lateralis		X			Anterolateral aspect of thigh, lateral to the rectus femoris
Vastus medialis		X			Anteromedial aspect of the lower third of the thigh, medial to the rectus femoris
Posterior					
Biceps femoris	X		X		Lateral aspect of posterior surface of knee
Semimembranosus	X			X	Tendon is beneath gracilis and semitendinosus at the knee
Semitendinosus	X			X	Medial aspect of posterior surface of the knee
Sartorius	X			x	At the anterior superior iliac spine
Gracilis	X			x	Medial aspect of posterior surface of knee, anterior to the semitendinosus tendon
Popliteus	x			X	Cannot be palpated

C. Muscles Acting at the Ankle, Foot and Toe Joints

Muscles and Location	Ankle		Foot				Toes		Where to Palpate
	Dorsi-flexion	Plantar Flexion	Dorsi-flexion	Plantar Flexion	Supination Inversion and Adduction	Pronation Eversion and Abduction	Flexion	Extension	
Anterior aspect of leg									
Tibialis anterior	X		X		X				Anterior surface of leg, just lateral to tibia
Extensor digitorum longus	X		X			x		X	Anterior surface of ankle and dorsal surface of foot, lateral to tendon of extensor hallucis longus
Extensor hallucis longus			X					X great toe	Dorsal surface of foot and great toe
Peroneus tertius	X		X			X			Dorsal surface of foot close to base of fifth metatarsal
Posterior aspect of leg									
Gastrocnemius		X							Calf of leg and back of ankle
Soleus		X							Slightly lateral to and below the lateral bulge of the gastrocnemius
Tibialis posterior				X	X				Cannot be palpated
Flexor digitorum longus				x	x		X 4 lesser toes		Cannot be palpated
Flexor hallucis longus				x	x		X great toe		Medial border of calcaneal tendon close to calcaneus
Lateral aspect of leg									
Peroneus longus				X		X			Lateral surface of upper half of leg (belly) and lateral surface of lower half of leg and just above and behind lateral malleolus
Peroneus brevis				x		X			Lateral margin of foot just posterior to base of fifth metatarsal

TABLE E–3. Muscles Acting on the Head and Trunk
A. At the Head and Neck Joints
B. At the Thoracic and Lumbar Joints

A. Muscles Acting at the Head and Neck Joints

Muscles and Location	Head and Neck (Cervical)					Where to Palpate
	Flexion	Extension	Lateral Flexion	Rotation Same side	Rotation Opposite side	
Anterior						
Prevertebral muscles	X					Cannot be palpated
Hyoid muscles	x					Suprahyoids just below the jaw bone. Infrahyoid cannot be palpated
Lateral						
Three scaleni	x neck		X neck			On the side of the neck between the sternocleid-omastoid and upper trapezius
Sternocleidomastoid	X		X		X	On the side of the neck just under the ear and at the junction of the clavicle and sternum
Levator scapulae			X			Cannot be palpated
Posterior						
Splenius capitis and cervicis		X	X	X		On back of the neck lateral to the trapezius and posterior to the sternocleidomastoid above the levator scapulae
Suboccipitals		X	X	X		Cannot be palpated
Erector spinae Capitis and cervicis portions		X	X	X		Cannot be palpated
Semispinalis capitis and cervicis		X	X			Cannot be palpated

B. Muscles Acting at the Thoracic and Lumbar Joints

Muscles and Location	Thoracic and Lumbar Spine					Where to Palpate
	Flexion	Extension	Lateral Flexion	Rotation Same side	Rotation Opposite side	
Anterior and Anterolateral						
Rectus abdominis	X					Front of the abdomen from pubis to the sternum
External oblique	X		X		X	At the side of the abdomen
Internal oblique	X		X	X		Side of the abdomen beneath external oblique when the latter is relaxed
Lateral						
Quadratus lumborum			X lumbar			Lateral to the erector spinae in the lumbar region
Psoas	?		X lumbar			See A. Muscles Acting at the Hip Joint
Posterior						
Erector spinae Thoracis and lumborum portions		X	X	X		Lumbar and thoracic region of the back, in two broad ridges on either side of the spine
Semispinalis thoracis		X	X thoracic		X thoracic	Cannot be palpated
Deep posterior muscles		X	x		X	Cannot be palpated

APPENDIX F

CHECK LISTS FOR THE MUSCULAR ANALYSIS OF MOVEMENTS OF THE MAJOR BODY SEGMENTS

These check lists were originally devised for the recording of the muscular actions identified in the palpation experiments described in the section headed Demonstrations and Laboratory Exercises at the end of Chapters 12 through 19. For the most part only the basic movements of individual body segments were used in these exercises. Although it is recognized that the palpation method is not as accurate as the electromyographic method for ascertaining muscular actions, the palpation method is invaluable as a method for studying muscular activity and for supplementing book study.

In addition to their use in identifying the actions of muscles in basic movements, the check lists are useful for the recording of the muscular analyses of postural and conditioning exercises and of the typical motor skills of familiar sports, gymnastic and tumbling events, dance techniques, and so on. For this purpose an ample number of duplicate copies of the lists should be available inasmuch as a complete set may be needed *for each phase* of a movement that involves the entire body. It would be helpful if spaces were provided on these for the student's name and the name of the motor skill being analyzed.

For developing skill in analyzing movements anatomically, much practice is needed. It is therefore suggested that the student start as soon as feasible to make such analyses and that he progress from the basic movements to more complex motor skills as rapidly as he is able. The following suggestions may prove helpful.

*Procedure for Making a Kinesiologic Analysis of a Movement**

1. Have someone demonstrate the movement to be analyzed both before and at frequent intervals throughout the analysis. In lieu of this, motion pictures (preferably slow motion ones shown on a projector which can be stopped at will) are an excellent substitute. If these are not available, a series of still shots or even a single photograph or sketch is helpful.

2. Divide the movement into logical phases, such as:
   a. Essential act or propulsive phase; b. return movement or recovery phase. Appropriate for calisthenic exercises, swimming strokes, and other two-part movements.
   a. Preparatory movement; b. essential act; c. follow through or recovery. Appropriate for throwing, striking and kicking activities.

3. Consider the starting position of the body (vertical, horizontal—prone, supine, side, or other) and the means of its support (ground, water, suspension apparatus, none). In this connection consider the effect of gravity on the muscular action.

4. Consider the nature of the movement, whether fast or slow, ballistic or nonballistic, against or not against resistance, and so on. Consider the effect of this on the muscular action.

5. Identify the movement of each body segment and analyze the joint actions. These may be recorded on the check lists by placing a check in the appropriate spaces across the top of the check list.

6. Considering all of the essential factors, analyze the muscular action and record on the check list.

---

*See Appendix G for illustrations of conditioning and postural exercises which serve as material for practice in making kinesiologic analyses.

Elementary method. Place a check mark in the appropriate space for each muscle that contributes positively to the movement.

Advanced method

(1) To differentiate between principal and assistant muscles use P and A, or X and x.

(2) To differentiate between concentric (shortening), eccentric (lengthening), and static contraction, use different colored pencils.

7. After completing the muscular analysis consider the following questions:

a. Are there any clear-cut examples of the neutralizing or of the mutually neutralizing action of muscles? If so, identify and explain.

b. Are there any clear-cut examples of stabilization of a segment of the body by muscular action? If so, identify and explain.

c. Are there any pertinent mechanical aspects or principles which should be taken into consideration in this exercise? If so, identify and explain.

Check lists follow

Check List for Muscular Analysis of Movements of the Arm on the Body*

	Sideward Elev. of Arm	Sideward Depr. of Arm	Fwd. Elev. of Arm	Fwd. Depr. of Arm	Bkwd. Elev. of Arm	Hor. Bkwd. Swing of Arm	Hor. Sideward Fwd. Swing	Outwd. Rot'n of Arm	Inwd. Rot'n of Arm	Elev. of Shoul. Gird.	Depr. of Shoul. Gird.	Abd. of Scap.	Add. of Scap.
SHOULDER GIRDLE													
Subclavius													
Pectoralis minor													
Serratus anterior													
Levator scapulae													
Trapezius I													
Trapezius II													
Trapezius III													
Trapezius IV													
Rhomboids													

*The check lists in Appendices B and F may be reproduced for class use without specific permission.

Check List for Muscular Analysis of Movements of the Arm on the Body (Continued)

	Side-ward Elev. of Arm	Side-ward Depr. of Arm	Fwd. Elev. of Arm	Fwd. Depr. of Arm	Bkwd. Elev. of Arm	Hor. Bkwd. Swing of Arm	Hor. Side-ward Fwd. Swing	Outwd. Rot'n of Arm	Inwd. Rot'n of Arm	Elev. of Shoul. Gird.	Depr. of Shoul. Gird.	Abd. of Scap.	Add. of Scap.
SHOULDER JOINT													
Deltoid: middle													
Deltoid: anterior													
Deltoid: posterior													
Supraspinatus													
Pect. major: clavicular													
Pect. major: sternal													
Coracobrachialis													
Subscapularis													
Latissimus dorsi													
Teres major													
Infrasp. & teres minor													

Check List for Muscular Analysis of Movements of Forearm at Elbow and
Radioulnar Joints

	Flexion	Extension	Supination	Pronation
MUSCLES OF ELBOW AND FOREARM:				
Biceps				
Brachialis				
Brachioradialis				
Pronator teres				
Pronator quadratus				
Supinator				
Triceps				
Anconeus				
MUSCLES OF WRIST:				
Flexor carpi radialis				
Flexor carpi ulnaris				
Palmaris longus				
Extensor carpi radialis longus				
Extensor carpi radialis brevis				
Extensor carpi ulnaris				

Check List for Muscular Analysis of Movements of the Hand at the Wrist

	Flexion	*Extension*	*Ulnar Flexion*	*Radial Flexion*
MUSCLES OF WRIST				
Flexor carpi radialis				
Flexor carpi ulnaris				
Palmaris longus				
Extensor carpi radialis longus				
Extensor carpi radialis brevis				
Extensor carpi ulnaris				
MUSCLES OF THUMB AND FINGERS				
Flexor digitorum superficialis				
Flexor digitorum profundus				
Extensor digitorum				
Extensor indicis				
Extensor digiti minimi				
Flexor pollicis longus				
Extensor pollicis longus				
Extensor pollicis brevis				
Abductor pollicis longus				

Check List for Muscular Analysis of Movements of the Fingers

	Metacarpophalangeal				Interphalangeal	
	Flex.	Ext.	Abd.	Add.	Flex.	Ext.
ON FOREARM						
Flexor digitorum superficialis						
Flexor digitorum profundus						
Extensor digitorum						
Extensor indicis						
Extensor digiti minimi						
IN HAND						
Lumbricales						
Palmar interossei						
Dorsal interossei						
Abductor digiti minimi						
Flex. dig. minimi brev.						
Opponens digiti minimi						

Check List for Muscular Analysis of Movements of the Thumb

	Carpometacarpal					Metacarpophalangeal		Interphalangeal	
	Flex.	Ext. & Hyp. Ex.	Abd.	Add. & Hyp. Add.	Opp.	Flex.	Ext.	Flex.	Ext.
ON FOREARM									
Fl. pol. long.									
Ext. pol. long.									
Ext. pol. brev.									
Abd. pol. long.									
IN HAND									
Fl. pol. brev.									
Abd. pol brev.									
Opponens pol.									
Adductor pol.									

Check List for Muscular Analysis of Movements of the Pelvic Girdle

	Increased Inclination	Decreased Inclination	Lateral Tilt	Rotation
Rectus abdominis				
External oblique				
Internal oblique				
Erector spinae				
Quadratus lumborum				
Psoas				
Gluteus maximus				
Gluteus medius and minimus				
Tensor fasciae latae				
Others:				

Note: Because of the numerous two-joint muscles found in the lower extremity, the check list for the muscular analysis of movements of the hip is combined with that for the knee. See following page.

Check List for Muscular Analysis of Movements
of the Thigh and Leg

	Hip						Knee			
	Flex.	Ext.	Abd.	Add.	Out. Rot.	Inwd. Rot.	Flex.	Ext.	Out. Rot.	Inwd. Rot.
Iliopsoas										
Sartorius										
Pectineus										
Tensor fasciae latae										
Gluteus maximus										
Gluteus medius										
Gluteus minimus										
Six deep rotators										
Adductor magnus										
Adductor longus										
Adductor brevis										
Gracilis										
Biceps femoris										
Semitendinosus										
Semimembranosus										
Rectus femoris										
Vastus intermedius										
Vastus lateralis										
Vastus medialis										
Popliteus										
Gastrocnemius										

Check List for Muscular Analysis of Movements
of Ankle, Foot and Toes

	Ankle		Foot				Toes	
	Dorsi-flex.	Plant. Flex.	Dorsi-flex.	Plant. Flex.	Inv. & Adduc.	Evers. & Abd.	Flex.	Ext.
Tibialis anterior								
Ext. halluc. long.								
Ext. digit. longus								
Peroneus tertius								
Peroneus longus								
Peroneus brevis								
Tibialis posterior								
Gastrocnemius								
Soleus								
Flexor hal. long.								
Flex. digit. long.								

Check List for the Muscular Analysis of Movements of the Head and Neck

	Flexion	Extension	Lateral Flexion	Rotation Same Side	Rotation Opposite Side
ANTERIOR:					
Prevertebral muscles					
Hyoid muscles					
LATERAL:					
Three scaleni					
Sternocleidomastoid					
Levator scapulae					
POSTERIOR:					
Splenius					
Suboccipitals					
Erector spinae					
Semispinalis					
Deep poster. muscles					
OTHER:					

Check List for the Muscular Analysis of Movements
of the Thoracic and Lumbar Spine

	Flexion	Extension	Lateral Flexion	Rotation Same Side	Rotation Opposite Side
ANTERIOR:					
Rectus abdominis					
Ext. oblique abd.					
Int. oblique abd.					
LATERAL:					
Quad. lumborum					
POSTERIOR:					
Erector spinae					
Semispinalis thoracis					
Deep. post. muscles					
OTHER:					

Check List for the Muscular Analysis of the Movements Involved in Respiration

	Normal Inhalation	Vigorous Inhalation	Vigorous Exhalation
MUSCLES OF RESPIRATION:			
Diaphragm			
External intercostals			
Internal intercostals, anterior			
Internal intercostals, posterior and lateral			
Levatores costarum			
Serratus posterior superior			
Serratus posterior inferior			
Transversus thoracis			
Transversus abdominis			
MUSCLES OF THE SPINE:			
Sternocleidomastoid			
Three scaleni			
Thoracic extensors			
Rectus abdominis			
External oblique			
Internal oblique			
MUSCLES OF THE SHOULDER GIRDLE AND JOINT:			
Pectoralis minor			
Trapezius I			
Levator scapulae			
OTHERS:			

APPENDIX G

EXERCISES FOR KINESIOLOGIC ANALYSIS

These exercises, intended as laboratory material for the student, are presented for kinesiologic analysis (major joint and muscle action) of movements commonly used to develop strength, increase flexibility, and improve posture. In most instances the exercises are organized according to the major body segments (the upper and lower extremities and the trunk-head-neck). Many of the exercises are illustrated by three views: (1) the starting position, (2) the movement, and (3) the return to the starting position. The calisthenic and gymnastic exercises were selected on the basis of their use in (1) most physical fitness and posture programs, in (2) conditioning programs for improving athletic performance, and in (3) tests for assessing strength and muscular endurance. The exercises are organized in the following series:

Series 1   Weight Training Exercises (barbells and weighted pulleys)
Series 2   Calisthenic and Gymnastic Exercises
Series 3   Isometric Tension Exercises (singly and with partners)
Series 4   Flexibility Exercises
Series 5   Posture Exercises

The exercises within each series are numbered consecutively in the following manner: The first exercise in Series is numbered 1–1, the second, 1–2. The first exercise in Series 2 is numbered 2–1, followed by 2–2, and so on in similar fashion.

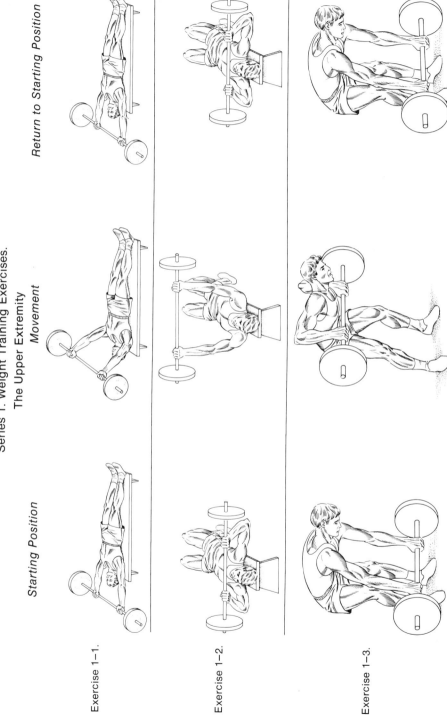

Series 1. Weight Training Exercises.
The Upper Extremity

Starting Position

Movement

Return to Starting Position

Exercise 1–1.

Exercise 1–2.

Exercise 1–3.

Series 1. Weight Training Exercises.
The Upper Extremity

Starting Position   *Movement*   *Return to Starting Position*

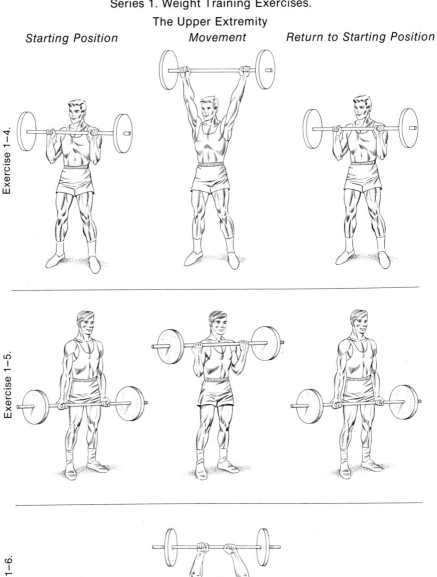

Exercise 1–4.

Exercise 1–5.

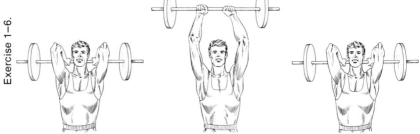

Exercise 1–6.

Series 1. Weight Training Exercises.
The Upper Extremity

Starting Position   *Movement*   *Return to Starting Position*

Exercise 1–7.

Exercise 1–8.

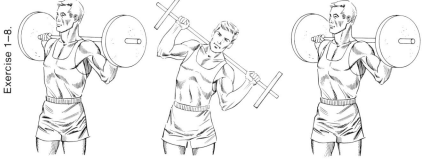

Series 1. Weight Training Exercises.
The Lower Extremity

Starting Position   *Movement*   *Return to Starting Position*

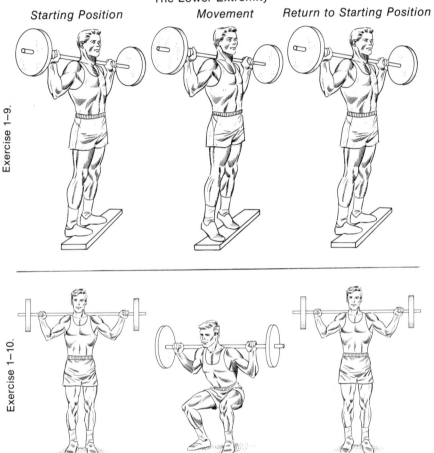

Exercise 1–9.

Exercise 1–10.

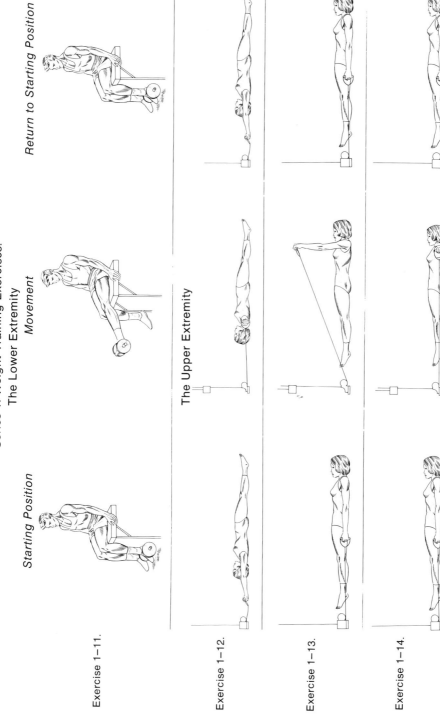

Series 1. Weight Training Exercises.
The Lower Extremity

Starting Position   Movement   Return to Starting Position

Exercise 1–11.

The Upper Extremity

Exercise 1–12.

Exercise 1–13.

Exercise 1–14.

Series 1. Weight Training Exercises.
The Upper Extremity
Movement

Starting Position

Return to Starting Position

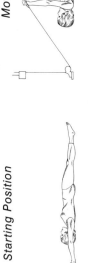
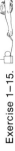

Exercise 1–15.

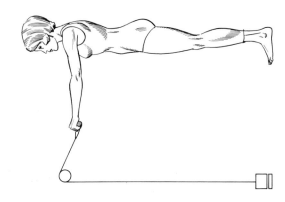

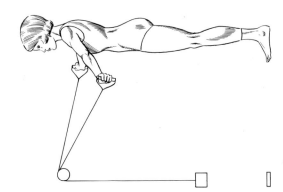

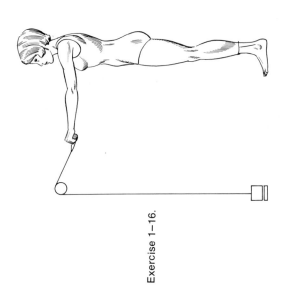

Exercise 1–16.

Series 1. Weight Training Exercises.
The Upper Extremity

Starting Position

Movement

Return to Starting Position

Exercise 1–17.

Return to Starting Position

Series 2. Calisthenic and Gymnastic Exercises.
The Upper Extremity
Movement

Starting Position

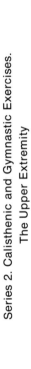

Exercise 2–1.
Dip and
push-up on
the parallel
bars.

Series 2. Calisthenic and Gymnastic Exercises.
The Trunk

Starting Position   Movement   Return to Starting Position

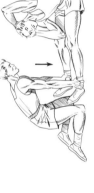
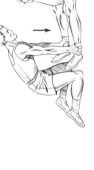
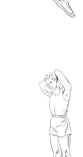
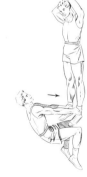

Exercise 2–2.
Twist sit-up
with legs
extended.

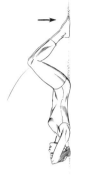
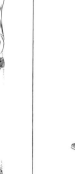
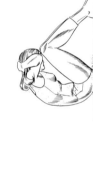
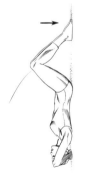

Exercise 2–3.
Sit-up with
knees
flexed.

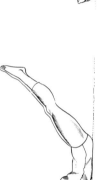
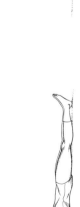
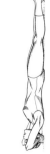

Exercise 2–4.
Sit-up with
double leg
lift.

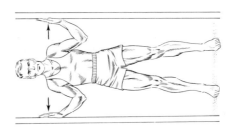

Exercise 3–3.
Push Out

Series 3. Isometric Tension Exercises.
The Upper Extremity

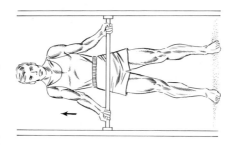

Exercise 3–2.
Pull Up

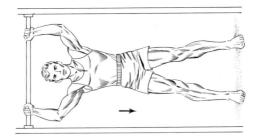

Exercise 3–1.
Pull Down

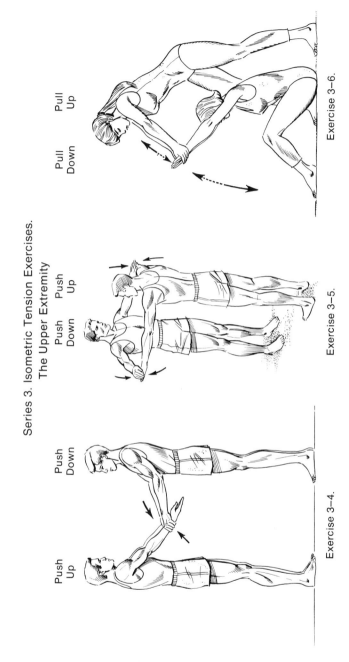

Series 3. Isometric Tension Exercises.
The Upper Extremity

Push Up   Push Down

Exercise 3-4.

Push Down   Push Up

Exercise 3-5.

Pull Up   Pull Down

Exercise 3-6.

Series 3. Isometric Tension Exercises.
The Lower Extremity and Trunk

Push Up

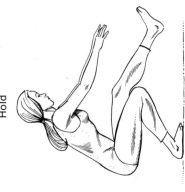

Exercise 3–7.

Hold

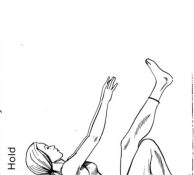

Exercise 3–8.

Pull Leg Down

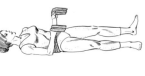

Exercise 3–9.

Press Lumbar
Spine Back

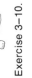

Exercise 3–10.

The Trunk—Head—Neck

Push Down   Pull Up

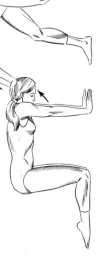

Exercise 3–11.

Pull Up   Push Down

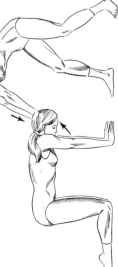

Exercise 3–12.

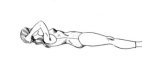

Exercise 3–13.
Pull neck
backward.

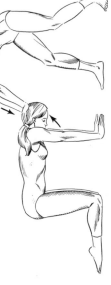

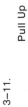

Series 4. Flexibility Exercises for Major Joints.

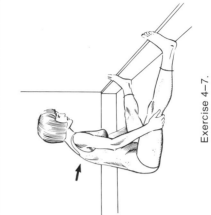

Exercise 4–4.

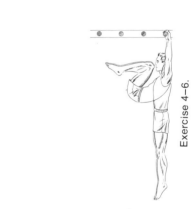

Exercise 4–7.

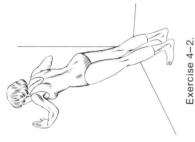

Exercise 4–3.

Exercise 4–2.

Exercise 4–6.

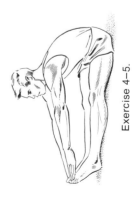

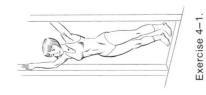

Exercise 4–1.

Exercise 4–5.

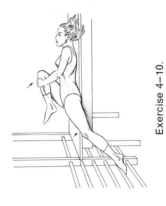

Exercise 4–10.

Series 4. Flexibility Exercises for Major Joints.

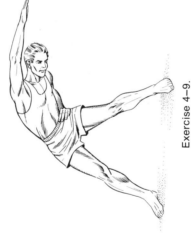

Exercise 4–9.

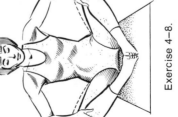

Exercise 4–8.

Series 5. Posture Exercises.

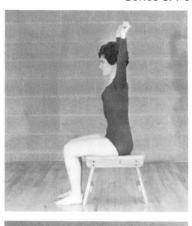
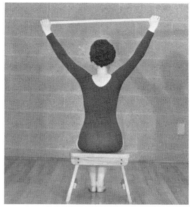
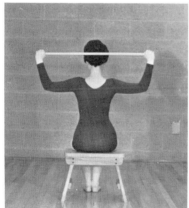
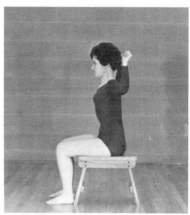

Exercise 5–1.
(Photographs taken from Wells, K. F.: Posture Exercise Handbook: A Progressive Sequence Approach. The Ronald Press Company, New York, 1963.)

Series 5. Posture Exercises.

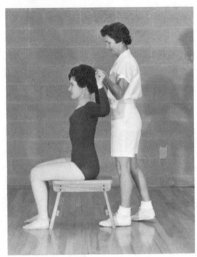

Exercise 5–2.

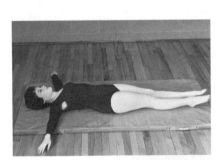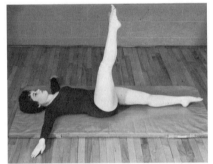

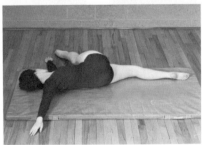

Exercise 5–3.

Series 5. Posture Exercises.

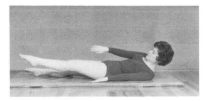
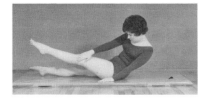

Exercise 5–4.

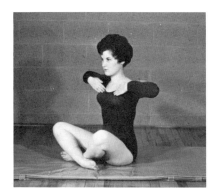
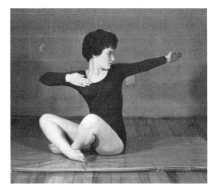

Exercise 5–5.

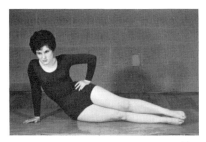
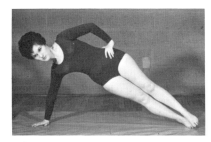

Exercise 5–6.

Series 5. Posture Exercises.

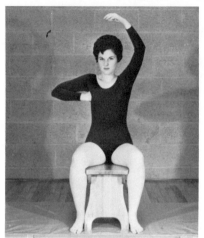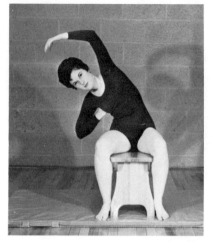

Exercise 5–7.

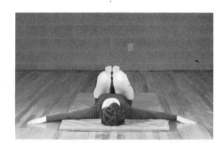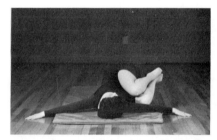

Exercise 5–8.

INDEX

Research Studies Cited or Summarized

Part I

Center of gravity and line of gravity of human body: relationships to stance and alignment of weight-bearing segments
 Croskey et al., 20 (Ref. #1, p. 21)
 Crowley, 20 (Ref. #8, p. 21)
 Cureton and Wickens, 20 (Ref. #2, p. 21)
 Hellebrandt et al., 19 (Ref. #3, p. 21)
 Hellebrandt and Franseen, 20 (Ref. #4, p. 21)
 Johnston, 20 (Ref. #8, p. 21)
 Palmer, 20 (Ref. #6, p. 21)
Joints: electrogoniometry
 Adrian, 28 (Reg. #5, p. 32)
 Karpovich, 28 (Ref. #5, p. 32); 149 (Ref. #1, p. 151)
Joints: range of motion and measurement studies
 Glanville and Kreezer, 31 (Ref. #7, p. 32)
 Van Horn, 31 (Ref. #10, p. 33)
 Wells, 28, 30, 31 (Unpublished)
Muscle strength in relation to cross section
 Morris, 104 (Ref. #3, p. 108)

Part II

Muscle tonus
 Basmajian, 171 (Ref. #1, p. 176)
 deVries, 171 (Ref. #2, p. 176)
 Ralston and Libet, 171 (Ref. #15, p. 176)
Regional anatomic studies
 Upper extremity: Shoulder region
 Freedman and Munro, 206 (Ref. #5, p. 211)
 Inman et al., 203 (Ref. #8, p. 211)
 Shevlin et al., 203 (Ref. #12, p. 211)
 Wiedenbauer and Mortenson, 205 (Ref. #14, p. 211)
 Forearm (elbow and radioulnar joints)
 Basmajian and Latif, 224 (Ref. #1, p. 226)
 Downer, 223 (Ref. #4, p. 226)
 Larson, 224 (Ref. #5, p. 226)
 McCraw, 225 (Ref. #6, p. 226)
 Provins and Salter, 224 (Ref. #8, p. 226)
 Rasch, 224 (Ref. #9, p. 226)
 Lower extremity: Thigh (hip joint)